Childhood, Pain and Emotion

Situated between the history of pain, history of childhood and history of emotions, this innovative work explores cultural understandings of children's pain, from the 1870s to the end of the Second World War. Focusing on British medical discourse, Leticia Fernández-Fontecha examines the relationship between the experience of pain and its social and medical perception, looking at how pain is felt, seen and performed in contexts such as the hospital, the war nursery and the asylum. By means of a comparative study of views in different disciplines – physiology, paediatrics, psychiatry, psychology and psychoanalysis – this work demonstrates the various ways in which the child in pain came to be perceived. This context is vital to understanding current practices and beliefs surrounding childhood pain, and the role that children play in the construction of adult worlds.

LETICIA FERNÁNDEZ-FONTECHA is a historian, writer, and poet. She is a Visiting Assistant Professor at Washington and Lee University.

Childhood, Pain and Emotion

A Modern British Medical History

Leticia Fernández-Fontecha

Washington and Lee University

CAMBRIDGE
UNIVERSITY PRESS

CAMBRIDGE
UNIVERSITY PRESS

Shaftesbury Road, Cambridge CB2 8EA, United Kingdom

One Liberty Plaza, 20th Floor, New York, NY 10006, USA

477 Williamstown Road, Port Melbourne, VIC 3207, Australia

314–321, 3rd Floor, Plot 3, Splendor Forum, Jasola District Centre, New Delhi – 110025, India

103 Penang Road, #05-06/07, Visioncrest Commercial, Singapore 238467

Cambridge University Press is part of Cambridge University Press & Assessment, a department of the University of Cambridge.

We share the University's mission to contribute to society through the pursuit of education, learning and research at the highest international levels of excellence.

www.cambridge.org
Information on this title: www.cambridge.org/9781009558730

DOI: 10.1017/9781009558723

When citing this work, please include a reference to the DOI 10.1017/9781009558723

First published 2025

A catalogue record for this publication is available from the British Library.

Library of Congress Cataloging-in-Publication Data
Names: Fernández-Fontecha, Leticia, 1985- author
Title: Childhood, pain and emotion : a modern British medical history / Leticia Fernández-Fontecha, University of North Carolina, Chapel Hill.
Description: Cambridge, United Kingdom ; New York, NY : Cambridge University Press, 2024. | Includes bibliographical references and index.
Identifiers: LCCN 2024042987 (print) | LCCN 2024042988 (ebook) | ISBN 9781009558709 paperback | ISBN 9781009558730 hardback | ISBN 9781009558723 ebook
Subjects: LCSH: Pain in children–Great Britain–History | Children–Health and hygiene–Great Britain–History | Child health services–Great Britain–History | Pain in children–Great Britain–Psychological aspects
Classification: LCC RJ365 .F47 2024 (print) | LCC RJ365 (ebook) | DDC 618.92/0472–dc23/eng/20241003
LC record available at https://lccn.loc.gov/2024042987
LC ebook record available at https://lccn.loc.gov/2024042988

ISBN 978-1-009-55873-0 Hardback

For Ángel González García

Contents

List of Figures — *page* viii
Acknowledgements — x

Introduction — 1
1 The Language of Children's Pain — 21
2 Infant Pain Denial — 57
3 Articulating Mental Pain — 79
4 The Nervous Child — 110
5 The Pain of Separation — 152
Conclusion — 197

Bibliography — 204
Index — 242

Figures

1.1 Oscar Reijlander and Herr Kindermann, *Fold-out plate of weeping children and babies from Chapter VI, Expression of Suffering,* by Charles Darwin, *The Expression of the Emotions in Man and Animals,* J. Murray, London (1872). Opp page 148, Pl. 1. Wellcome Library, General Collections. *page* 26

1.2 Oscar Reijlander, *Child crying*, from Charles Darwin, *The Expression of the Emotions in Man and Animals,* J. Murray, London (1872). Facing page 148, Tab. I, Figure 1. Wellcome Library, General Collections. 27

1.3 Photographer unknown, *Outpatients* (c. 1920), B-INT 01989, Great Ormond Street Archives. 43

1.4 Photographer Unknown, *Dresden Ward* (c. 1910), B-INT 00478D, Great Ormond Street Archives. 43

1.5 Langley & Sons, *Dresden Ward* (c. 1910), B-INT 00237, Great Ormond Street Archives. 44

1.6 *Dresden Postcard* (c. 1900), B-INT 00478D, Great Ormond Street Archives. 45

1.7 Robert Faulkner & Co, *Nellie Wallace* (c. 1875), Hospital for Sick Children Fundraising Album, Great Ormond Street Archives. 47

1.8 Robert Faulkner & Co, *Nellie Wallace* (c. 1875), Hospital for Sick Children Fundraising Album, Great Ormond Street Archives. 48

1.9 Robert Faulkner & Co, *Sidney Jones* (c. 1875), Hospital for Sick Children Fundraising Album, Great Ormond Street Archives. 49

1.10 Robert Faulkner & Co, *Annie Eastland* (c. 1875), Hospital for Sick Children Fundraising Album, Great Ormond Street Archives. 50

5.1 Cecil Beaton, *Copy negative made from vintage print. Eileen Dunne, aged three, sits in bed with her doll at the Great Ormond Street Hospital for Sick Children, after being injured during an air raid on London in September 1940* (1940), MH 26395, Ministry of Information Second World War Official Collection, Imperial War Museum. 161
5.2 Cecil Beaton, *Children in hospital series* (c. 1940), GOS_01 jpg Cecil Beaton 2, Great Ormond Street Archives. 165
5.3 Photographer unknown, *Evacuated children from London dance happily on the lawn at the country mansion of a well-known peer. The house was given over entirely to the children* (c. 1940), HU 69020, Ministry of Information Second World War Press Agency Print, Imperial War Museum. 169

Acknowledgements

I began researching the history of childhood pain ten years ago when I was a PhD student living in London, trying to come to terms with the pain of my own childhood. Many things have happened since then. I finished my PhD and moved to New York, hoping to secure an academic position. I experienced the fear that comes with academic precarity and found other ways to keep writing. I then moved to Iowa City to pursue an MFA in Spanish Creative Writing, where I met my husband in a poetry seminar. Less than a year after we first met, we got married in a parking lot in the middle of a pandemic. Soon after, I became pregnant, and nine months later, we welcomed our first child. At the end of this journey, I returned to this project and realised it needed to become a book. I worked on it during the last months of my pregnancy and the first months of my child's life. During those nights of writing, I came to realise how much I had grown and learned while working on this project, and how much this book has given me over the years.

First of all, I wish to express my gratitude to this project for everything I have learned about myself and others through it. I am also grateful to many of the authors whose work I read while researching this book. They taught me so much about what it means to be human, what it means to be in pain, how to understand myself better in the world and, in many ways, how to be a better person. They gave me the tools I needed to become a historian, to tell this story and – by looking at it so closely – finally to move beyond the realm of pain. While it is impossible to list all the people who played a role in the process of writing this book, I do not wish to leave unmentioned those who have been particularly important.

I am deeply indebted to Matthew Eddy and Tom Tweed for championing this book. Special thanks to Rob Boddice for his generosity – his support has meant so much to me – and for his valuable comments on the manuscript. Thanks to Joanna Bourke for her early support of this project and for being such a great example of what it means to be a committed historian. I am also grateful to Lucy Rhymer for believing in this book and to the wonderful team at Cambridge University Press for their help throughout the publishing process. My thanks also go to the two anonymous readers of the manuscript.

My heartfelt thanks to Paul Davies for reading this book with such care and for his generosity and patience; he has made this process feel less lonely. Special thanks to my friend Beatriz Pichel, with whom I shared many muffins while reflecting on this topic at the Wellcome Trust. I am indebted to Ángel González García, who believed in me and whom I dearly miss. Many people have shared their research with me, sometimes without even knowing me, showing me the importance of what I call 'academic generosity' – to all of them, many thanks. I am also deeply grateful to Dolores Martín Moruno, Rosa Medina Doménech, Stephanie Olsen and David Konstan for their invaluable support, whether through advice, conference invitations or reference letters.

I spent four years immersed in the vibrant and enriching atmosphere of the Wellcome Library in London. A researcher's life can sometimes be solitary – especially when living away from one's home country – so I am grateful to the Wellcome Trust for offering me a space that felt like home. Special thanks to Danny Rees for his kindness. I am also thankful to Nick Baldwin from the Great Ormond Street Archives for his invaluable assistance. Various universities and grants have supported me throughout the development of this project. I am grateful to the University of Greenwich, Columbia University, the University of Iowa, the Iowa Arts Fellowship, the Juan de la Cierva Postdoctoral Scholarship, the Instituto Interuniversitario López Piñero and the University of North Carolina at Chapel Hill.

I would like to express my deep gratitude to my mother, Patricia Rumeu, who supported me through many years of academic uncertainty. To my friends and family, thank you for your love and encouragement.

I started working on this book when I was pregnant with my child Ignacio. Thank you, Iggy, for showing me what love is every day. I am so grateful that you chose me to be your mother. I am also immensely thankful to my husband Kevin, who has created a home with me, and who has taught me that I can be myself, always. You are my broom.

Introduction

On 18 February 1871, six-year-old Edward Lee was taken ill with 'pain in the foot, then in knees and back'. Little Edward had been 'the healthiest of the family' until about two years earlier, when he had been an in-patient at Great Ormond Street Hospital for Sick Children in London, with 'abscess on the Heel, & pains in limbs & joints'.[1] He made a good recovery and had remained well until this new bout of pain. After being sick for three days – 'hot and feverish, especially at night', when he was restless and 'in great pain'[2] – his father took him back to the Hospital for Sick Children, where the institution's founder, the physician Dr Charles West, diagnosed him with acute rheumatism and pericarditis. In September 1874, the ten-year-old girl 'S.T.' started complaining of 'severe pain at the epigastrium'.[3] 'S.T.' had always been healthy until three months before the doctor was sent for, when she had started to suffer 'of the same pain once or twice a week', a pain that progressively worsened. The pain was so severe that the girl 'soon became sallow', developed an 'abdominal aspect' and 'became quite unable to walk', eventually succumbing to convulsions and screaming fits.[4] S.T.'s symptoms led the British doctor William H. Spurgin to diagnose hysteria. Almost seventy years later, in March 1941, four-year-old Patrick, 'of pleasing appearance, well built and rather big for his age', was sent to the Hampstead War Nurseries.[5] Soon after his mother left, separation became intolerable for Patrick. He refused to eat, play and speak and had to be moved around like an automaton. After a few days, he was reduced to a state of 'compulsive formula and symptomatic actions'. Finally, Patrick entered a state of nervous compulsion, with a weak and rapid pulse, with no interest in the outside world and 'with an absolutely

[1] GOS/10/12, Dr Charles West casenotes, 1871–72, Great Ormond Street Archives.
[2] GOS/10/12, Dr Charles West casenotes, 1871–72, Great Ormond Street Archives.
[3] William H. Spurgin, 'Case of hysteria in a child aged ten years', *British Medical Journal* (2 October 1875), 555.
[4] Spurgin, 'Case of hysteria', 555.
[5] Anna Freud and Dorothy T. Burlingham, *War and Children* (Medical War Books, New York, 1943), 26.

tragic expression on his face'.[6] For the psychoanalyst Anna Freud, who was among the first to document how children suffered when separated from their parents during the Second World War, Patrick's symptoms were directly related to 'the pain of separation'.

Even though children were often deemed incapable of being able to articulate the nature and characteristics of their own suffering, the archives are full of children in pain. Children who cry out to us from the hospital, the asylum, the therapy session, the nursery and from the bombed cities of the Second World War. Their voices and the accounts of the physicians and scientists who diagnosed and treated them provide insights into the experiences of children from the past and provoke numerous questions about the perception, experience and treatment of pain in childhood. How did ideas of pain in childhood change between the 1870s and the middle of the twentieth century (the period covered by this book) and how do these shifts reflect the cultural beliefs, scientific disciplines and emotional worlds of those times? How and why did the physical and emotional discomfort of a child become understood and accepted historically, and how did this understanding lead to different kinds of clinical treatment? Which cultural elements configured the expression of children's pain? And what were the cultural conditions that made those experiences possible in the first place? This book explores these questions historically, examining the forms of objectification of painful experience and the rhetorical modalities that have enabled the cultural understanding of childhood pain, with a focus on British medical discourse from the dawn of Darwinism until the advent of the welfare state. It covers the period from the 1870s, when Darwin published his *A Biographical Sketch of an Infant* (1877), thereby opening the door to the scientific study of childhood,[7] to the end of the Second World War, when there was an major shift in the way that the environments of children's pain – the institution, the home, the street – were conceived.[8] It is, therefore, a contribution to current knowledge about both the experience of pain and the experience of childhood.

The cases of Edward, S.T. and Patrick show how, during the period under discussion, children's pain became an unstable object that acquired different properties and meanings within different clinical and scientific disciplines. In this way, similar symptoms received radically different diagnoses and treatments, so that what was seen as 'rheumatism' in the late nineteenth century was viewed as 'anxiety phenomena' by the middle of the twentieth. This book also exemplifies how the shifts in the medical concepts of pain

[6] Freud and Burlingham, *War and Children*, 26.
[7] Charles Darwin, 'A biographical sketch of an infant', *Mind*, 2 (1877), 1.
[8] On this shift, see Mathew Thomson, *Lost Freedom: The Landscape of the Child and the British Post-War Settlement* (Oxford University Press, Oxford, 2013), particularly chapter 3.

accompanied radical alterations in the experience and the sense-making of children's pain. Pain, therefore, does not just have a body – it also has a history.[9]

The Child in Pain

The proliferating historical analyses of medical and physiological constructions related either to suffering or to the remedies that prevent and treat it confirm that pain has become an important topic within the historiography of experience and emotions. However, despite the abundant and still-growing body of literature on the human relationship with pain, very little has been written about the historical experience of pain in children, possibly because of the methodological difficulties a history of a subjective phenomenon must confront. When the subject is studied not only as a *locus* of pain but also as a *child in pain*, this negative consideration of subjectivity is doubled: very few

[9] Numerous works providing a cultural perspective on pain have been written by scholars across various disciplines, including the following key texts: Rachel Ablow, *Victorian Pain* (Princeton University Press, Princeton, NJ, 2017); Sara Ahmed, 'The contingency of pain', *Parallax*, 8 (2008), 17–34; Lucy Bending, *The Representation of Bodily Pain in Late Nineteenth-Century English Culture* (Clarendon Press, Oxford, 2000); David Biro, *The Language of Pain: Finding Words, Compassion, and Relief* (Norton, New York, 2010); Rod Boddice (ed.), *Pain and Emotions in Modern History* (Palgrave Macmillan, Basingstoke, 2014); Rob Boddice, *Knowing Pain: A History of Sensation, Emotion, and Experience* (Polity Press, Cambridge, 2023); Joanna Bourke, 'The art of medicine: languages of pain', *The Lancet*, 379 (2012), 2420–21; Joanna Bourke, *Pain and the Politics of Sympathy: Historical Reflections, 1760s to 1960s* (Utrecht University, Utrecht, 2011); Joanna Bourke, *The Story of Pain: From Prayers to Painkillers* (Oxford University Press, Oxford, 2014); Sarah Coakley and Kay Kaufman Shelemay (eds.), *Pain and Its Transformations: The Interface of Biology and Culture* (Harvard University Press, Cambridge, MA, 2007); Esther Cohen, *The Modulated Scream: Pain in Late Medieval Culture* (University of Chicago Press, Chicago, 2010); Esther Cohen, 'The animated pain of the body', *American Historical Review*, 105 (2000), 36–68; Esther Cohen, 'Towards a history of European physical sensibility: pain in the later middle ages', *Science in Context*, 8 (1995), 47–74; Cathy Gere, *Pain, Pleasure and the Greater Good* (University of Chicago Press, Chicago, 2017); Thomas Dormandy, *The Worst of Evils: The Fight against Pain* (Yale University Press, New Haven, CT, 2006); Arthur Kleinman, *The Illness Narratives: Suffering, Healing and the Human Condition* (Basic Books, New York, 1988); David Le Breton, *Anthropologie de la Douleur* (Métailié, Paris, 1995); Ronald Melzak and Patrick D. Wall, *The Challenge of Pain* (Penguin, London, 1982); Javier Moscoso, *Pain: A Cultural History* (Palgrave Macmillan, Basingstoke, 2012); David Morris, *The Culture of Pain* (University of California Press, Berkeley, 1991); Elaine Scarry, *The Body in Pain: The Making and Unmaking of the World* (Oxford University Press, Oxford, 1985); Roselyne Rey, *The History of Pain* (Harvard University Press, Cambridge, MA, 1995); Susan Sontag, *Regarding the Pain of Others* (Hamish Hamilton, London, 2003); Susan Sontag, *Illness as Metaphor* (Allen Lane, London, 1979); Andrew Wear, 'Perceptions of pain in seventeenth century England', *Society for the Social History of Medicine Bulletin*, 36 (1985), 7–9; and Lisa Wynne Smith, 'An account of an unaccountable distemper: the experience of pain in early eighteenth century England and France', *Eighteenth-Century Studies*, 41 (2008), 459–80.

scholars of science have attempted to approach children's subjectivity and recognise its irreducible autonomy.[10]

Under similar coordinates, the ostensible referent of pain might seem doomed to invisibility – children are deemed incapable of properly articulating the nature and characteristics of their suffering. By exploring the attribution of meaning to children's pain from a historical perspective, this book contributes to historiographical debates about the experience of harm. Situated between cultural history and the history of science, this study asserts that the persuasive forms used to relate to others' experiences of pain are especially important in cases of individuals who either lack the ability to speak (such as animals) or who lack verbal dexterity (such as children).[11] To cover this difficult topic, the study explores the physical, emotional and performative dimensions of pain from a cultural perspective – that is, it seeks to explore the relationship between the experience of pain in childhood and the social perception of that experience. This approach enables the understanding of how and why the physical and emotional discomfort of a child became understood and accepted historically, and how it led to clinical treatment and, in some cases, financial support. Through an analysis of written narratives and visual culture, this book emphasises the performative nature of pain as it was enacted in different contexts such as the hospital, the war nursery and the asylum. The drama of pain twists and turns behind and around the child in pain – usually a secondary subject of inquiry – and the sympathetic, impassive or oblivious onlookers, as each of them imbued pain with different meanings, values and emotions, thereby presenting pain as a by-product of a heterogeneous activity. For

[10] A notable exception is Matthew Daniel Eddy, who has framed the voice of the child in archival studies of infant writing. See Matthew Daniel Eddy, *Media and the Mind: Art, Science, and Notebooks as Paper Machines, 1700–1830* (University of Chicago Press, Chicago, 2023). See also 'The child writer: graphic literacy and the Scottish educational system, 1700–1820', *History of Education*, 45 (2016), 695–718; 'The interactive notebook: how students learned to keep notes during the Scottish Enlightenment', *Book History*, 19 (2016), 87–131; 'The shape of knowledge: children and the visual culture of literacy and numeracy', *Science in Context*, 26 (2013), 215–45.

[11] For a discussion on animal pain, see: Bernard E. Rollin, *The Unheeded Cry: Animal Consciousness, Animal Pain and Scientific Change* (Oxford University Press, Oxford, 1989) especially chapters 5, 6, and 7; Rob Boddice, *Humane Professions: The Defense of Experimental Medicine, 1876–1914* (Cambridge University Press, Cambridge, 2021). On animal pain and anaesthesia, see: Rob Boddice, 'Species of compassion: aesthetics, anaesthetics and pain in the physiological laboratory', *Interdisciplinary Studies in the Long Nineteenth Century*, 15 (2012), 1–22; Tarquin Holmes and Carrie Friese, 'Making the anaesthetised animal into a boundary object: an analysis of the 1875 Royal Commission on Vivisection', *History and Philosophy of the Life Sciences*, 42 (2020), 1–28; Tarquin Holmes, 'Science, sensitivity and the sociozoological scale: constituting and complicating the human–animal boundary at the 1875 Royal Commission on Vivisection and beyond', *Studies in History and Philosophy of Science*, Part A, 90 (2021), 194–207; Shira Shmuely, *The Bureaucracy of Empathy: Law, Vivisection, and Animal Pain in Late Nineteenth-Century Britain* (Cornell University Press, Ithaca, NY, 2023).

instance, in the children's nurseries of the Second World War, the child in pain became a symbol of national resistance and courage in the face of the Blitz. If, as David Morris argues, pain is subjected to historical changes, this book addresses the nature of these shifts and how they are configured.[12]

In looking at the figure of the child through the topic of pain, this book offers an approach informed by the history of medicine, the history of childhood and the history of science, yet it is also grounded in the history of emotions and the history of people's experiences. In these already interdisciplinary fields, scholars theorise about the relationships between power, materiality and inequality in the making of cultural worlds. Taken together, these different areas of study provide indispensable tools for critical thought that can confront the cultural domination of existing hierarchies. Indeed, this book would not be possible without the already massive body of work of theorists who have articulated how the facts, institutions, technologies and meanings that comprise our bodies and worlds simultaneously exert power and exist in a situation of fluid contingency.[13] In looking at the history of childhood through pain, one can see how children's experiences become the locus of ideological and disciplinary battle. Supplementing the most frequent methods that historians of science have used to shed light on hidden subjectivities, the present study draws on theoretical resources from interdisciplinary work. The objective is to bring childhood into the heart of discussions concerning the construction of historically situated cultural assumptions about human nature, medicine and the nature of suffering. Consequently, I juxtapose scientific figurations of the child in pain with those of other cultural contexts.[14] By engaging in a comparative study between different disciplines – physiology, paediatrics, psychiatry, psychology, and psychoanalysis – this book studies the various ways in which the child in pain came into being as a figure, as well as the many forms this figure has then generated. The construction of medical and scientific

[12] See Morris, *Culture of Pain*, 1–9.

[13] The approaches of several writers have proved particularly useful in informing my approach. In the first instance is Foucault's work on power and knowledge, in particular *Discipline and Punish*, and his work on the birth of the clinic. See Michel Foucault, *Discipline and Punish: The Birth of the Prison* (Allen Lane, London, 1977) and Michel Foucault, *The Birth of the Clinic* (Taylor & Francis, Abingdon, 2002). More relevant has been the work of other authors who, though taking their lead from Foucault, have worked in this particular direction. Ian Hacking's reflections on the philosophical uses of history, especially the insightful model offered in *Historical Ontology* (2002), has aided my efforts to understand the historicity of core epistemological referents such as 'objectivity', 'demonstration' and 'explanation'. See Ian Hacking, *Historical Ontology* (Harvard University Press, Cambridge, MA, 2002). For more on this topic, see also: Ian Hacking, *Mad Travelers: Reflections on the Reality of Transient Mental Illnesses* (Harvard University Press, Cambridge, MA, 2002); Ian Hacking, *Rewriting the Soul: Multiple Personality and the Sciences of Memory* (Princeton University Press, Princeton, NJ, 1998).

[14] This concept was developed by Claudia Castañeda. See Claudia Castañeda, *Figurations: Child, Bodies, Worlds* (Duke University Press, Durham, NC, 2002).

models of childhood pain reflects and creates a series of paradoxes and tensions in relation to the emergence and consolidation of the various scientific disciplines. The book also advances a strong claim: that the disciplines of physiology, paediatrics, psychiatry, psychology and psychoanalysis never agreed on a standard and unified theory of the child in pain. Instead, the interests of each individual discipline prefigured the way it explained and represented this figure.

This book examines the politics of diagnosis, through which the institution of medicine ascribes meaning or value to different states of pain and suffering, which in turn makes it possible to unveil or reconstruct the sense-making experiences of patients. In other – more explicitly Foucauldian – terms, the examination of authoritative medical discourses allows the framing of specific biopolitics that affect children in situations of harm, while the disciplinary archaeology operating within the margins of an interdisciplinary historical examination constitutes a taxonomy of bodies of knowledge that adopts a critical stance towards those institutionalised practices. At the same time, this approach opens a window that empowers the contemporary subject to deconstruct the often invisible discourses on the nature of pain, suffering and healing. The central argument is that, on the basis of the same symptoms or expressive signs, each discipline constructed its own figurations of childhood: the child without pain, the sick child, the insane child, the nervous child and the uprooted child. These different figurations, in turn, played a unique and constitutive role in the adult construction of worlds, particularly the worlds of nature and culture. To put it simply, the approach adopted in each chapter follows two lines. First, it describes the constellation of practices, materialities and knowledge through which a specific figure arises and is consolidated in the context of disciplines and epistemic communities. Second, it unveils how that figure contributes to broader cultural claims, both within and beyond the disciplinary realms.

One of the justifications for this book's focus on the perceptions and practices of physicians and scientists regarding pain is that there are few surviving narratives of children's personal experiences of pain. The detailed examination of the ways in which leading British physicians understood pain does not imply any wish to downplay or invalidate the experiences of pain suffered by the patients themselves. Rather, I suggest, understanding how medical professionals viewed their little patients' pain is a valid and worthy subject in its own right, particularly because their understanding of pain played an important role in influencing their treatments and in making decisions about their patients, including whether any intervention was necessary.

In a book that covers different disciplines over nearly a century, it is not possible to adopt a uniform approach to sources or their modulations. The subject of this book – pain in childhood – is addressed by a loose community of 'scientists' that includes evolutionary theorists, physiologists, medical doctors, public-health officials, political gurus, eugenicists, psychiatrists and psychoanalysts. What unites the disparate band is an interest in the scientific study of childhood. I suggest that the diversification of knowledge about the human body and its treatment that took place during the nineteenth century and that was consolidated in the twentieth century turned children's pain into an unstable object that was invested with different properties and meanings in each discipline: pain as a sign of illness, as a symptom of an organic lesion, as an element of a child's emotional development and even as an aspect of a nation's fortitude. In all cases, the study and understanding of pain follows the same sequence: examining the subject as a sign, taking it as evidence and finally considering it as a fluctuating object of a new science. A similar process can be observed in the intellectual understanding of pain, whether in science, medicine, philosophy, the social sciences or religion. While to the general scientist, pain might be a series of complex neural circuits, a medical professional might see the patient's experience of pain more than a mere electrical sensation, while the historian or social scientist might focus on how humankind's views of pain have changed from the idea that it is something that might be good for us (whether to build character, to encourage a change of behaviour or to build up our defences to cope with stronger pain), and whether today the lack of a 'meaning' in pain has reduced our ability to cope with it. In this context, I suggest that the figure of the child in pain appears in medical, scientific and popular discourses both in its own right and as a bodily theatre through which other stories are told. In so doing, I also suggest that the history of childhood is important not only with respect to children's experiences but also as a way to understand how adult worlds are created and to deepen our understanding of the history of medicine and the emotions.[15] Asking how and why the figure of the child in pain has been used and categorised for wider cultural endeavours makes the child the focus of an analysis about how it has been deployed and valued in adult discourses.

[15] For a discussion on how the history of childhood might influence the history of emotions see Stephanie Olsen, 'The history of childhood and the emotional turn', *History Compass*, 15 (2017), e12410. See also Kristine Alexander, Stephanie Olsen and Karen Vallgårda, *Voices and Sources: Lessons from the History of Childhood, Digital Handbook of the History of Experience* (Research Council of Finland's Centre of Excellence in the History of Experiences (HEX), 2023), https://researchprofiles.ku.dk/en/publications/voices-and-sources-lessons-from-the-history-of-childhood. Stephanie Olsen, 'The limits of experience? A case study on children's dreams', *Digital Handbook of the History of Experience* (2022), https://researchportal.tuni.fi/en/publications/the-limits-of-experience-a-case-study-on-childrens-dreams. For a discussion on the role of emotions in researching children in the archives see Jack Hodgson, 'Historians, emotions, and children's trauma in the archives', *Qualitative Inquiry*, https://journals.sagepub.com/doi/full/10.1177/10778004231200265

Just as pain is a concept that does not have a single universal meaning, childhood has been seen differently across cultures and periods. The age at which 'children' are deemed to become 'adults' varies, and across the world today much variation can still be seen, both in legal terms and in practical ways.[16] In the period covered in this book, childhood was valued in terms of personal maturation, initially in a physical sense dominated by 'biological benchmarks', but increasingly regarding psychological transformation into adulthood.[17] For the purposes of this book, childhood covers the period from birth to puberty or adolescence.[18] The guiding principle here is drawn from medical treatises that make a distinction between childhood and puberty based on sexual development, which gives rise to a series of illnesses that are not suffered by children. However, this frontier is culturally bound and fuzzy, as the sexual element in puberty can be stimulated or deflected vis-à-vis the cultural conditions of a particular moment.[19] More generally, childhood is far from being a stable essentialised concept, as the extensive variations and partial overlaps between English words for non-adults show ('child', 'kid', 'infant', 'baby' and so on).[20]

Several recent historical studies of children have highlighted the fact that the adult population had a vested interested in the development of 'normal' healthy children for the continuation of national economic and political status, focusing on the significance of children as future citizens of the British Empire.[21] An analysis of the motivating factors shaping approaches to pain in childhood supports this argument to a degree. It was often a reason publicly

16 For a discussion of age as a category of historical analysis, see Anna Davin, 'What is a child?', in Anthony Fletcher and Stephen Hussey (eds.), *Childhood in Question: Children, Parents and the State* (Manchester University Press, Manchester, 1999), 14–36; and the first edition of *Journal of the History of Childhood and Youth* 1 (2008), particularly: Steven Mintz, 'Reflections on age as a category of historical analysis', 91–94; Leslie Paris, 'Through the looking glass: age, stages, and historical analysis', 106–13, Peter Stearns, 'Challenges in the history of childhood', 35–42.

17 For further analysis of this aspect of childhood see Castañeda, *Figurations*.

18 The term adolescence is historically imprecise and only began to gain prominence in the late nineteenth century, culminating in G. Stanley Hall's formalization of the concept in his seminal work, Adolescence: Its Psychology and Its Relations to Physiology, Anthropology, Sociology, Sex, Crime, Religion and Education (D. Appleton and Company, New York, 1904).

19 Sally Shuttleworth, *The Mind of the Child: Child Development in Literature, Science, and Medicine, 1840–1900* (Oxford University Press, Oxford, 2010), 10.

20 Davin, 'What is a child?'.

21 For an account on the significance of children as future citizens, see: Anna Davin, 'Imperialism and motherhood', *History Workshop Journal*, 5 (1978), 9–65; Deborah Dwork, *War Is Good for Babies and Other Young Children: A History of the Infant and Child Welfare Movement in England, 1898–1918* (Tavistock, London, 1987); Bernard Harris, *The Health of the Schoolchild: A History of the School Medical Service in England and Wales* (Open University Press, Buckingham, 1995); Harry Hendrick, 'Child labour, medical capital, and the school medical service, c.1890–1918', in Roger Cooter (ed.), *In the Name of the Child: Health and Welfare 1880–1940* (Routledge, London, 1992), 45–71; Stephanie Olsen, *Juvenile Nation: Youth,*

presented by different individuals and groups as their source of concern, particularly in the earlier decades of the twentieth century, when issues of eugenics and social hygiene were still prominent.[22] Harry Hendrick suggests that one defining characteristic of the category of children is that they have no political significance.[23] While it is true that individual children did not have the power to vote, this study aims to show that children were of immense political significance, and not only when adults debated child labour policy in the industrial West. In seeking to analyse historical variations in the notions of childhood, Anna Davin has argued that the attainment of adult status and adult authority is confirmed through control and/or support of children. In addition, adults have had the power to set the terms of childhood according to their priorities in the present and for the future.[24] This study confirms this view by showing that, in many cases, the agents placing emphasis on the health of children in relation to the future of the UK often had different agendas, with alternative motivations, as they used the issue of child health and welfare for political or professional advancement.

Since the early 1990s, the historiography of childhood has swelled. Historians have engaged in the continuing study of the evolution of childhood as a concept, mapping out the social, cultural, economic and political context of the 'birth of the modern child'.[25] These efforts have highlighted the absence

Emotions and the Making of the Modern British Citizen, 1880–1914 (Bloomsbury Academic, New York, 2014); Michal Shapira, *The War Inside: Psychoanalysis, Total War, and the Making of the Democratic Self in Post-War Britain* (Cambridge University Press, Cambridge, 2013); and G. R. Searle, *The Quest for National Efficiency: A Study in British Politics and Political Thought, 1899–1914* (University of California Press, Berkeley, 1971).

22 For the general context of early eugenicists, see Daniel Pick, *Faces of Degeneration: A European Disorder, c.1848–c.1918* (Cambridge University Press, Cambridge, 1989), 216–21 and Alison Bashford and Phillipa Levine (eds.), *The Oxford Handbook of the History of Eugenics* (Oxford University Press, Oxford, 2010). For further reviews of the field, see: Peter Bowler, *The Mendelian Revolution: The Emergence of Hereditarian Concepts in Modern Science and Society* (Athlone, London, 1989); Frank Dikötter, 'Race culture: recent perspectives on the history of eugenics', *American Historical Review*, 103 (1998), 467–78; Pauline M. H. Mazumdar, *Eugenics, Human Genetics and Human Failings: The Eugenics Society, Its Sources and Its Critics in Britain* (Routledge, London, 1992); Robert A. Nye, 'The rise and fall of the eugenics empire: recent perspectives on the impact of biomedical thought in modern society', *Historical Journal*, 36 (1993), 687–700; G. R. Searle, *Eugenics and Politics in Britain, 1900–1914* (Noordhoff International, Leyden, 1976); Richard Soloway, *Demography and Degeneration: Eugenics and the Declining Birthrate in Twentieth-Century Britain* (University of North Carolina Press, Chapel Hill, 1990); Mathew Thomson, *The Problem of Mental Deficiency: Eugenics, Democracy, and Social Policy in Britain c.1870–1959* (Oxford University Press, Oxford, 1998); and Marius Turda, 'Recent scholarship on race and eugenics', *Historical Journal*, 51 (2008), 1115–24.

23 Harry Hendrick, *Children, Childhood and English Society* (Cambridge University Press, Cambridge, 1997), 3.

24 Davin, 'What is a child?'.

25 Academic studies on the historical development of the concept of childhood include: Hugh Cunningham, *Children and Childhood in Western Society since 1500* (Longman, London,

of adequate representations and understanding of children's experience in the historic forms of medical and scientific disciplines.[26] The effect of these varied ideas of childhood on the lives of children has been the focus of recent work on the history of childhood and the history of emotions.[27] Nonetheless, the question of the child has rarely been considered in wider theoretical debates, and theorists have paid limited attention to the function and roles of the figurations of childhood in the making of adult worlds, resulting in consequences that conflict with the interests of those the category purports to represent.[28] As Claudia Castañeda has pointed out, this lack of attention to childhood is significant because it means that children are not placed at the centre of social, political and cultural concerns.[29] I align myself with this approach and attempt to reveal the processes grounded in scientific figurations and artistic representations that have shaped the cultural understanding of children's experience of pain.

Although the category 'child' includes actual children and their experiences, this book does not specifically address that relationship. Although I am convinced that these assumptions affected children, it is not my aim to explain how this might have occurred. This book is, rather, about the creation of different figures of the child in pain and their multiple uses across various cultural sites. It argues that the study of the different categories of children's pain provides an important context for understanding the emergence of other discourses on childhood in the nineteenth and twentieth centuries. It also offers an opportunity to explore the boundaries of psychiatry, physiology, paediatrics, psychology and psychoanalysis during this period. The scientific texts

1995); Hugh Cunningham, *The Invention of Childhood* (BBC Books, London, 2006); Lloyd De Mause (ed.), *The History of Childhood: The Untold Story of Child Abuse* (Psychohistory Press, New York, 1974); Colin Heywood, *A History of Childhood: Children and Childhood in the West from Medieval to Modern Times* (Polity Press, Cambridge, 2001); Hendrick, *Children, Childhood and English Society*; Allison James and Alan Prout, *Constructing and Reconstructing Childhood: Contemporary Issues in the Sociological Study of Childhood* (Routledge, London, 1997); Peter Stearns, *Childhood in World History* (Routledge, London, 2009); Shuttleworth, *Mind of the Child*; Carolyn Steedman, *Strange Dislocations: Childhood and the Idea of Human Interiority, 1780–1930* (Virago Press, London, 1995); and Joseph L. Zornado, *Inventing the Child: Culture, Ideology, and the Story of Childhood* (Routledge, Oxford, 2006).

[26] A notable exception is Hannah Newton, *The Sick Child in Early Modern England, 1580–1720* (Oxford University Press, Oxford, 2012).

[27] See: Stephanie Olsen, *Childhood, Youth and Emotions in Modern History: National, Colonial and Global Perspectives* (Palgrave Macmillan, Basingstoke, 2015); Olsen, *Juvenile Nation*; Ute Frevert, Pascal Eitler, Stephanie Olsen, et al., *Learning How to Feel: Children's Literature and the History of Emotional Socialization, 1870–1970* (Oxford University Press, Oxford, 2014).

[28] For exceptions, see: Castañeda, *Figurations*; Jacqueline Rose, *The Case of Peter Pan, or the Impossibility of Children's Fiction* (Macmillan, London, 1984); Shapira, *The War Inside*; Olsen, *Juvenile Nation*; and Steedman, *Strange Dislocations*.

[29] Castañeda, *Figurations*, 4.

analysed in this book lead us to an important issue in the history of science, which is also a methodological problem that arises when practising interdisciplinary studies: the lack of scientific unity.[30] A radical epistemology would see the object of study of each discipline as a disconnected entity: the infant brain of neurology, the infant body of paediatrics and the infant mind of psychology would find no common ground and no common language.

Rather than insisting on the historical disagreements between the disciplines, this book seeks to advance the understanding of the contemporary construction of the relationship between the mind and the body by uncovering the different meanings of children's pain in the traditions of scientific and medical discourse. It may be surprising to modern readers – who might assume that there is a clear distinction between organic and psychological processes – that there was a considerable overlap between body and mind in much medical thinking in the nineteenth and early twentieth centuries. It is, for example, quite difficult to clearly separate the late nineteenth century speciality of neurology from the earlier discipline of 'physiological psychology'.[31] Thus, this study illustrates how the variety and complexity of concepts of children's pain transcended the simple dualistic perspective that treats mind and body as separate entities.

By placing the child in pain at the centre of the debate, this book draws attention to the importance of age as a category in modern medicine. Historians of pain have often overlooked age as a category, concentrating instead on gender as the organising principle of modern medicine. Martin Pernick has shown how, following the great 'Chain of Feeling', certain social groups – identified by race, class and gender – were seen as being relatively insensitive to pain.[32] Many scholars have since engaged with this idea, debating the politics of gender in relation to pain.[33] This book argues that gender – though evidently crucial in medical perceptions of adults – was far less significant in the representation of the bodies and minds of children, a point similar to that made by Hannah Newton in her study of early modern England. When they described the constitution of children and the cause of their pain, doctors did not usually distinguish between boys and girls. The reason why gender rarely

[30] For a discussion on whether science is unified or disunified, see Mario Biagoli and Peter Galison, *The Disunity of Science: Boundaries, Contexts, and Power* (Stanford University Press, Stanford, CA, 1996).

[31] See Chapter 3.

[32] Martin Pernick, *A Calculus of Suffering: Pain, Professionalism, and Anesthesia in Nineteenth-Century America* (Columbia University Press, New York, 1985).

[33] For instance, Javier Moscoso's discussion on the pain of childbirth in Moscoso, *Pain*, 96–104. See also Whitney Wood, '"When I think of what is before me, I feel afraid". Narratives of fear, pain and childbirth in late Victorian Canada', in Rob Boddice (ed.), *Pain and Emotions*, 187–203; Joanna Bourke and Whitney Wood, 'Conceptualizing gender and pain in modern history', *Gender & History*, 32 (March 2020), 8–12.

appears in the medical and scientific observations and treatments of children is probably that the characteristics that define children in medical opinion are largely related to puberty. This argument cuts against the current historical picture regarding children's gendered identities, which suggests that gender was of considerable importance across the whole life cycle, from the moment of birth and – in particular – after the age of about seven.[34] In making this argument, I am not seeking to suggest that gender did not affect other areas of children's lives,[35] but that, as this book demonstrates, in the context of children's pain, the most important variable was age and the least important seems to have been gender.

Histories of Childhood and of Pain

Those interested in the existential significance of history – that which Nietzsche claimed as history for life[36] – cannot ignore the importance of the historical study of childhood. Unlike many historical examinations that have an internal vision of periodisation and accuracy, the studies of many practising historians of childhood have a retroactive interest: they are concerned with the world in which they live and feel the urge to explain it through the yet untold 'history of childhood'.[37]As with the histories of sexuality, the emotions and the body, the history of childhood has also become a medium used to cast light on present-day situations, most notably situations of violence and abuse

34 Sara Mendelson and Patricia Crawford, *Women in Early Modern England, 1550–1720* (Oxford University Press, Oxford, 2003), 77–78. This has also been supported by Heywood, *A History of Childhood*, 103, and Elizabeth Foyster, *Manhood in Early Modern England: Honour, Sex, and Marriage* (Longman, London, 1999), 39. Other works that explore the gendering of childhood include: Anthony Fletcher, *Growing Up in England: The Experience of Childhood 1600–1914* (Yale University Press, London, 2008); Elizabeth Foyster, 'Boys will be boys? Manhood and aggression, 1660–1800', in Tim Hitchcock and Michele Cohen (eds.), *English Masculinities, 1660–1800* (Longman, London, 1999), 151–66; Brigitte Glaser, 'Gendered childhoods: on the discursive formation of young females in the eighteenth century', in Anja Müller (ed.), *Fashioning Childhood in the Eighteenth Century: Age and Identity* (Ashgate, Aldershot, 2006), 189–98; and Linda Pollock, '"Teach her to live under obedience", the making of women in the upper ranks of early modern England', *Continuity and Change*, 4 (1989), 231–58.

35 Historians such as Brigitte Glaser have convincingly shown how the way that boys and girls were brought up was often very different. See Glaser, 'Gendered childhoods'. Likewise, in the recent volume *Learning How to Feel*, several authors discuss the intersection of gender and the socialisation of children in different emotional realms. In her article 'Piggy's Shame', Ute Frevert shows how transformations in the uses and valuations of shame and shaming reveal and sustain changes in gender prescriptions, notions of authority, and childhood ideals. See Ute Frevert, 'Piggy's shame' in Ute Frevert, Pascal Eitler, Stephanie Olsen, et al., *Learning How to Feel*, 134–54.

36 Friedrich Nietzsche, *On the Advantage and Disadvantage of History for Life* (Hackett Publishing Company, Oxford, 1980).

37 Hugh Cunningham, 'Histories of childhood', *American Historical Review*, 103 (1998), 1195.

committed against children.[38] It is not surprising therefore that it was precisely the revolution in approaches to history heralded by the French historical magazine *Annales* that led to a recovery of the child as an object of historical research and to the production of the first significant work on the history of childhood, Philippe Ariès's *Centuries of Childhood*.[39] This 'new' history, in approaching areas that had not previously been explored and in investigating the way in which different levels of society experienced the events of daily life, took into consideration social groups that until then had been little regarded and converted them into the preferred subjects of investigation. In the specific case of childhood, it can be said that Ariès's study led to a surge in publications that have made the subject so fashionable today.

In the last two decades, the history of childhood has expanded considerably. As concerns about children have increased, stories about children of the past have proliferated. Despite these notable developments, the themes of childhood pain and medicine have rarely entered the historiography. Since the 1992 publication of *In the Name of the Child: Health and Welfare 1880–1940* – Roger Cooter's landmark collection of essays – there have been some advances in the historiography of children's health.[40] Themes that have been addressed (sometimes including consideration of the topic of pain) include children's hospitals and health, disability and mental deficiency and mental health.[41] Hannah Newton's *The Sick Child in Early Modern England, 1580–1720*, published in 2012, addressed and developed the issue of the sick child, raised by Cooter in his introduction to the 1992 essay collection, thereby filling one of the gaps in the historiography of child health.[42] My own project also emerges from one of Cooter's observations and reflects on how, where and why the 'concept of childhood became far more socially homogeneous by virtue of its reconstruction in predominantly psycho-medical terms'.[43] I take a new perspective on the history of childhood health and welfare by focusing on an issue that has been a neglected but integral part of the life sciences since

[38] Adrian Bingham, Lucy Delap, Louise Jackson and Louise Settle, 'Historical child sexual abuse in England and Wales: the role of historians', *History of Education*, 45 (2016), 411–29.

[39] See Philippe Ariès, *Centuries of Childhood: A Social History of Family Life* (Alfred A. Knopf, New York, 1962).

[40] Cooter, *In the Name of the Child.*

[41] An important publication, which has been recognised as the successor to Cooter for its influence, is *Cultures of Child Health in Britain and the Netherlands in the Twentieth Century*, ed. Marijke Gijswijt-Hofstra and Hilary Marland and published in 2003. Exploring advances in the history of children's health that had taken place in the years after Cooter's book was published, this volume highlights the importance of seeing children's health in a wider social and cultural context. Marijke Gijswijt-Hofstra and Hilary Marland, *Cultures of Child Health in Britain and the Netherlands in the Twentieth Century* (Rodopi, New York, 2003). Another important volume is *Childhood, Literature and Science: Fragile Subjects*, ed. Jutta Ahlbeck, Päivi Lappalainen, Kati Launis, and Kirsi Tuohela (Routledge, London, 2017).

[42] Newton, *The Sick Child.* [43] Cooter, *In the Name of the Child*, 2.

antiquity: children's pain, its negotiation in medical and psychological practices and the underlying philosophical and political debates about the status of children.

Another of the objects of this new history is pain. Despite the recent proliferation of research about the way in which class, race and gender shape an individual's experiences of pain, the child in pain has also been largely absent from the history of medicine. Joanna Bourke argues that the reluctance of historians 'to tackle the history of pain' results from its subjective character.[44] Such subjectivity is doubled if the object of study is a child in pain. An extensive and still-growing body of literature in the humanities has been produced devoted to the subject of the human relationship with pain, but there has been hardly any serious discussion in the history of science and medicine about the systematic reliance on the bodies of children who suffer illness and pain as a source of knowledge about the normal child. Elissa N. Rodkey and Rebecca Pillai Riddell, who devoted an article to the subject in 2013, concluded that despite the importance of the historical record for studying medical assumptions of children's experiences of pain, few published works have reviewed this history.[45] The phenomenon of infant pain denial – which characterised many medical approaches to children during much of the twentieth century – can be seen as, in part, a consequence of the invisibility of the subject and the consequent lack of investigative focus on children's experience of pain.

Although the history of children's pain has stayed hidden to scholars until recently, earlier manifestations of theoretical interest in the history of child medicine cannot be neglected, as they include some insights on the nature of child pain from within specific disciplinary boundaries. From the start of the twentieth century, various paediatricians wrote histories of their specialism, of which the most famous are John Ruhrah's *Pediatrics of the Past* (1925) and George Frederic Still's *The History of Paediatrics: The Progress of the Study of Diseases of Children* (1931).[46] The subtitle of Still's book indicates the style

[44] Joanna Bourke, 'The history of medicine as the history of pain', *History Today*, 61 (2011), 56–57.

[45] Elissa N. Rodkey and Rebecca Pillai Riddell, 'The infancy of infant pain research, the experimental origins of infant pain denial', *The Journal of Pain*, 14 (2013), 339.

[46] John Ruhrah, *Pediatrics of the Past* (P. B. Hoeber, New York, 1925) and George Still, *The History of Paediatrics: The Progress of the Study of Diseases of Children up to the End of the 18th Century* (Hodder & Stoughton, Oxford, 1931). Other histories of paediatrics include: Isaac Abt and Fielding Garrison (eds.), *History of Paediatrics* (W. B. Saunders Company, London, 1965); Boyd M. Berry, 'The first English paediatricians and Tudor attitudes towards childhood', *Journal of the History of Ideas*, 35 (1974), 561–77; Thomas E. Cone, *History of American Pediatrics* (Little Brown & Co, Boston, 1979); C. B. Mahnke, 'The growth and development of a specialty: the history of pediatrics, *Clinical Pediatrics*, 39 (2000), 705–14; B. L. Nichols, A. Ballabriga, and N. Kretchmer (eds.), *History of Pediatrics 1850–1950* (Nestlé Nutrition,

of these works, which were written to celebrate the rise of modern paediatrics. They thus tend to be teleological in structure, attempting to uncover the past origins of current medical knowledge and to identify the 'real condition' behind the diagnosis. In opposition to the condescending view on past practices, this book explores historical medical views on children's pain in their own terms, examining the coherence and logic of the medical ideas, however irrational they might seem from a modern perspective.

The child in pain is also mentioned in another context, that of current scientific and psychological articles of research into infant pain. Important articles in this line of research include those by David Chamberlain, who reviews twentieth-century infant pain research from an anti-circumcision perspective; Laura M. Carpenter who explores masculinity and circumcision pain from a sociological perspective; Patrick McGrath, who considers the history of infant pain research in the 1980s; Emilia Pabis, Anita Unruh and colleagues, who review ancient and medieval views of infant pain; and the already cited Elissa N. Rodkey and Rebecca Pillai Riddell, who investigate the origins of infant pain denial.[47] The history of childhood pain has not been neglected entirely by historians. Hannah Newton's *The Sick Child in Early Modern England, 1580–1720* deals with pain in the context of children's illnesses. In a similar way, Joanna Bourke's *The Story of Pain* (2014) examines the history of child pain and calls attention to the way that

New York, 1991); and Samuel X. Radbill, 'Pediatrics', in Allen G. Debus (ed.), *Medicine in Seventeenth Century England* (University of California Press, London, 1974), 237–82.

[47] David B. Chamberlain, 'Babies don't feel pain: a century of denial in medicine', *The Journal of Prenatal and Perinatal Psychology and Health*, 14 (1999), 145–68; Laura M. Carpenter, 'If you prick us: masculinity and circumcision pain in the United States and Canada, 1960–2000', *Gender & History*, 32 (2020), 54–69. Patrick McGrath, 'Science is not enough: the modern history of pediatric pain', *Pain*, 152 (2011), 2457–59; E. Pabis, M. Kowalczyk, and T. B. Kulik, 'Pain in children in historical perspective', *Anestezjol Intens Ter*, 42 (2010), 37–41; Anita Unruh, 'Voices from the past: ancient views of pain in childhood', *The Clinical Journal of Pain*, 8 (1992), 247–54; Rodkey and Riddell, 'The infancy of infant pain research', 338–50. Recent scientific publications on infant pain include: K. J. Anand, 'Effects of perinatal pain and stress', *Progress in Brain Research*, 122 (2000), 117–29; K. Andrews, D. Desai, H. K. Dhillon, D. T. Wilcox and M. Fitzgerald, 'Abdominal sensitivity in the first year of life: comparison of infants with and without prenatally diagnosed unilateral hydronephrosis', *Pain*, 100 (2002), 35–46; K. Andrews and M. Fitzgerald, 'Cutaneous flexion reflex in human neonates: a quantitative study of threshold and stimulus-response characteristics after single and repeated stimuli', *Developmental Medicine and Child Neurology*, 41 (1999), 696–703; K. Andrews and M. Fitzgerald, 'The cutaneous withdrawal reflex in human neonates: sensitization, receptive fields, and the effects of contralateral stimulation', *Pain*, 56 (1994), 95–101; R. E. Grunau, 'Early pain in preterm infants: a model of long-term effects', *Clinics in Perinatology*, 29 (2002), 373–94; C. C. Johnston, J. M. Collinge, S. J. Henderson and K. J. Anand, 'A cross-sectional survey of pain and pharmacological analgesia in Canadian neonatal intensive care units', *Clinical Journal of Pain*, 13 (1997), 308–12; M. Fitzgerald, C. Millard and N. MacIntosh, 'Cutaneous hypersensitivity following peripheral tissue damage in newborn infants and its reversal with topical anaesthesia', *Pain*, 39 (1989), 31–36; and Gayle Giboney Page, 'Are there long-term consequences of pain in newborn or very young infants?', *Journal of Perinatal Education*, 13 (2004), 10–17.

the understanding of children's pain has been revised. Bourke argues that for most of the twentieth century 'many scientists and clinicians [claimed] that infants were almost totally insensible to pain'.[48] However, the argument advanced in the current book is that this theoretical perspective describes only partially the medical, physiological and psychological theories and practices relating to children's pain that existed in the United Kingdom at the end of the nineteenth century and in the early twentieth century.

Pain and Emotion

The Austrian philosopher Ivan Illich has drawn attention to the central role that culture plays in providing ways to experience, express and understand pain: 'Precisely because culture provides a mode of organizing this experience, it provides an important condition for health care: it allows individuals to deal with their own pain.'[49] It is through society's norms and values that pain is culturally obtained and placed.[50] It is not difficult to identify extreme cases in which cultural norms dictate what are unacceptable and acceptable pains. Certain pains, such as menstrual pain or some forms of psychological pain, are expected to remain unvoiced, while others, such as grief and mourning, are required to be displayed in public. As Joanna Bourke has pointed out, even when they are suffering, 'people adhere to societal norms, rituals, and stories'.[51] One could thus say that there is no such thing as 'pain': there are only 'people in pain', who are joined to a specific society through their feelings and emotions. Thus, pain is not just a physical experience: it is an embodied experience to which meaning is attached through culturally validated and rhetorical artefacts, including societal classifications and norms, codified

[48] Bourke, *Story of Pain*, 214. In his recent book *Knowing Pain*, Rob Boddice briefly discusses the pain of infants. See Boddice, *Knowing Pain*, chapter 3.

[49] Ivan Illich, *Medical Nemesis: The Expropriation of Health* (Calder & Boyars, London, 1975), 101.

[50] This has been given several expressions from within the world of pain science. See Robert J. Gatchel, Yuan Bo Peng, Madelon L. Peters, Perry N. Fuchs, and Dennis C. Turk, 'The biopsychosocial approach to chronic pain, scientific advances and future directions', *Psychological Bulletin*, 133 (2007), 581–624 and Geoff MacDonald and Lauri A. Jensen-Campbell (eds.), *Social Pain, Neuropsychological and Health Implications of Loss and Exclusion* (American Psychological Association, Washington, DC, 2011). The study of neurosciences in history offers great potential for the exploration of these claims. See: Daniel Lord Smail, *On Deep History and the Brain* (University of California Press, Berkeley, 2008), 112–56; Jeremy Trevelyan Burman, 'History from within? Contextualizing the new neurohistory and seeking its methods', *History of Psychology*, 15 (2012), 84–99; Lynn Hunt, 'The experience of revolution', *French Historical Studies*, 32 (2009), 671–78. From a cultural historical point of view, the contextual experience of pain has already been extensively explored. See: Cohen, *Modulated Scream*; Bourke, *Story of Pain*; Boddice, *Knowing Pain*; and Moscoso, *Pain*.

[51] Bourke, *Pain and the Politics of Sympathy*, 6.

identities and even moral taboos.[52] There is no single and universally accepted meaning of pain. People who suffer pain appeal to all kinds of different value systems to frame their suffering with meaning.[53] Similarly, susceptibility to pain has been taken as an indication of civilisation and sensitivity, while pain has also been dismissed as a mere product of neurology. In other words, pain has been read by people in many very different ways as they attempt to make sense of what they feel and to explain these feelings within a coherent worldview.

However, tacit and explicit social norms on what is proper, just and decorous are not the only masters of pain and its sense-making. The ways we express pain are very much influenced by the various theories – medical, religious and concerning the body – that are current at the time in which we live.[54] Therefore, experiences of pain differ between individuals and from one social group to another, and they change according to geography and time. Contrary to the notion that the experience of pain is timeless, the meaning of pain arises from cultural and social interactions.

Rather than infecting the phenomenon of painful experiences with the virus of relativism, sociocultural determination opens the door to the work of historians and cultural theorists who can delve into the specifics of cultural manifestations at a given time. Hannah Newton has argued in *The Sick Child* that research on the experiences of illness and pain in childhood can be undertaken by studying their expressive metaphors.[55] In *The Story of Pain*, Joanna Bourke also argues that sufferers in the past used metaphors as a way of conveying their pain, which gives scholars of pain some insight into the subjective experiences of historical individuals.[56] In contrast, in *The Body in Pain* (1985), Elaine Scarry asserts that the experience of pain cannot be shared because of its essentially private nature. For Scarry, pain's subjective nature borders on solipsism: it 'does not simply resist language but actively destroys it'.[57] Following a quite radical interpretation of modern theories of knowledge and perception, she argues that physical pain 'has no referential content. It is not of or for anything, [and] resists objectification in language'.[58] Despite opposition and criticism, this theory of an insubstantial, noumenal pain has encouraged a new line of scholarship in which the focus has moved away from pain as an entity towards exploring the narratives of 'people in pain'. Theorists have had to wrestle with the problem that words often seem inadequate for expressing pain, with Virginia Woolf's essay 'On

[52] Bourke, 'History of medicine', 57.
[53] Louise Hide, Joanna Bourke and Carmen Mangion, 'Introduction: perspectives on pain', *19, Interdisciplinary Studies in the Long Nineteenth Century*, 15 (2012), 1.
[54] Hide et al., 'Introduction', 7. [55] Newton, *The Sick Child*, 196–97.
[56] Bourke, *Story of Pain*, 214. [57] Scarry, *Body in Pain*, 4. [58] Scarry, *Body in Pain*, 27.

Being Ill' often cited as evidence: 'The merest schoolgirl, when she falls in love, has Shakespeare, Donne, Keats to speak her mind for her; but let a sufferer try to describe a pain in his head to a doctor and language at once runs dry.'[59]

In *The Representation of Bodily Pain in Late Nineteenth-Century English Culture (2000)*, Lucy Bending challenges this point of view and argues that 'physical pain does not entirely resist linguistic expression' – or at least not to any greater extent than any other sensation or emotion.[60] In fact, Moscoso's *Pain: A Cultural History* (2012) reveals that pain experiences and their cultural meaning are based and built upon science, art and legislation. Moscoso sees pain as what Victor Turner in *The Anthropology of Performance* calls a 'social drama', a form of human experience that follows the ritual structure of rites of passage. In his view, the cultural historian should analyse the objectified forms of this subjective experience, together with the rhetorical means employed to relate experiences and expressions.[61] Joanna Bourke shifts the focus from 'illness' to the 'body-in-pain'. While Elaine Scarry argues that pain and language are refractory, Bourke assumes that – either directly or indirectly – embodied suffering becomes entangled in social behaviour – whether in observing or adhering to social norms, in reluctance to follow them, or in outright disagreement with them – but always around the complex language of socialisation. According to this approach, certain kinds of pain – notably chronic pain – do not fracture language but rather generate a wide range of linguistic manifestations. Bourke, examining narratives of pain from a historical perspective, argues that it is possible to develop a historical understanding of pain and the different ways in which 'people-in-pain' handle it and continue to live meaningful lives.[62]

This book shares the view endorsed by Bending, Moscoso and Bourke that there are linguistic conventions in both fiction and nonfiction for discussing both subjective pain and the pain of others. One of the main goals of this book is to identify how these conventions function in specific historical moments in the discourses of doctors, scientists and in public discourses, thus contributing to the construction of the intersubjective level of discourse on pain – where intersubjective does not refer to the horizontal, dialogical negotiation of sense among subjects with exchangeable positions, but rather to the institutionalised and normalised patterns for determining states and subjects of pain, which are then inherited in exchanges among subjects. Since the methodologies offered by Moscoso and Bourke have not proved helpful for the study of children's pain – precisely because they are constituted around metaphors and

[59] Virginia Woolf, *On Being Ill* (Paris Press, Ashfield, MA, 2002), 3.
[60] Bending, *Representation of Bodily Pain*, 1–5.
[61] Moscoso, *Pain*, 1–8. [62] Bourke, *Story of Pain*.

language – this book addresses the more difficult question of what happens in the case of historical subjects, such as children, who either lack verbal dexterity or do not have a recognisable cultural voice. Focusing on how certain adults – the paediatrician, the psychiatrist and the psychoanalyst – approached the experience of pain of their little patients, this study also explores the larger problem of how the historian can approach the past experiences of a person in pain.

As Bourke, Moscoso and Rob Boddice have shown, pain and its understanding as a phenomenon worthy of study beyond the life sciences is embedded in the literature on emotions and experience, and their importance for understanding historical processes. As Boddice argues, 'as a form of experience, pain is affectively produced'.[63] Although pain may not be merely an emotion, the experience of pain cannot be separated from its affective component. A child's expression of a painful experience – whether it be a scream or an outburst of tears – is an emotional experience, closely related to the scene where it takes place and dependent on the child's repertoire of expression and their own accumulated experiences. This book stands alongside other scholarship that convincingly argues that to treat emotions as entirely natural and independent of the self would, in Monique Sheer's words, 'depoliticize emotions by naturalizing them and endowing them with fundamental autonomy, thus denying their social and historical contingency'.[64] As Bourke and historian Keith Wailoo have argued, pain is a political practice.[65] Building on this politics of emotion, this book traces how over time the powerful question of children's pain became a recurrent site for disciplinary and political conflict. In these battles, as we shall see, theories of children's pain – medical, physiological, psychological and other views on children's suffering – become a tool of social and professional power.

Finally, while writing this book, I have encountered some surprising reactions from those around me. These reactions suggest that the topic of the child in pain invites much conjecture. Like David Morris in his book *The Culture of Pain*, I was repeatedly struck by the consistency with which I was asked, over and over: *Are you writing about children's physical pain or emotional pain?* This uniform reaction convinced me that Morris is right in his description of the 'Myth of Two Pains' in saying that we live at a time when many people have a deep and unexamined belief that physical and mental pain are separate

[63] Boddice, *Knowing Pain*, 5.

[64] Monique Sheer, 'Are emotions a kind of practice (and is that what makes them to have a history)? A Bourdieuian approach to understanding emotion', *History and Theory*, 51 (May 2012), 209–17.

[65] Bourke, *Story of Pain*, 18. Keith Wailoo, *Pain: A Political History* (Johns Hopkins University Press, MD, 2014).

entities, imagining that there is a huge gulf between them.[66] However, different sources of pain do not necessarily imply different pains. One of the purposes of this book is to support those who want to reject the artificial division of human pain into categories labelled 'physical' and 'mental'.[67]

[66] See Morris, *Culture of Pain*, 9.

[67] Boddice, *Pain and Emotion*; Boddice, *Knowing Pain*; Bourke, *Story of Pain*.

1 The Language of Children's Pain

For some people, the mere mention of the words 'children' and 'pain' will bring to mind Oscar Rejlander's photographs of children crying that Charles Darwin (1809–82) used in his work *The Expression of the Emotions in Man and Animals*. One of these illustrations, which bears the title 'Mental Distress' in the book but became known to the public as 'Ginx's Baby',[1] met with such success that Rejlander ended up selling 250,000 *cartes de visite* based on it.[2] The photograph shows what Darwin claimed was the characteristic physiognomy of a baby 'weeping or crying': the eyes closed, 'so that the skin round them is wrinkled, and the forehead contracted into a frown'; the mouth open with the lips 'retracted in a peculiar manner', and the teeth 'being more or less exposed'. For Darwin, the 'violent and prolonged screams' of children were emotional expressions associated with 'pain, moderate hunger, or discomfort'.[3] But how, in fact, can we then know *why* this particular child is crying? Is 'Ginx's Baby' a representation of pain, hunger frustration or – as it appears in Darwin's book – 'mental distress'? Does 'Ginx's Baby' have anything to tell us from a medical point of view? For many medical professionals in the late nineteenth century, the answer would undoubtedly have been in the affirmative.

As a research subject, the child in pain – which combines the previously separate fields of the history of childhood and the history of medicine – has been little investigated by historians.[4] Works that have reviewed the history of childhood pain – written mostly by psychologists – suggest that beliefs about the sensitivity of children and infants underwent huge changes during the

1 The title for the photograph was taken from a novel about an orphaned boy, by John Edward Jenkins (1838–1910).

2 Jonathan Smith, *Charles Darwin and Victorian Culture* (Cambridge University Press, Cambridge, 2006), 226; Phillip Prodger, 'Rejlander, Darwin, and the evolution of 'Ginx's Baby'", *History of Photography*, 3 (1999), 260–68.

3 Charles Darwin, *The Expression of Emotions in Man and Animals* (John Murray, London, 1872), 147.

4 See Introduction. For works that provide a cultural perspective on pain, see footnote 9. For a recent literary review on the subject of the sick child, see Newton, *The Sick Child*, 1–30.

second half of the nineteenth century.[5] This chapter develops Joanna Bourke's argument in *The Story of Pain* that children's pain was subject to a re-evaluation that concluded in the first half of the twentieth century with 'many scientists and clinicians claiming that infants were almost totally insensible to pain'.[6] By developing this line of argument and extending it to the field of the history of paediatrics, I explore how the emotional expression of children's suffering (mainly cries and screams) was interpreted differently by the various professional bodies with the power to shape its meaning.[7]

Two key questions emerge about the communication of children's pain. First, are children's expressions of pain and suffering capable of communicating certain states, conditions and emotions? If so, is there a univocal correspondence between expressions and their internal referents that justifies a scientific programme of description, classification and analysis? Anthropologists (or proto-anthropologists) tended to frame childhood within an evolutionary perspective – interpreting infant emotions as stages of development in a linear notion of progress – while paediatricians tried to decode the language of children to treat and heal them. The second – more radical – question emerged from the widespread belief that infants are mechanically programmed to cry: beyond the communicational use of screams and cries to relate to adults nonverbally, are children capable of feeling pain?

This chapter explores how the nonverbal and verbal expression of children's suffering was framed by different research programmes, understood from various theoretical angles and interpreted differently, depending on which professional body was shaping its meaning. The emerging life sciences, such as embryology and psychology, often claimed children were essentially insensitive to pain, while paediatricians – who faced the practical challenge of diagnosing and treating children – saw screams and cries as proof of the existence of pain and used such expressions to diagnose children's illnesses or injuries. Darwin tried to connect children's expressions to their emotions, while physiologists linked pain to the nervous system. Thus, the child's scream and cry created significantly different 'emotional bodies' in paediatric and experimental contexts. To shed light on this issue, it is important to investigate what physiologists, psychologists, doctors and paediatricians considered to be

[5] Chamberlain, 'Babies don't feel pain'; McGrath, 'Science is not enough'; Pabis et al., 'Pain in children in historical perspective'; Unruh, 'Voices from the past'; Rodkey and Riddell, 'The infancy of infant pain research'.

[6] Bourke, *Story of Pain*, 214.

[7] I have further developed this topic in Leticia Fernández-Fontecha, 'The language of children's pain (1870–1950)', in Dolores Martin Moruno and Beatriz Pichel (eds.), *Emotional Bodies: Studies on the Historical Performativity of Emotions* (University of Illinois Press, Urbana-Champaign, 2019), 77–96.

the causes of pain in children and, where appropriate, to explore their reasons for believing that such pain did not exist.

In addition to examining scientific sources previously analysed in published works about infant-pain experiments, my research for this chapter included an extensive literature search for medical and paediatric publications on infant pain, beginning with the Institute of Child Health (University College, London) Library Historical Collections on the History of Paediatrics and extending to vernacular medical texts. The study of paediatrics textbooks and journal articles illustrates changes in medical ideas about children's pain and shows how these shifts affected popular understanding of the body. With this aim in mind, this chapter concludes with an examination of Great Ormond Street Hospital's *cartes de visite*, which were used in fundraising. Photographs of children in pain – in the laboratory, the sickbed and the fundraising photograph – are useful tools for unravelling the complex social and political meanings of pain.

On Darwin, or Emotional Expressions as Reflex Actions

The subject of Darwin's 1877 'biographical sketch' was his own son 'Willy'. The article began in the following way:

> During the first seven days various reflex actions, namely sneezing, hickuping, yawning, stretching, and of course sucking and screaming, were well performed by my infant. On the seventh day, I touched the naked sole of his foot with a bit of paper, and he jerked it away, curling at the same time his toes, like a much older child when tickled.[8]

With the aim of evaluating the distinct behaviours and reactions of the child, Darwin focused on the realm of the instincts, differentiating the innate from the acquired and, at the same time, adopting an approach according to which development implied a process of hierarchy, with a gradual increase in the complexity of behaviour. Thus, throughout the text, two polarities are woven together: that of the child as an adult-in-training – which, in the Darwinian perspective was linked to the evolution from animals to humans – and that of the adult as a person of will. Four paragraphs below, Darwin describes Willy's first visit to the zoo, at the age of two. While the contemplation of known animals, such as the antelope and the deer, produced great enthusiasm in the child, the vision of the 'beasts in houses' provoked much concern and alarm in the little one. Not being able to explain the child's fear on the basis of previous

[8] Darwin, 'A biographical sketch', 1. For analysis and critique of Darwin's approach, see Michael Lewis and Alan Slater, 'A brief history of infancy research', in A. Slater and M. Lewis (eds.), *Introduction to Infant Development* (Oxford University Press, Oxford, 2002), 5–7.

experiences, Darwin asked if his son's vague but real fear might not be 'the inherited effects of real dangers and abject superstitions during ancient savage times?'[9]

The importance of this question and the repercussions of Darwin's publication lie both in its content and in the identity of the author. Inspired by the publication of *L'Acquisition du langage chez l'enfant et dans l'espèce humaine* by French philosopher Hippolyte Taine, the father of the theory of evolution decided to make use of the notes in his notebooks 'M' and 'N' about the development of his son William.[10] Darwin's publication took place during the middle of the nineteenth century, at a time when the first systematic studies of human development – the so-called biographies of babies – started to appear.[11] In Darwin's narration, as in other biographies of the same subject, the child appears as an object of knowledge through which the history of human development, or of humanity to come, is told: a universal figure seen through the example of a specimen. Chapter 2 of this study, taking the child as a symbol whereby research could mount a diachronic investigation of the human species would become a cornerstone for Darwinist anthropologists and representatives of the child study movement.

The observations on the physical and mental development of Willy – articulated around expression and including rage, fear, affection, and moral sense – set in motion the investigation that culminated in the publication of *The Expression of the Emotions in Man and Animals* (1872).[12] Darwin considered childhood the only natural – rather than culturally formed – stage of life, a blank page that hid two potentialities: the possibility of moulding the future adult and (which Darwin considered more important) the possibility of finding the ancestors of the modern human being in the behaviour and expressions of the child. In not granting the child the human attributes of freedom and free will, Darwin classified it alongside animals and automata. Despite the fact that

[9] Darwin, 'A biographical sketch', 1.

[10] Marjorie Lorch and Paula Hellal, 'Darwin's "natural science of babies"', *Journal of the History of the Neurosciences*, 19(2) (2010), 140.

[11] For a clear account of the 'advice to parents' industry see Christina Hardyment, *Dream Babies: Childcare Advice from John Locke to Gina Ford* (Frances Lincoln, London, 2007).

[12] On Darwin and the expression of emotions see Daniel M. Gross, 'Defending the humanities with Charles Darwin's *The Expression of the Emotions in Man and Animals* (1872)', *Critical Inquiry* 37 (2010), 49. The misapprehension of Darwin's overall approach to the changeability of emotions, in *Expression and Descent of Man*, is evidenced in the following: Paul Ekman and Wallace Friesen, 'Constants across cultures in the face and emotion', *Journal of Personality and Social Psychology*, 17 (1971), 124–29; Paul Ekman and Wallace Friesen, *Pictures of Facial Affect* (Consulting Psychologists Press, Palo Alto, 1976); Paul Ekman, *Emotions Revealed: Recognizing Faces and Feelings to Improve Communication and Emotional Life* (Times Books, New York, 2003). Ekman also wrote the introduction to a recent edition of Charles Darwin's *The Expression of Emotions in Man and Animals* (Oxford University Press, Oxford, 2002).

the body of the child contained the same muscles that permitted adults to express their emotions, the absence of both conscious control and conditioning proper to experience allowed one to see in the child the instinctive expressions of human beings and the traits shared with animals.[13] This child in pain, seen as a bodily theatre through which expressions of human history can be observed, is reinforced through the distribution of the chapters and the illustrations of *The Expression*. Darwin used these images not only as research material but also as a visual strategy that established a hierarchy of man and animal. While representations of animals appear only in the first half of the book (and only in the form of traditional woodcuts), pictures of humans are found in the second half of the book, from infants to older children and adults, and predominantly in the form of photographs.[14]

For Darwin, the child's emotional expressions illustrated human history. He considered a child's crying to be central to his investigations of expression, as it was one of the first and most common expressions. While other habits, such as laughing and weeping, were acquired gradually, 'the art of screaming [...] from being of service to infants, has become finely developed from the earliest days'.[15] Considered an innate expression, screaming proved ideal for studying the similarities between human and animal behaviour. Unsurprisingly, then, the first photographs of the chapter 'Special expressions of man: suffering and weeping' – which marks the narrative's transition from animals to humans – are of babies screaming and crying (Figure 1.1). Foremost among these was the one entitled 'Mental Distress' – taken by the Victorian artistic photographer Oscar Rejlander and which became famous as 'Ginx's Baby' (Figure 1.2) – which Darwin claimed illustrated the characteristic physiognomy of a baby 'weeping or crying'. According to the naturalist, the 'violent and prolonged screams' of children were emotional expressions associated with 'pain, moderate hunger, or discomfort'.[16] Nevertheless, within the context of the evolutionary process they became reflex actions strengthened by custom and, as a result, they were not reliable as indicators of pain.[17]

'A biographical sketch of an infant' launched a new field of observation and experimentation – the child in his or her early months – and would ultimately allow a naturalisation of the experimentation of childhood pain in the so-called century of the child.[18] Following the publication of Darwin's *On the Origins of Species* (1859), and more specifically through the emergence of evolutionary

[13] Phillip Prodger, *Darwin's Camera: Art and Photography in the Theory of Evolution* (Oxford University Press, Oxford, 2009), 105; Smith, *Charles Darwin*, 226; Prodger, 'Rejlander, Darwin', 260–68.

[14] Prodger, *Darwin's Camera*, 155.

[15] Darwin, *Expression of Emotions*, 210.

[16] Darwin, *Expression of Emotions*, 147.

[17] Rodkey and Riddell, 'The infancy of infant pain research', 338–50.

[18] Ellen Key, *The Century of the Child* (G. P. Putnam's Sons, New York, 1909).

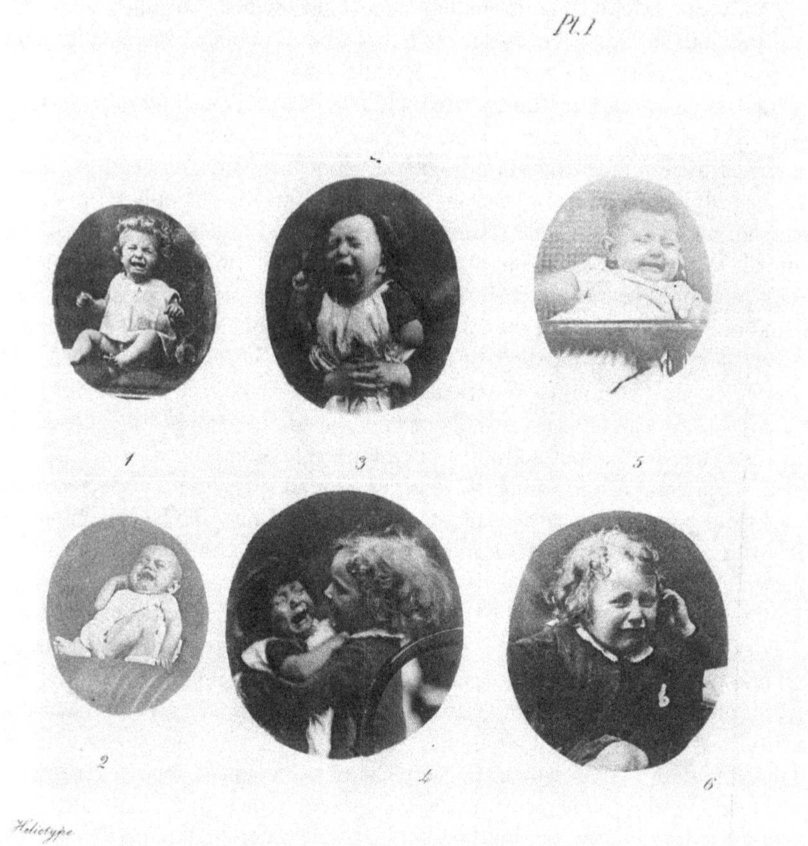

Figure 1.1 Oscar Reijlander and Herr Kindermann, *Fold-out plate of weeping children and babies from Chapter VI, Expression of Suffering,* by Charles Darwin, *The Expression of the Emotions in Man and Animals,* J. Murray, London (1872). Opp page 148, Pl. 1. Wellcome Library, General Collections.

psychology and psychiatry, there were pronounced displacements in the construction of childhood. Scientific validation for the idea of the child as an animal or savage could be found in the theories of recapitulation, which claimed that the child was a mirror that reflected the ancestral forms – both animal and human – of the species.[19] Furthermore, Darwin's interest in infant senses and the organising of responses into reflexes and instinct was an

[19] Shuttleworth, *Mind of the Child*, 4.

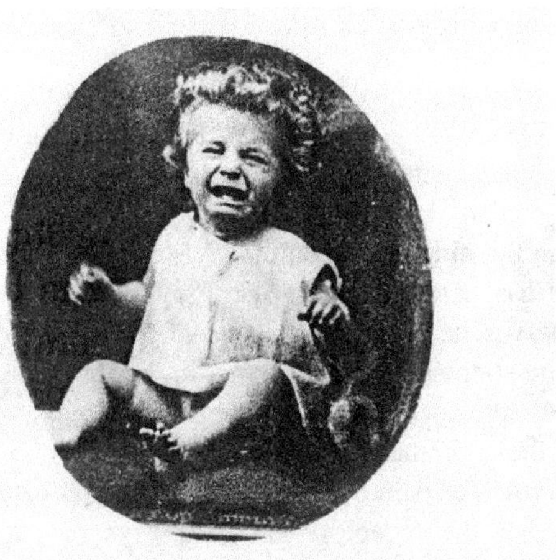

Figure 1.2 Oscar Reijlander, *Child crying*, from Charles Darwin, *The Expression of the Emotions in Man and Animals,* J. Murray, London (1872). Facing page 148, Tab. I, Figure 1. Wellcome Library, General Collections.

important influence on later experimental investigations that superimposed a preconceived interpretation of gestural language as a symbol of the biological past.[20]

German Contributions to Child Research: Experimental Tests of Infant Pain Sensitivity

Darwin was one of various authors who converged in the configuration of research programmes in which children's pain, or children's expressions of pain, were fixed as a representation of something else – whether the primitive past of the species or some kind of 'common sense' superstition. Many of the contributions to what would consolidate in the twentieth century as the theories of infant pain denial came from Germany, where the emergence of university science programmes coincided with an interest in the psychophysical and encouraged the growth of the new discipline of experimental physiology. This new physiology set out to understand the nature of the nervous system with an approach imbued in methodological scepticism and experimental caution. The experimental practices of prominent continental scientists, including Alfred Genzmer, Traugott Kroner and Silvio Canestrini, are framed within the development of the new physiology, which emerged in Germany around

[20] See Chapter 2.

the figure of Johannes Müller (1801–58). This new body of knowledge proposed an empirical programme for the study of vital functions and was greatly dependent on the development of new theoretical lines of investigating pain.[21]

Ernst Weber (1795–1878) investigated tactile thresholds and localisation but did not venture into the mechanisms of pain.[22] Nonetheless, his research on the senses and their perceptual thresholds was an important influence on psychophysics research in the nineteenth century.[23] Müller and other professionals – including Richard Bright, Maximilian von Frey, and Arthur Goldschneider – emphasised the nerves in their descriptions of the physiology of pain. As a result, an ever-more sophisticated understanding of the human nervous system emerged. However, the incomplete nature of knowledge about the nervous system prevented the attainment of a consensus about important points. Thus, scientists debated whether pain depended on the central or peripheral nervous systems and whether the receptors and pathways of pain served only to perceive pain or whether, on the contrary, they had more general functions.[24] Finally, they tried to settle the question of which theory described the physiology of pain with greater certainty: the theory of specificity (according to which the body perceives pain via a differentiated sensory system) or the pattern theory (pain receptors are shared with other senses).[25]

The development of experimental embryology strengthened the theoretical framework and enabled researchers to apply it to the understanding of the nervous system and the experience of pain. In 1872, Paul Emil Flechsig (1847–1929), Special Professor of Psychiatry at Leipzig University, started an investigation with sections of the brains of infants and children. His analysis of the brain sections led to the discovery that nerve fibre myelination had different rhythms during different states of development. While the newly born had both myelinated and unmyelinated fibres, only the myelinated ones were completely functional. The conclusion was that the demyelination of the newly born ensured that sensory stimuli, such as pain, were not completely functional and that a child at birth might have only simple sensations.[26]

In 1859, nearly two decades before Darwin's book, German internist Adolf Kussmaul (1822–1902) published his experimental studies of child behaviour titled *Untersuchungen über Das Seelenleben des Neugeborenen Menschen* (*Investigations of the Mental Life of the Newborn Child*). In the same year

[21] Moscoso, *Pain*, 122.

[22] See Stanley Finger, *Origins of Neuroscience: A History of Explorations into Brain Function* (Oxford University Press, Oxford, 1994), 134.

[23] Rey, *The History of Pain*, 194.

[24] Rey, *The History of Pain*, 135.

[25] See Bourke, *Story of Pain*, 10; Melzack and Wall, 'Pain mechanisms', 971–79.

[26] The Paul Flechsig conference, summarised by Frederick W. Mott, can be found in 'Cerebral development and function', *British Medical Journal*, 1, 3145 (1921), 529, cited in Bourke, *Story of Pain*, 216.

that Darwin paved the way for the anthropological interpretations of children with 'A biographical sketch of an infant', Kussmaul was analysing the 'normal' development of childhood to understand the adult mind's constitution. Inscribed in the tradition of the New German Physiology, his report about the behaviour and sensory repertoire of the newborn can be considered a work of experimental psychiatry, in which children became privileged subjects for conducting laboratory research.[27] Discussions about normal development during early childhood were an essential part of Kussmaul's psychiatric classes at the University of Heidelberg, and it was precisely his dissatisfaction with existing books that pushed him to carry out his own experiments.[28] His investigation centred on the function of the senses, including touch and sensitivity to temperature, and he performed experiments about smell, sight, audition, pain, muscular sensitivity and 'air hunger'.[29] Unlike the rest of the book, however, the section on sensitivity to pain was merely anecdotal and did not include experimental results. Kussmaul's reticence here stemmed from the fact that his attempts to carry out experiments on pain appeared to cause discomfort to the baby: trial experiments with tartaric acid were met with cries and discomfort, which led him to cancel this line of investigation.[30]

The first to combine Darwin's and Kussmaul's approaches and carry out experiments on infants' pain sensitivity was Alfred Genzmer (1851–1912) who, as a doctoral candidate in medicine and surgery at Halle-Wittenberg University, published *Investigations on the Psychic Function of the Newborn* in 1873.[31] The dissertation is a critical study of Kussmaul's work.[32] But if Kussmaul's discussion, like that of Darwin, was based on observations that were more incidental than experimental, Genzmer deliberately produced pain in children, pricking them with pins in the nose, the upper lip, and the hands. Even though the intensity of the stimulus was such that 'small drops of blood oozed from these openings', he claimed that the children 'gave no evidence of discomfort – not even a slight quivering'. However, he recognised that the stimulus was followed by an expression: 'the wetness of their eyes' increased

[27] Alfred Kussmaul, *Untersuchungenüber das Seelenleben des Neugeborenen Menschen* (Winter, Leipzig, 1859), cited in Rodkey and Riddell, 'The infancy of infant pain research', 343.

[28] Wolfgang G. Bringmann, Norma J. Bringmann, and William D. G. Balance, 'Experimental approaches to developmental psychology before William Preyer', in G. Eckardt (ed.), *Contributions to a History of Developmental Psychology: International William T. Preyer Symposium* (Mouton, Berlin, 1985), 159.

[29] Bringmann et al., 'Experimental approaches', 160.

[30] Bringmann et al., 'Experimental approaches', 160.

[31] Rodkey and Riddell, 'The infancy of infant pain research', 343.

[32] Alfred Genzmer, *Untersuchugen Ueber die Sinneswahrhehumugen des Neugeborenen Menschen*, Inaugural Dissertation (Plötzche Buchhandlung, Halle, 1873), cited in Rodkey and Riddell, 'The infancy of infant pain research', 343.

when the pins were placed in the children's faces. From all of this, he concluded that pain was 'exceptionally poorly developed in the neonate'.[33] In Genzmer's work, pain is presented as a tool of the experimental method, and children are objects of experimentation linked to the investigation of the development of organic functions.

Genzmer's work was continued by disciples including Traugott Kroner (1854–99), who in 1882 delivered an inaugural lecture at the University of Breslau that tackled the same subject,[34] and Silvio Canestrini, who in 1913 experimented with a group of seventy children and concluded that infantile touch showed a surprisingly light reaction to painful stimuli and a limited electrical excitability of the nervous system.[35] However, Genzmer's work remained obscure to the point it would most likely not have been remembered were it not for William Thierry Preyer who cited it in an 1882 work that was published in Germany, which explicitly merged Genzmer's research programme with Darwin's theories.[36]

In 1882, the English physiologist William Thierry Preyer (1841–97) published in Germany *Die Seele des Kindes* (later translated as The Mind of the Child), which summarised his observation of the development of his son Axel during his first three years, as well as the discoveries of many other investigators, making reference to recent empirical work in physiology and child psychology, including that carried out by Genzmer and Darwin.[37] Strongly influenced by the theory of evolution, Preyer understood development as a trajectory in which language and assertive action gradually took the place of instinct and reflex.[38] The rigour and meticulousness of Preyer's biography of his son – which was the most complete observational record of child development up until that time – opened a new period of studying the child.[39]

Even though Preyer had full confidence in Genzmer as an authority on the study of newborn infants, in the section dedicated to 'Unpleasant feelings in

[33] Genzmer, *Untersuchugen Ueber die Sinneswahrhehumugen*, 344, cited in Rodkey and Riddell, 'The infancy of infant pain research', 343.

[34] Traugott Kroner, 'Uber die sinnesempfindungen der neugeborenen', *Separat-Abzug aus der Breslauer arztl. Zt.*, 4 (1882), 14, cited in Florence Maater, *Child Behavior: A Critical and Experimental Study of Young Children by the Method of Conditioned Reflexes* (The Gorham Press, Boston, 1918), 20.

[35] Maater, *Child Behavior*, 20.

[36] William Preyer, *The Mind of the Child: The Development of the Intellect* (Arno Press, New York, 1889).

[37] Preyer's initial findings were published in the German journal *Deutsche Rundschau* as 'The mental development of man during the first few years of life' in May 1880. This preceded the publication of his more widely read *The Mind of the Child*, which was published in German as *Die Seele des Kindes* in 1882.

[38] Christine von Oertzen, 'Science in the cradle: Milicent Shinn and her home-based network of baby observers, 1890–1910', *Centaurus*, 55 (2013), 176.

[39] See von Oertzen, 'Science in the cradle', 175–95.

general', the psychologist wrote: 'It is an error to maintain that the very young child is not yet capable of having the genuine feeling of pain or even a high degree of unpleasant feeling', arguing that 'he who can enjoy must also be able to suffer, otherwise he could not enjoy'.[40] Although Preyer admitted that the newborn child is less sensitive to painful impressions than adults, he added that 'it would be a mistake to infer from this a condition of anaesthesia or analgesia'.[41] Noting that his son Axel 'reacted by movements upon the slightest touches of his face',[42] Preyer thought that babies showed indications of experiencing pain and declared that it was something 'unmistakable for every diligent observer. Above all, crying is characteristic: it is piercing and persistent in pain'.[43]

Preyer interpreted Genzmer's results in the light of the latest knowledge on nerve development and argued that if infants did not respond to a stimulus, it was not necessarily because they were insensitive to pain but could be explained by the painful stimuli affecting only a few nerves. So Preyer comes to a conclusion that may seem contradictory. On the one hand, he denies that babies experience pain to the degree that adults do; on the other hand, he insists that this does not mean that they do not actually experience pain because 'screaming and movements can be elicited from children and animals just born [...] by pinching the skin'.[44] However, he also expressed a view commonly held at the time: 'It would be of great interest to draw up a list, as complete as possible, of the reflex movements of the newly-born'.[45] Such a list would have made it possible to distinguish between merely mechanical movement and 'personal action'.

The belief that a child's external features reveal its inner qualities emerged during the eighteenth-century Enlightenment. Thus, it became possible to consider the child as more than 'an object of aesthetic contemplation' and to see it also from the point of view of scientific curiosity.[46] During the nineteenth century, evolutionary theories that showed the link between humans and animals provoked a change in concepts of human development, presenting this as a dynamic process rather than a series of static events.[47] From this perspective, children were seen as an embodiment of a primitive past and a link to the natural world, which could be studied to reveal the processes behind the formation of adult capacities.

[40] Preyer, *The Mind*, 147. [41] Preyer, *The Mind*, 147. [42] Preyer, *The Mind*, 106.
[43] Preyer, *The Mind*, 147. [44] Preyer, *The Mind*, 97. [45] Preyer, *The Mind*, 223.
[46] Donna Varga, 'Look – normal: the colonized child of developmental science', *History of Psychology*, 14 (2011), 140.
[47] Michael Wertheimer, 'The evolution of the concept of development in the history of psychology', in G. Eckardt, W. G. Bringmann and L. Sprung (eds.), *Contributions to a History of Developmental Psychology: International William T. Preyer Symposium* (Mouton Publishers, New York, 1982), 13–26.

This approach was notably advocated by George Romanes (1848–94), a prominent Darwinist and pioneer of comparative psychology. In his book *Mental Evolution in Man* (1888), Romanes wrote: 'The emotional life of animals is so strikingly similar to the emotional life of man – and especially young children – that I think the similarity ought to be taken as direct evidence of a genetic continuity between them.'[48] He argued that by studying the 'psycho-genesis of a child' it was possible to ascertain if there were a difference in kind between human self-consciousness and the emotions displayed by animals. The child was considered to be the ideal embodiment of the concept that 'ontology repeats phylogeny' – that each living organism goes through the evolutionary stages of its genus.[49] In the manner of the baby biographies, he took an incident where his own child knocked his head against a table.[50] On asking where he was hurt, the child 'immediately touched the part of his head in question – i.e., indicated the painful spot'. Now, Romanes asks, 'will it be said that in doing this the child was predicating the seat of injury?'[51] If so, he continues, 'all the distinctive meaning which belongs to the term predicating [. . .] is discharged'.[52] The 'gesture-signs' that are 'abundantly employed' by animals would have to be regarded in a similar way because 'they differ in no respect from those of the still speechless infant'.[53]

The clinical and academic interest in the functioning of reflex actions and the nervous system, the development of the scientific method and the Darwinist vision of the infant as an inferior primitive being and the child as an adult in training contributed to the generation of a mechanistic vision of childhood: a perspective that allowed a naturalisation of the experimentation of childhood pain.[54] Nonetheless, it is surprising how, just as science started to take a significant interest in childhood, both childhood itself and childhood pain seemed to disappear as autonomous subjects. All these detailed scientific annotations about the first movements and expressions of children and their reactions to sensation and pain did not stem from an interest in the child itself, but from its function as an index of evolutionary development. In all these narratives, the child is key to understanding the mind of the adult and the appearance of self-consciousness. By seeing the child's body as embodying the animal and the savage, Preyer and Darwin contributed to the naturalisation of experiments on childhood pain and to the consequent denial of the child's

[48] George Romanes, *Mental Evolution in Man: Origin of Human Faculty* (Kegan Paul, London, 1888), 7.

[49] Steedman, *Strange Dislocations*, 83.

[50] For Romanes' experiments with his child and the chimpanzee see Rob Boddice, 'Vivisecting major: a Victorian gentleman scientist defends animal experimentation, 1876–1885', *Isis*, 102 (2011), 215–37.

[51] Romanes, *Mental Evolution in Man*, 324.

[52] Romanes, *Mental Evolution in Man*, 324.

[53] Romanes, *Mental Evolution in Man*, 324.

[54] See Chapter 2.

dignity as a locus of recognition and sympathy. While these two approaches converged, there is a marked contrast between Darwin's account of the child as the embodiment of the long-lost savage and the scientific practices of Genzmer and Canestrini. By deliberately producing pain in the laboratory – pricking infants with pins in the nose, lips and hands, for instance – as part of an experimental method that led to infant pain denial, these two scientists ended up creating a very different kind of body: that of the child in pain, with its performative dimension.[55]

The Sick Child in Paediatrics

With the emergence of dedicated children's hospitals in Britain in the mid-nineteenth century, these institutions soon became the primary locations of observation and clinical practice on ill children and the main source of specialised research published in respected journals throughout Europe. However, where the experimental caution and methodological scepticism of physiologists and evolutionists had doubted the authenticity of children's language for communicating pain, the construction of the sick child as an object of study ran parallel with the programme of decoding the meaning of the gestural language of pain in infants.

In 1833, in a review of a pioneering French text about childhood illness, a contributor to *The Lancet* recognised that, in spite of medicine's general progress, children's illnesses had been ignored or attributed to teething, to the presence of worms, or to a vague notion of 'growth'.[56] Even though earlier doctors had recognised a series of illnesses that were either very common during childhood or that were considered exclusive to children, the study of pathologies proper to this period of life developed as a medical speciality only in the second half of the century. A series of concomitant factors explains this development. The search for professional recognition by anaesthetists at the end of the nineteenth century and the interest of physiology and evolutionary psychology in the development of the child coincided with the aspirations for legitimacy of another professional group: children's doctors. Thus, this medical speciality, based on the scientific construction of the child/adult dichotomy, started to organise the care of childhood in more scientific ways.[57]

[55] For recent discussions on pain as a kind of practice, see Dolores Martín Moruno, 'Pain as practice in Paolo Mantegazza's science of emotions', *Osiris*, 31 (2016), 137–68; In a similar line, historian Joanna Bourke has described pain as 'a type of event': Bourke, *Story of Pain*, 5–9.

[56] Westminster Medical Society, Saturday, 23 November, 1833. Mr. Pettigew in the Chair, *The Lancet*, 21 (1833), 367.

[57] On the history of paediatrics, see: A. R. Colón and P. A. Colón, *Nurturing Children: A History of Pediatrics* (Greenwood Press, Westport, CT, 1999); F. Garrison and A. Abt, *Abt-Garrison*

Given these conditions, the first hospitals dedicated exclusively to the care of sick children were created in various European cities during the nineteenth century. In 1802, the world's first independent children's hospital was opened in Paris: the *Maison Royale de l'Enfant-Jésus*, which later became the *Hôpital des Enfants-Malades*.[58] The arrival of paediatric hospitals and specialist institutions in the United States and the United Kingdom came much later, encountering considerable resistance on the part of the medical guild and public opinion, which insisted that children did not need to be subjects of hospital care. In London, the Great Ormond Street Hospital for Sick Children opened in February 1852 as the first specialist hospital for children in England. The hospital has been described many times as the realisation of the vision and dream of one man, Dr Charles West. Trained as a 'Physician Accoucheur' – in modern terms somewhere between a male midwife and a gynaecologist – West had gained interest in child health via women's health and through direct experience of children's hospitals in France and Germany and maternity hospitals in Dublin, where he trained.[59] West had the fortune of counting among his friends the British novelist Charles Dickens, who wrote an article in the widely read magazine *Household Words* to draw attention to the hospital when it opened.[60] So, although the hospital was at first treated with suspicion, little by little, its fame began to spread across the whole city.

Five years before Great Ormond Street opened its doors to the public, West delivered a series of lectures to students at the Middlesex Hospital about the illnesses of infants and children,[61] which already contained the seeds of what would be his future paediatric practice.[62] The text, like many others of the period, opens with the debate about whether children can communicate their emotions and their pain in a credible way. The difficulties faced by practitioners when diagnosing children's diseases and pains were such that many writers believed that children were unable to provide a reliable account of their own

History of Paediatrics, with New Chapters on the History of Paediatrics in Recent Times (W. B. Saunders, Philadelphia, PA, 1965).

58 Garrison and Abt, *Abt-Garrison History*, 289; Elizabeth Lomax, *Small and Special: The Development of Hospitals for Children in Victorian Britain*, *Medical History*, 16 (Wellcome Institute for the History of Medicine, London, 1996).

59 Andrea Tanner, 'Too many mothers? Female roles in metropolitan victorian children's hospital', in J. Henderson and A. Pastore (eds.), *The Impact of Hospitals* (Peter Lang, Oxford, 2007), 136.

60 For an elucidation on Charles Dickens's advocacy for the hospital see Jules Kosky, *Mutual Friends: Charles Dickens and Great Ormond Street Hospital* (Weidenfeld & Nicolson, London, 1989).

61 Charles West, *Lectures on the Diseases of Infancy and Childhood* (Longman, Brown, Green & Longmans, London, 1852).

62 Filippo Festini and Edward Alan Glasper, 'The contribution of Dr. Charles West to the development of contemporary health care for sick children', *Comprehensive Child and Adolescent Nursing*, 39 (2016), 84–93.

experiences. Already in 1849, A. Hess had described paediatrics as the most arduous of medical specialities 'arising from the inability or the unwillingness of children to give a proper description of their feelings, or owing to their fretfulness, shyness, and resistance to the proceedings of the physician'.[63] West passionately believed that, in spite of the significant barriers that young doctors faced when they came to examine children, the latter demonstrated their pain both through their behaviour and physiologically, providing sufficient proof to be correctly recognised by any decent doctor whose praxis was not based on folklore or on ancient forms of diagnosis. 'You cannot question your patient', explained West. Their lack of response, he said, could be explained by the absence of verbal abilities at early ages and by the paralysis provoked by fear. As a result, doctors had to rely on obtaining information from how a child expressed itself and behaved, which was not always an easy thing to accomplish. 'The child is fretful and will not be looked at, you endeavour to feel his pulse, he struggles in alarm: you try to auscultate his chest, and he breaks out in a violent fit of crying.'[64] Some doctors, not familiar with treating children, showed themselves incapable of learning how to examine and diagnose their youngest patients. West insisted that they try and that, although still speechless, a child 'has a language of its own, and that language must be your object to learn'.[65] With these words, West not only showed the difficulties that faced those who were interested in treating childhood illness but also emphasised the importance and necessity of the figure of the paediatrician.

West compared the children's doctor with an explorer who expects the inhabitants of a country to speak an already known language but finds that they speak a completely foreign tongue.[66] While some professionals never overcame this difficulty – and for them children's illnesses became a closed book – the 'good' doctor dedicated himself patiently to study 'a new semiotics, a new pathology and a new therapy', gaining access through this new language to an understanding of the child and his illness.[67] West, who used the metaphor of the explorer to express the lack of a first-person account from the patient, argued that those who did not cultivate their powers of observation would never be able to learn the language of childhood. He went further still, telling his students that doctors who did not appreciate young children would not be able to learn this language, 'for they soon make up their minds as to who loves them, and when ill they will express their real feelings, whether by words or

[63] A. Hess, 'On the necessity of practical instruction in the treatment of diseases of children', *The Lancet*, 10 (1849), 341.

[64] West, *Lectures*, 1–3.

[65] West, *Lectures*, 1–3.

[66] See J. Gillis, 'Not just small adults: the metaphors of paediatrics', *Archives of Disease in Childhood*, 92 (2007), 946–47.

[67] West, *Lectures*, 1–3.

signs, to no one else'. Those who were interested in the 'practical' or 'theoretical' study of children's illnesses not only had to be disposed to listen to and understand their patients; they also had to love them. The metaphor of the explorer (with all its implications of empire) persisted throughout the second half of the nineteenth century. Thus, in his 1891 presidential address to the American Pediatric Society, Thomas Rotch, the first chair in paediatrics at Harvard, spoke in words similar to West, telling his colleagues: 'We have entered upon the especial investigation of and research in this branch of anthropology with the keen interests of explorers in an almost unknown country.'[68]

The dominant view, until well into the nineteenth century, was that sick children were better off being looked after within their families than in institutions dedicated to their care.[69] So, it is not so strange that the accounts of these doctors, like those in many other treatises of the period, serve not only as a guide for those interested in the conditions proper to childhood but also as an exaltation of the qualities of paediatrics and the vindication of its existence. The discourses of Charles West and Thomas Rotch took place during the consolidation of the paediatric specialism, which happened within the wider battle for the legitimisation of new professional bodies and institutions that could strengthen this legitimisation. With the persistence of high levels of infant mortality in the cities, the role of hospitals as suitable places for sick children was gradually accepted.[70] Their defenders believed that children's hospitals had beneficial effects – both physical and moral – for patients, and the hospital wards were seen as middle-class homes beyond the strictly domestic sphere, promoting good behaviour and making working-class children more respectable.[71] With the recognition of the children's hospital as the ideal scenario for social change came the validation of the figure of the paediatrician, whose importance lay not only in his being a healer of the body, but also in being a trainer of the spirit.

The Diagnostic Power of Crying

As the narratives of West and Rotch show, the correct diagnosis of children's illness was a challenge for many doctors, which meant that pain was a subject

[68] Thomas Rotch, 'Iconoclasm and original thought in the study of pediatrics', *Archives of Pediatrics*, 7 (1891), 811.

[69] Lomax, *Small and Special*, 12.

[70] M. J. Daunton, 'Health and housing in Victorian London', *Medical History*, Suppl. 11 (1991), 126.

[71] Andrea Tanner, 'Choice and the children's hospital: Great Ormond Street Hospital patients and their families, 1855–1900', in A. Borsay and P. Shapely (eds.), *Medicine, Charity and Mutual Aid: The Consumption of Health and Welfare in Britain, c.1550–1950* (Ashgate, Aldershot, 2007), 136–37.

treated with great seriousness by doctors who were interested in the field of children's health. They reclaimed the diagnostic value of pain, which the scientific community had come to see as representing not much more than a symptom of disease or injury.[72] As early as 1842, the Irish doctor Richard Tonson Evanson had demonstrated the instrumental use of pain in the 'Diagnosis' section of his manual about children's diseases. For this doctor, it was essential to determine the existence of pain and its seat in the child or the cause that might make an infant cry, given that pain and the expressive gestures that accompanied it were the most direct manner of accessing childhood illness.[73] As West later indicated, the importance of children's physical signs and their translation into clinical signs could confer on them the status of a code that could be deciphered, allowing doctors to approach childhood pain. Doctors such as West and Evanson encouraged the screams and cries of the children not because they could not remedy them, but because they believed that in promoting the abundance of such signs they could arrive at a more accurate diagnosis of the illness.

This semiotic effort was a specific epistemological tool that the incipient discipline of paediatrics chose to adopt, and it marked a differentiated approach to the inclusion of pain in a body of scientific knowledge. Towards the end of the nineteenth century, paediatricians embraced the anatomo-clinical tradition and tried to connect signs of pain with organic injuries. Hence, a search for the most systematic tests for pain in children began expanding observations about childhood crying and examining the changes in children's facial expressions or sleeping habits under the effects of illness. The semantics of pain encountered many of the same problems that any scientific analysis of natural language needs to tackle, mainly homonymy (the same sounds having different meanings) and polysemy (the inability to connect each term to only one meaning, and only one meaning to each term), beginning with the polysemy of tears. The American doctor Louis Starr, who believed that healthy children rarely cried, noted that crying was a single means to communicate various meanings: 'Crying is the chief, if not the only means that the young infant possesses of indicating his displeasure, discomfort or suffering.'[74] Although crying seems to be the behaviour most often associated with pain, there were controversies over whether crying always indicated discomfort, pain or illness in a child. For this reason, doctors put their efforts

[72] See Hide et al., 'Perspectives on pain', 5; Bending, 'Pain and religion', 1–5.

[73] Richard Evanson, *A Practical Treatise on the Management and Diseases of Children* (Fannin & Co., Dublin; Renshaw and Longman, London, 1842), 63.

[74] Louis Starr, 'The clinical investigation of disease and the general management of children', in Louis Starr and T. S. Westcoote (eds.), *An American Text-Book of the Diseases of Children* (Saunders, Philadelphia, PA, 1985), 3.

into developing a scheme for evaluating children's pain based on different kinds of crying to distinguish the crying of pain from that caused by boredom, frustration or exercising the lungs. Evanson thought that crying that came from acute suffering 'is clear, loud, sounding and continuous', belonging more to exhalation than inspiration.[75] The paediatrician added to crying a series of complementary gestures, such as the position of the eyebrows and the hands, trying to construct an invariable connection between the sign and the anatomic injury. For Starr, the first professor of paediatrics at the University of Pennsylvania Medical School, a direct relationship could be established between different kinds of crying and specific illnesses and degrees of pain. While hydrocephalic crying consisted of a sudden, paroxysmal and loud cry which implied headache, 'loud brazen crying' was a precursor of spasmodic croup, and a child who cried during a coughing fit or soon afterwards – when the crying was accompanied by a distortion of the features – was suffering from pneumonia.[76]

The American paediatrician Luther Holt was particularly concerned that the pain of infants under two months of age should not be overlooked. In 1899, he argued that the absence of tears before this time should not be taken as an indication that the young baby did not feel pain. Holt divided children's cries into several functional groups according to whether the cause was hunger, indigestion, temper, weakness or exhaustion, discomfort, pain or habit. Holt suggested that children suffering extreme pain cried in a sharp and penetrating way, contracting their facial features, raising their legs and, sometimes, ending up falling into an exhausted sleep.[77] In his opinion, crying that resulted from less severe pain was more like moaning and less sharp in tone. Ralph Vincent, who founded the Infants' Hospital in Westminster in 1907, also affirmed that crying produced by an intense pain was characteristic: '[I]t is sharp and penetrating and is united with the contraction of the extremities and the features.' Some lines later he added: 'one of the cries which is often misinterpreted is that which results from the pain of indigestion. The cry itself is not as sharp as in the case of those that result from more intense pains and is closer to that of the cry of hunger.'[78] Just as for Darwin there was a direction relationship between emotions and their expression, for Starr too pain was always expressed through the same gestures and expressions. He described the facial expression of childhood pain and indicated how to infer the origin of the pain from these expressions – for instance, 'the contraction of the frown denotes

[75] Evanson, *Practical Treatise*, 108. [76] Starr, 'Clinical investigation', 6.

[77] Luther Emmett Holt, *The Diseases of Infancy and Childhood: For the Use of Students and Practitioners of Medicine* (Appleton, New York, 1899), 1–45.

[78] Ralph Vincent, *The Nutrition of the Infant*, 4th ed. (Bailliere, Tindall and Cox, London, 1913), 198.

headache', the stretching of the nasal cavities indicated 'chest pain, and the raising of the upper lip pointed to abdominal pain'.[79]

However, not all authors agreed with Starr's interpretation. Although the manuals about childhood conditions published in the second half of the nineteenth century never questioned the diagnostic value of pain, authors such as the American John Forsyth Meigs, one of the pioneers of the study of childhood illness, criticised the belief that the origin of pain could be localised through the response of the patient.[80] Those doctors who repudiated the concept that associated specific pathologies with their expressive signs underlined the importance of obtaining a good history. Thus, James Carmichael, physician at the Royal Hospital for Sick Children, advised the doctor to

> talk to the mother or nurse and learn the history of the present and previous illnesses, the number of children, and where the patient comes in the family; the number and health of those living; the causes of death of any which are dead; the mother's health during pregnancy; the nature of the confinement, and of any difficulties or abnormalities at birth; the number of miscarriages, and the mode of feeding.[81]

Carmichael recommended practising these investigations before exploring any concrete illness, given that parents could suppose that they could seek to ascribe the cause of the said illness to a life circumstance or the previous history of the family. Although, like many of his colleagues, this doctor believed that heredity played a major role in certain illnesses, he did not consider it advisable to mention this to the family and thought that it could even be considered 'unkind' to do so, given that 'ready as a parent may be to transmit disease to the child, there is a natural objection to taking the blame thereof'.[82] In this, Carmichael was not alone.

The diagnostic method used by Charles West follows a similar line, as explained in his book *Lectures on the Diseases of Infancy and Childhood*, and it was applied in an almost literal form by all the paediatricians at the Great Ormond Street Hospital.[83] On this occasion, as on the others, the case notes register the doctor's first impressions of the child and its family, and they cover the territory relating to the pregnancy, the method of weaning, and the sobriety and the health of the mother. Children's hospitals had a contradictory vision of the mothers of their patients. On the one hand, the institutions needed parental consent, without which no patient could be admitted; for this reason, it was

[79] Starr, 'Clinical investigation', 3–4.
[80] John Forsyth Meigs, *A Practical Treatise on the Diseases of Children* (Lindsay and Blackiston, Philadelphia, PA, 1853), 23.
[81] James Carmichael, *Disease in Children: A Manual for Students and Practitioners* (Pentland, Edinburgh, 1892), 3.
[82] Carmichael, *Disease in Children*, 3.
[83] Charles West, nineteen volumes of case notes (1838–80) are stored in the archives at The Hospital for Sick Children, Great Ormond Street.

important to sell the hospital services to the families. On the other hand, there was a conviction that maternal incapacity was partly responsible for childhood illnesses.[84] Despite this lack of confidence, the information the doctor obtained about the state of the child before its entry into the hospital almost always came from the mother, so the maternal account was another of the methods used to diagnose childhood illness.[85]

Regarding these case notes, it is striking that, despite the disputes about the credibility of children's accounts of their own suffering, children's voices are indeed reported in relation to pain through their mother's accounts. Henry Ashby refers to the case of a child 'of nine years of age was suddenly seized (22 April 1881) with pain in the abdomen while at school, followed by the passage of blood and mucus by the bowel'. Some pages later he describes the case of John C., nine years old, who 'one day complained of pain in the belly, and vomited the same evening. He continued to vomit five or six times a day till his admission to hospital (under Dr Hutton), on the fifth day of illness [. . .] He complained of paroxysms of pain in the abdomen'.[86] The clinical cases reproduced in paediatric books were taken from the personal case notes of different doctors. In all of these case notes, we find the same situation. Every time a reference is made to the child's experience, it is in relation to its pain. Thus, we find the case of Ada Smith who, during the afternoon of 10 January, 'came to Nurse complaining of pain in the front of the chest (over sternum) and of feeling sick'.[87] Another case was Sarah Bennett, a four-year-old child from Camden Town who, having contracted pneumonia, returned one June day complaining of 'being cold & having a pain in the right side'.[88]

Paediatricians working at the Great Ormond Street Hospital clearly had considerable sympathy with their child patients, and they sought to encourage a similar attitude in society at large, believing that the public could ally itself to the cause of caring for sick children if the work of the hospital was communicated effectively.

The Visual Limits of Pain

Although Darwin had used photography to support his claim of the universality of most expressions, subsequent paediatric treatises contained few photographs. Photography was nonetheless used in the field of children's health – extensively in fundraising and as a support for medical practice. This section

[84] Tanner, 'Too many mothers', 55. [85] Tanner, 'Too many mothers', 55.
[86] Henry Ashby, *The Diseases of Children: Medical and Surgical* (Longman Green, New York, 1900), 120.
[87] GOS/10/11, Dr Charles West casenotes, 1870, Great Ormond Street Archives.
[88] GOS/10/11, Dr Charles West casenotes, 1870, Great Ormond Street Archives.

does not look at clinical photography, but rather at what can be considered a visual culture of the sick child, usually identified in art, media coverage, public health campaigns and activist images.[89] While clinical photographs served well to demonstrate unusualness, irritating appearances and irregular symptoms, fundraising photographs and the little patients campaign focused on the faces and the individuality of the sick children, to proclaim the importance of the new hospital and of the emerging field of paediatrics.[90]

Like all Victorian philanthropic creations, the Great Ormond Street Hospital had to compete for attention and funds in a market that was saturated with good causes. As would be the case with later children's hospitals, Great Ormond Street Hospital came into being thanks to the work of a strong and determined medic – West – who was supported by a group of private patrons.[91] Its dependence on patronage meant that there was a constant struggle to raise funds and to maintain a high profile in the eyes of the public. Unlike certain specialist institutions – such as St Mark's Hospital for Fistula, also in London and supported by Dickens – the children's hospitals' generalist approach granted them a potentially instantaneous entrée into the Victorian heart through the tales of their small patients, which filled many columns in the general and religious press. Engravings of the wards and of visitors to the hospital were used to illustrate these pieces, showing idealised images of the quasi-domestic atmosphere of the institution, with bouncing, happy children and the respectable adults who cared for them. Almost from the very beginning, Great Ormond Street Hospital was taken up by the press and social reformers as a symbol for campaigns to improve sanitation and to rescue children from the effects of poverty and deprivation.[92] They described the hospital and West's principles of paediatric care in terms of an approach to childhood that was largely characterised by middle-class values and sentimentalism.[93] West and his hospital, indeed, encouraged such attitudes, not least in the materials used for fundraising purposes.

In the late 1860s and early 1870s, the hospital needed to raise funds for two projects: the acquisition of a convalescent home in the country and the building of a completely new hospital on the Great Ormond Street site. The latter

[89] The photographic representation of the sick child has been studied in the context of Canadian hospitals, see Anne Marie Adams, David Theodore, and Patricia McKeever, 'Pictures of health: sick kids exposed', in Loren Lerner (ed.), *Depicting Canada's Children* (Wilfrid Laurier, Waterloo, 2009).

[90] I have further developed this topic in Leticia Fernández-Fontecha, 'Little patients: photography and the configuration of the sick child in Victorian Britain', in Jutta Ahlbeck, Paäivi Lappalainen, Kati Launis and Kirsi Tuohela (eds.), *Childhood, Literature and Science: Fragile Subjects* (Routledge, London, 2017), 110–27.

[91] Katharina Boehm, *Charles Dickens and the Sciences of Childhood: Popular Medicine, Child Health, and Victorian Culture* (Palgrave Macmillan, London, 2013), 81.

[92] Boehm, *Charles Dickens*, 82. [93] Steedman, *Strange Dislocations*, 66.

required a massive fundraising programme and the hospital turned to the relatively new medium of photography – which it already used to provide its supporters with images of its work – as one of its main tools. Two well-respected photographic companies – the Stereoscopic Company and Faulkner – were hired to take these images, which presented the hospital as a welcoming place for children, while giving little indication of medical technology or illness.[94] The photographs can be seen as falling into two categories: on the one hand, ward images depict the hospital as the place where heroic physicians used the latest medical knowledge to heal child patients who are portrayed as the frail and helpless beneficiaries of healthcare expertise; on the other hand, images of playfulness promote the institution as a place of social interaction and fun. These more positive images of hospital life portray sick children actively defying, through friendship and recreation, the seriousness of their circumstances and the fear and anxiety associated with illness.

Photographs of the hospital wards were produced and distributed in the form of postcards to raise funds.[95] These images did not focus on the sick child but, rather, showed the conditions in which these children lived at the hospital and documented the medical techniques, the healthcare environment and hospital life. Most of the extant images of the hospital were produced specifically for fundraising purposes. Some of the photographs show the 'bad' aspects of the hospital – crowded waiting rooms and stark corridors, for instance (Figure 1.3) – as a way of illustrating why it needed more money to become a better hospital. It was a difficult balancing act, as the images needed to show both that the institution was powerful and worthy of funding and that it lacked the funds it needed for the optimal performance of its role. So, there were also photographs that showed the 'good' aspects of the hospital, thereby demonstrating that money had been well invested. These images show an environment that is calm and orderly, where children walk around and play with toys, while those who are confined to beds lie in ordered rows between neatly tucked blankets and bright white sheets. The ward is light and airy, with high windows that are open, and a sense of home is created through the deployment of plants and toys. In these photographs, the only adults are usually women – the nurses (as surrogate mothers). These ward photographs show the hospital as clean, efficient and comforting for those inside, while also projecting an image of the institution as welcoming and urbane.

A remarkable series of photographs, produced by the Commercial & General Photographic Co. (c. 1870), shows the efficiency and antiseptic cleanliness of the hospital departments, featuring the white-clad nurses as almost angel-like healers of sick children (Figure 1.4). The children themselves

[94] GOS/1/2/12, Hospital Minutes, 22 February 1872, Great Ormond Street Archives.
[95] GOS/1/2/12, Hospital Minutes.

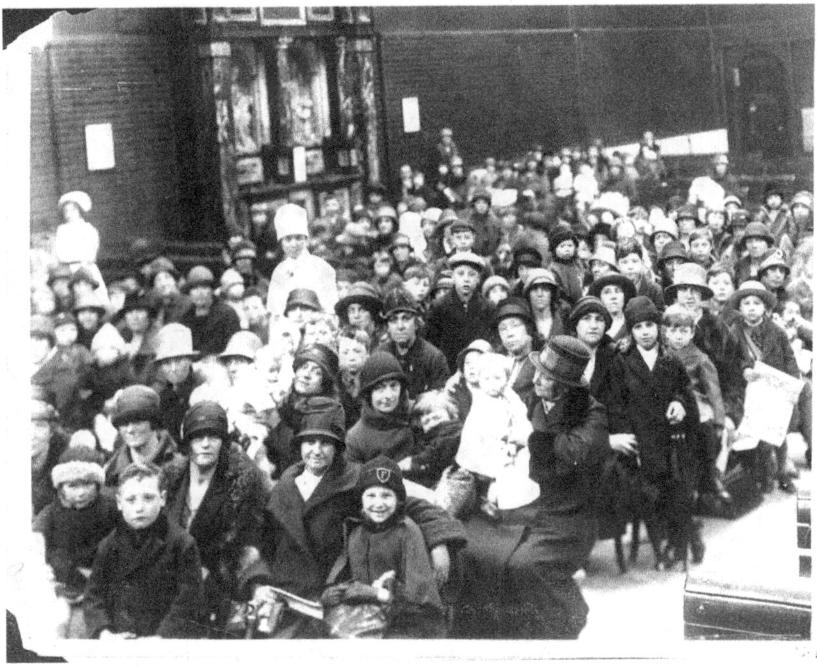

Figure 1.3 Photographer unknown, *Outpatients* (c. 1920), B-INT 01989, Great Ormond Street Archives.

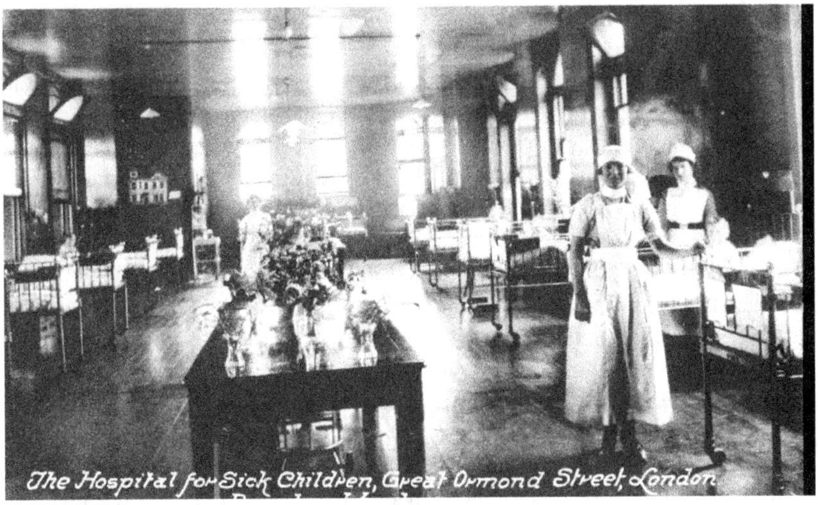

Figure 1.4 Photographer Unknown, *Dresden Ward* (c. 1910), B-INT 00478D, Great Ormond Street Archives.

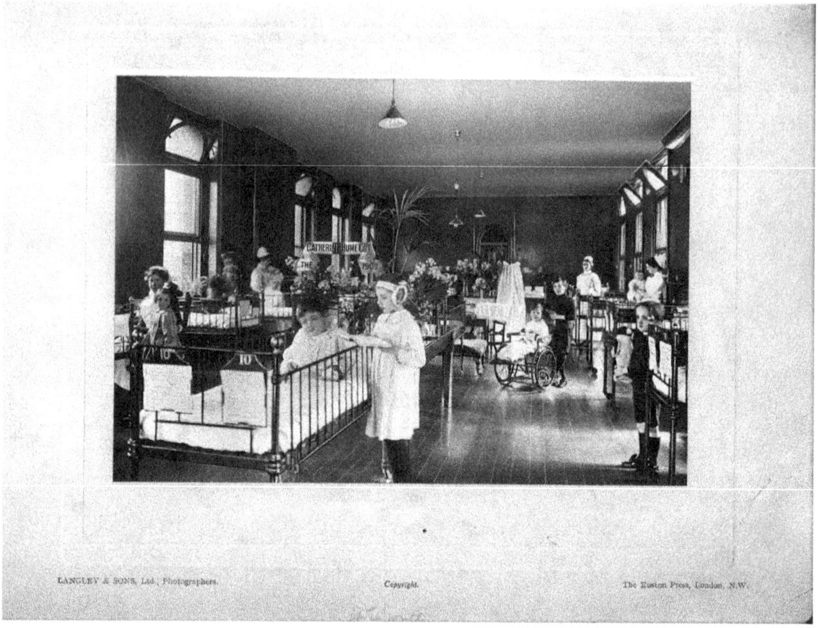

Figure 1.5 Langley & Sons, *Dresden Ward* (c. 1910), B-INT 00237, Great Ormond Street Archives.

are in their beds and appear to be still and vulnerable. Such images were designed to inspire hope in those who saw them, particularly those who might be willing to provide financial support to an institution that – long before the advent of state funding and national healthcare coverage – depended totally on patronage. Similarly, a photograph produced by the studio of Langley & Sons, Ltd., shows children in the ward, with two in the foreground, one reading a book to the other (Figure 1.5). Here, the hospital environment is turned into a school setting: health and education occupy the same space. The image also presents the architecture of the institution in a way that evokes associations with comforting places, such as a family home, a well-appointed hotel, or a church. The elegant wood panelling and carving convey the view that the child patients will be treated with dignity and respect in this hospital. Looking at these images in chronological order, one can see the changes at the hospital through the success of its fundraising efforts, such as the opening of new spaces and the deployment of new equipment.

However, these photographs also had a use beyond fundraising. They were an important means of communication between the hospital (represented by the ward sister) and the patients' parents. Visiting for family and friends was restricted to one afternoon a week, with the occasional Sunday afternoon

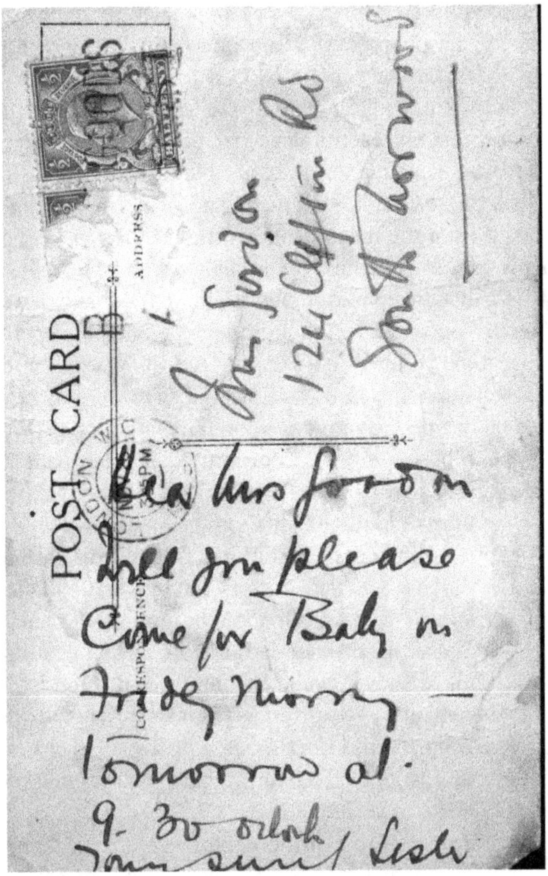

Figure 1.6 *Dresden Postcard* (c. 1900), B-INT 00478D, Great Ormond Street Archives.

known as 'Father's Day', and it was suspended completely during infectious outbreaks. These images became a precious means for families to keep track of their children's health. For parents living far from London, they might be the only news they had of their child until receiving the final letter, which would request their visit to take the child home. Cards were sent out each week, with a pencilled note, usually in large, cursive writing, reporting the patient's health during the previous seven days. The language is rather domestic: 'Baby is not so well this week' and 'baby is teething and sends you all a kiss' are two frequently sent messages (Figure 1.6).[96]

[96] Great Ormond Street Hospital B-INT 0478, ward postcards.

The photographs of children's hospitals are populated by happy and active children who smile for the photographer, despite their illnesses, injuries and physical limitations. Most of the patients at Great Ormond Street were from poor families, who did not have the means to contribute to a health insurance scheme, let alone pay a general practitioner when they were ill. These children lived in overcrowded and unsanitary conditions and their bodies displayed the marks of infectious disease, malnourishment and, very often, tuberculosis. They were a long way from the rosy-cheeked little cherubs so beloved of the engravers, which presented something of a challenge to the photographers. The hospital required that the photographs used in fundraising were sufficiently full of pathos to open the hearts and the wallets of the spectator, but they also had to present the children in a way that was sufficiently middle class to engender feelings of sympathy in those at whom they were directed.[97]

In 1870, the hospital decided to move beyond the photographs of the wards and to create a campaign based on images of individual child patients, which were sold as *cartes de visite*.[98] Two such photographs portray Nellie Wallace (Figures 1.7 and 1.8), admitted to the hospital on 29 June 1872 with problems with her knee (probably a tubercular condition). Despite recovering, Nellie was readmitted on 10 March 1873 and doctors removed part of the knee.[99] Another photograph shows Sydney Jones (Figure 1.9), admitted on 13 June 1873, whose diseased right knee led doctors to amputate his leg up to the thigh.[100] A third image shows Annie Kezia Eastland (Figure 1.10), who was admitted on 21 November 1870 suffering from necrosis.[101] Although all three children suffered from painful conditions and two of them underwent surgery, there is little visible sign of the pain of their illnesses and procedures they went through.

In attempting to reconstruct the historic experiences of children in pain, these photographs are important precisely because of the interplay between what is visible and invisible in them, as can be sometimes inferred from the patient histories reported below them. Because of their intended use, their main objective was to present the hospital's mission so that it could generate a sympathetic response from people and encourage them to donate money. However, photographers had to find new ways to display pain, disability and poverty while staying within the limits of certain moral conventions.

97 Andrea Tanner and Sue Hawkins, 'The sentimental hard sell: the role of early patient photography at Great Ormond Street Hospital', *Society for the Social History of Medicine Conference*, Durham University, July 2010, unpublished paper, 1–2.

98 GOS/1/2/12, Hospital Minutes.

99 GOS/9/1/2, 1865–72; GOS/9/1/3, 1872–78, Hospital's General Admissions Registers, Great Ormond Street Archives.

100 GOS/9/1/2, 1865–72; GOS/9/1/3, 1872–78.

101 GOS/9/1/2, 1865–72; GOS/9/1/3, 1872–78.

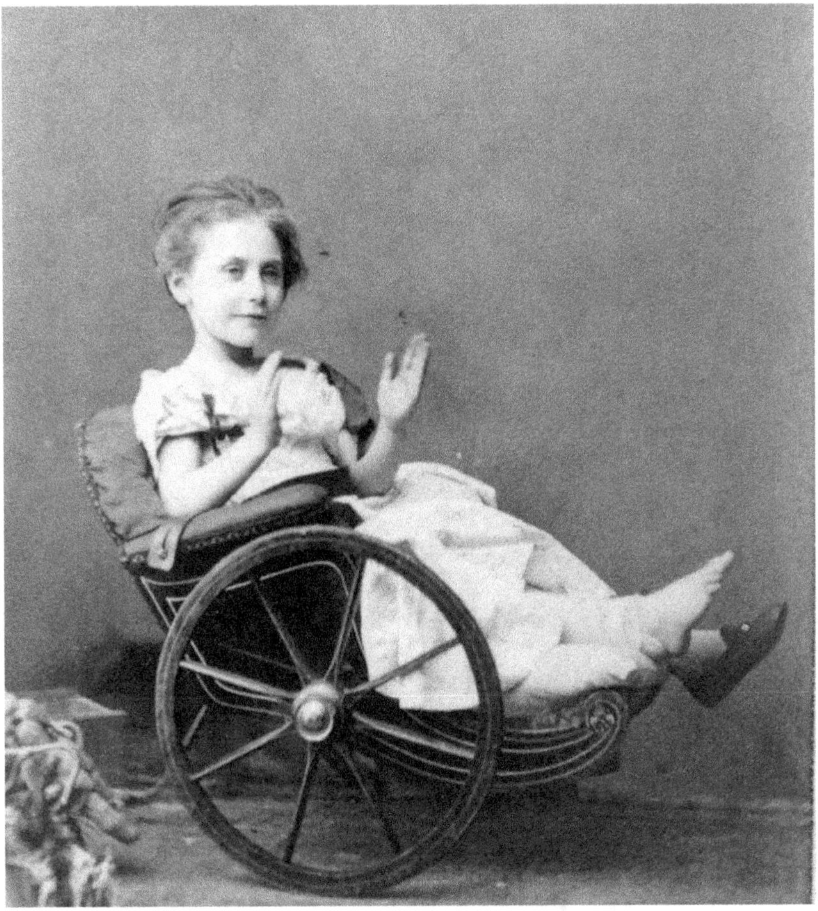

Figure 1.7 Robert Faulkner & Co, *Nellie Wallace* (c. 1875), Hospital for Sick Children Fundraising Album, Great Ormond Street Archives.

Nellie (otherwise Nelly or Ellen) Wallace, was admitted from her home in Hoxton (in London's East End) aged four and a half in 1872, suffering from a diseased knee. After three months, she was sent to the hospital's convalescent home in Highgate, where she contracted scarlet fever. She was readmitted in March 1873, when part of her knee joint was excised. In July, she was sent to Cromwell House, and then on to Brighton, to convalesce, although she returned for more surgery in November of that year and was finally discharged on 11 March 1874, once again pronounced fully recovered. Nellie's repeated stays at the hospital between the ages of four and seven seem to have made her a favourite of the hospital, and she was the subject of a short

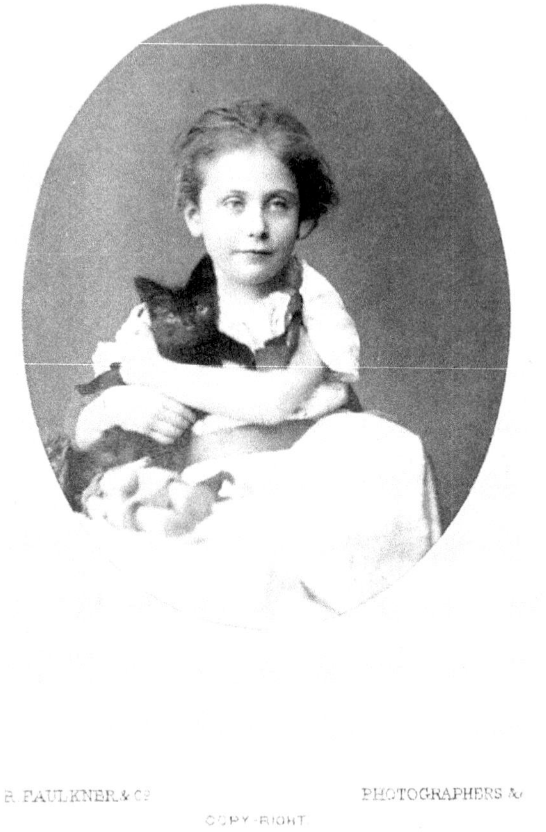

Figure 1.8 Robert Faulkner & Co, *Nellie Wallace* (c. 1875), Hospital for Sick Children Fundraising Album, Great Ormond Street Archives.

series of photographs, sitting in a rather grand, chariot-style, child's padded wheelchair and playing with Smut, the hospital cat. Her short hair is brushed back, to show her fine bone structure, and she is wearing what would appear to be a party dress, complete with ribbons and extensive ruching. It is possible that the photograph dates from after her brush with scarlet fever, as cutting off long hair 'to preserve strength' was a common strategy in cases of infectious fevers. There are toys strewn around the wheelchair, but no exotic

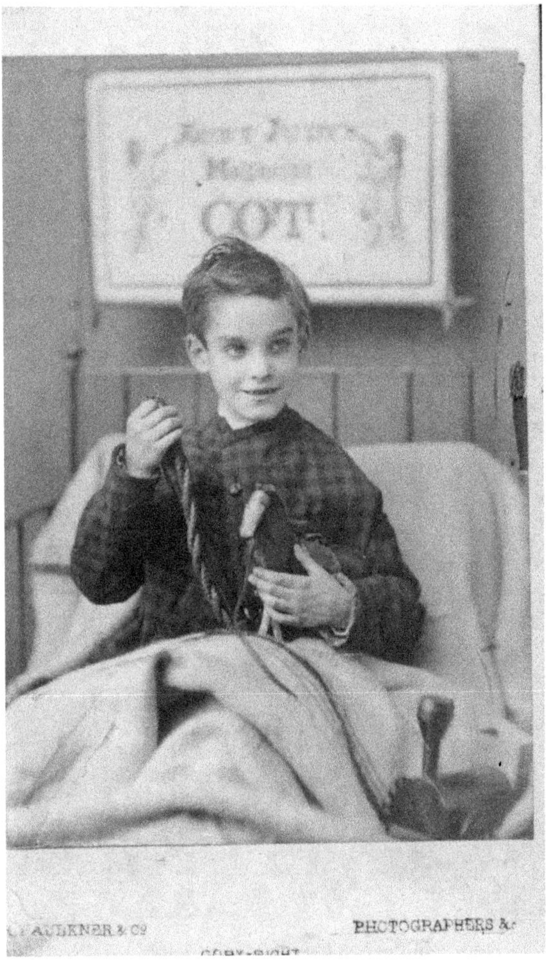

Figure 1.9 Robert Faulkner & Co, *Sidney Jones* (c. 1875), Hospital for Sick Children Fundraising Album, Great Ormond Street Archives.

backdrop, which would suggest that the images were taken in the hospital itself.[102]

Sydney Jones had been admitted suffering from 'disease of the knee' – probably tubercular – which was so severe that his leg required amputation.[103]

[102] GOS/9/1/2, 1865–72; GOS/9/1/3, 1872–78.
[103] GOS/9/1/2, 1865–72; GOS/9/1/3, 1872–78.

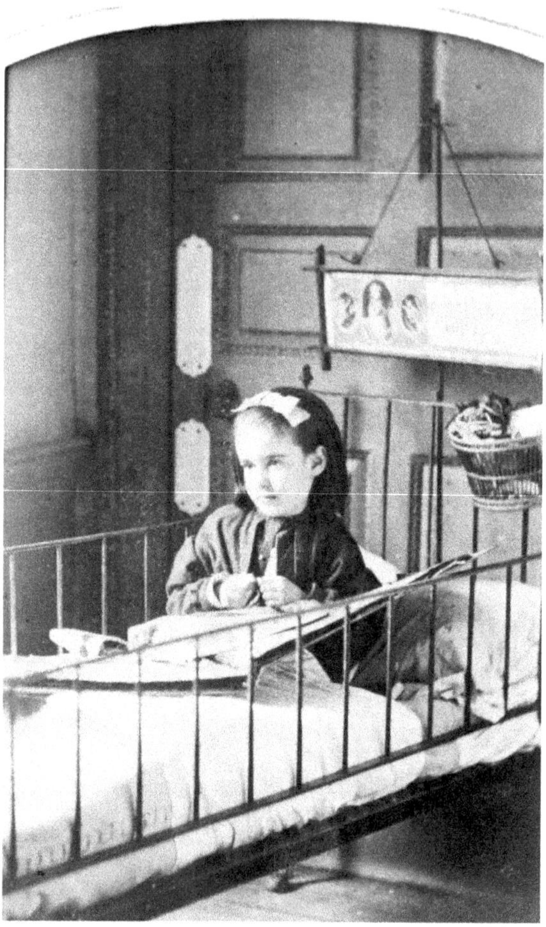

Figure 1.10 Robert Faulkner & Co, *Annie Eastland* (c. 1875), Hospital for Sick Children Fundraising Album, Great Ormond Street Archives.

The tenting of his blankets indicates it was probably his left leg that had been affected. Nevertheless, there he sits, looking cheerful and holding tightly onto his toy horse, with a wooden train tucked away to one side. His face is long, somewhat pinched and narrow, and his eyes may have a squint – it is possible that the reassuring toys and the checked smock serve as distractions from a face that is arguably older than its years and far removed from the chubbiness of the well-nourished eight-year-old. The photograph was taken by Robert Faulkner, a fashionable society photographer whose reputation largely rested on his child portraits.[104] His studio was in Baker Street, but this portrait was clearly taken at the hospital, and was probably commissioned either by *Aunt Judy's Magazine* or the Anglican magazine *Day of Rest*, which featured an article about the hospital and some of its inhabitants.[105] Faulkner did a lot of photography for the hospital *cartes des visites* but – curiously – retained the copyright of the images throughout. This image of an occupant of the *Aunt Judy's* Cot, the bed sponsored by the magazine, is professional and distinctive, with the patient looking towards the photographer, clutching a pull-along horse, with a toy steam engine on the bed.

Annie Kezia Eastland was nine years old when she was admitted to the Hospital for Sick Children on 21 November 1870, 'with a node on her tibia and a secondary diagnosis of necrosis'.[106] She was discharged more than six months later (on 15 June 1871), and it was said that her condition had been relieved. However, she was admitted to the hospital again on 25 August of that same year and 'with the same diagnosis'. The picture was probably taken for the sponsors of the Amy Louise Cot, and it shows Annie gazing wistfully into the distance, her long dark hair held back by a ribbon and wearing the hospital garibaldi jacket.

The images of Great Ormond Street suggest that the limits of the visually bearable were not – or, at least, not only – a matter of the external manifestations of pain. In a context where medical and scientific debates were concerned with the definition of its physical signs, pain could be represented in a variety of forms, and pictures like these could refer to experiences of pain without showing any apparent signs of it. This part of the chapter uncovers precisely the visual and material strategies that photographers such as Robert Faulkner followed to represent children in pain.[107]

Photographs are never disembodied images in a vacuum but material objects taken in particular circumstances. Shifting away from the visual content to the circumstances of their making, these staged photographs can easily be read as

[104] Several of his studies of children were published both as transparencies and as prints, which appeared in *Photographic News* (22 October 1880, 506–7) and which was said to have sold over 10,000 copies. Michael Pritchard, *A Directory of London Photographers, 1841–1908* (PhotoResearch, Watford, 1994), 59.

[105] GOS/1/2/12, Hospital's Committee of Management minute books, 1871–72, Great Ormond Street Archives.

[106] GOS/9/1/2, 1865–72; GOS/9/1/3, 1872–78.

[107] The adaption of methods from art history to visual history and their transformation towards an understanding of photography in its scientific application in the production of knowledge has been critically developed in recent historical scholarship. See: Jennifer Tucker, *Nature Exposed: Photography as Eyewitness in Victorian Science* (Johns Hopkins University Press, Baltimore, 2005); Lorraine Daston and Peter Galison, *Objectivity* (Zone Books, Cambridge, MA, 2007); Kelley Wilder, *Photography and Science (Exposures)* (Reaktion Books, London, 2009); Daniela Bleichmar, *Visible Empire: Botanical Expeditions and Visual Culture in the Hispanic Enlightenment* (University of Chicago Press, Chicago, 2012).

performative acts intended to provoke two actions in the viewing public: to feel compassion or pity for the suffering children and to donate money for their recovery. With these aims, the photographs were circulated as *cartes de visite* available for sale at the hospital for the price of sixpence, and they were published in journals such as *Aunt Judy*. The example of the children's magazine *Aunt Judy* sheds light on the ways in which pain was indirectly represented through objects rather than directly through expressions. This magazine, like foundations such as 'Kensington' or 'Mary H. West', sponsored a bed at the hospital. This served a double purpose: on the one hand, each month the magazine told the story of the patients that occupied the '*Aunt Judy's* Cot', describing their condition and evolution, as well as the facilities provided by the hospital. On the other hand, the cot served to channel donations. This is why it was so important that patients such as Sydney Jones were portrayed with the *Aunt Judy's* sign behind them. This sign not only identified the patient as someone whose story could be followed by readers, but it also helped to interpret his body as a suffering body. The description of the patients' conditions and the life at the hospital allowed readers to decode some objects in the pictures as part of the experience of pain. For example, many stories related that the patients had to spend several months in bed, usually because they had suffered the amputation of limbs.[108]

These images had to transmit a positive image of recovery. This is why another column related the story of a child, also suffering great pain after surgery, who had supposedly said 'Oh, I would be better if I only had *Aunt Judy's* label', as if being in *Aunt Judy's* cot would be a relief in itself.[109] Moreover, all these stories also stressed the presence of toys donated to the hospital by readers and the beneficial impact they had on children, especially at Christmas.[110] Sydney's portrait presents all these features: the bed suggests a painful condition, but the *Aunt Judy's* sign and the toys imply recovery. Precisely because these objects alluded to his pain, there was no need to express it with any physical signs.

Certain codes had to be followed to represent the body in pain. As fundraising tools, these images were intended to convey a sense of hope to the people who viewed them, especially those who were potential donors. It is important to bear in mind the extent to which hospitals and other medical institutions depended on patronage at a time before state funding of healthcare.[111] These images also needed to provide a positive image of recovery,

[108] Alfred Gatty, 'Report of the "Aunt Judy's Magazine Cots" at the Great Ormond Street Children's Hospital', in *Aunt Judy's Christmas Volume for Young People*, vol. 8 (Bell and Daldy, London, 1870), 447–749.

[109] Gatty, 'Report', 382–84. [110] Gatty, 'Report', 382–84.

[111] See Tanner, 'Too many mothers?', 135.

hence the emphasis on the presence of donated toys and their beneficial effect on child patients.[112] In Sydney's portrait, the boy's smile also transforms the hospital ward from a terrifying place of disease and death into an everyday environment typical of a happy childhood. In a photograph clearly designed to appeal to a middle-class audience, the boy wears a check smock and adopts a pose that echoes Victorian studio portraits of gentlemen. These children came from poor families, and their physical recovery was presented as also involving moral betterment.[113] The photograph – which presents Sydney as the living embodiment of the civilising influence of the hospital – seems to suggest how children *should* behave when in pain. Another example is the depiction of children using crutches. As one of the columns of *Aunt Judy* related, handling crutches was not an easy task for any child, who had to train for months before really being able to walk with them.[114] In this sense, the body of the child in these photographs showed how he had overcome difficulties and was able to stand up with the support of the crutches.

But these photographs worked not only because they displayed objects and bodies. A key factor in the success of these images was the action of the photographer, Robert Faulkner, renowned as a specialist in two fields: children's photography and backgrounds. The mastery of background became an essential element because the popular press stressed 'the cheerful and bright atmosphere of the ward' to a point that it seemed more like a nursery than a hospital.[115] Faulkner's technique was so good that he even patented it, and it was praised and explained in leading journals such as the *British Journal of Photography*.[116] According to these articles, his method produced graduated backgrounds that did not 'absorb the figure' but brought forward 'in a prominent manner the principal proportions of the figure', giving 'breadth, massiveness and harmony of effect'.[117] By means of these backgrounds, the portraits of sick children resembled those he had previously done for the bourgeoisie, facilitating the identification between the potential donors – who were mainly middle-class women – and the children. In the pictures of cots, the backgrounds emphasised the idea that the sponsored cots were places of relief.

But even more important was Faulkner's relationship with children. He was compared to the 'pied piper of Hamelin' by a contemporary commentator because he could do 'as he pleased with his little people [. . .] in his hands, they

[112] Gatty, 'Report', 177. [113] Boehm, *Charles Dickens*, 103. [114] Gatty, 'Report', 177.
[115] Boehm, *Charles Dickens*, 103.
[116] Robert Faulkner, 'Graduated backgrounds', *BJP* (25 October 1872), 513; 'Backgrounds: Mr. Faulkner's method of making them', *British Journal of Photography* (22 August 1873), 395; Robert Faulkner, 'Producing stippled grounds', *British Journal of Photography* (7 March 1873), 111.
[117] 'Backgrounds', 395.

are not only plastic as clay, but smiles and tears, humour and pathos are called up in the little faces at his bidding'.[118] This was a highly praised skill because getting the desired expression on children's faces was one of the most difficult tasks of photographers, as can be seen from debates in the photographic press. Children were compared to dogs as the most difficult subjects in photography, because they could not remain still.[119] Therefore Faulkner had developed a technique that allowed hiding the shutter, so its movement would not distract the children.[120]

In addition to the impact of these two techniques in the achievement of the images, there is another important element that is missing in the abovementioned narratives of Faulkner's work: the performance by the children themselves. As other accounts published in the photographic press relate, the best way to photograph children involved playing with them and allowing them to adopt the most comfortable poses.[121] In this context, the toys become not only signs to the viewers of the commodities at the hospital, but also traces of the prior play between the photographer and the children. Play adds another layer of meaning to these photographs. It suggests that these pictures were important not only because of their effect on the public but also because of the very act of photography. These photographic sessions were spaces in which children who had not moved from their beds in months could receive attention by engaging with toys and play. In this way, the moment of taking the picture could be something that the children enjoyed. Therefore, being in one of the sponsored cots could provide a momentary relief thanks to the privileges it involved, such as being portrayed photographically. This interpretation of the photographic act is consistent with Faulkner's method. As many articles in the photographic press pointed out, having a portrait taken caused anxiety to many sitters. Hiding the shutter not only avoided distractions but also allowed a more comfortable experience and an easier relationship between the photographer and the photographed person. These photographs thus allow us to reconstruct how photography engaged with medical and scientific debates on the nature of expressions of pain in children. Photographs served to communicate the hospital's aims and to construct social meanings of pain by means of their publication in journals. But besides the photographs, the very act of taking pictures also shaped the child patients' experiences of pain by introducing moments of relief.

[118] H. Baden Pritchard, 'Mr Robert Faulkner in Baker Street', in *The Photographic Studios of Europe* (Piper and Carter, London, 1882), 68–82.

[119] J. Wake, 'Babies', *British Journal of Photography* (26 April 1872), 195–96.

[120] 'How Mr Faulkner photographs children', *British Journal of Photography* (11 October 1872), 480–81.

[121] 'Lady Amateur', 'How I photograph my little ones', *BJP* (28 March 1872), 146–47.

Conclusion

The debate about childhood pain uncovers an important issue at the intersection of the history of science and the history of childhood: the lack of scientific unity and scientists' reflections on the definition, conceptualisation and treatment of pain.[122] The scientific and paediatric texts used in this chapter demonstrate the lack of scientific unity at the end of the nineteenth century and the varied renderings of the child body. By understanding development as a trajectory in which language and assertive action gradually took the place of instinct and reflex, the scientific texts by Darwin and Romanes show the story of human development. In biographical portraits, the child is presented as a developing body, an example of the 'human' that activates the exemplary observation of the history of humanity. In other words, the application of Darwinism to the interpretation of human development throughout each individual's lifespan contributed to the construction of a scientific theory: the notion that children and natural emotions represented past stages of human civilisation. In addition, scientific practices not only construct notions, they also constitute pragmatic devices for the generation of knowledge and experimental realities that include bodies. While the textual rendering of the child body produced the instinctual and emotional body, the practices of Gezmer and his followers generated the body of the child in pain.

The operationalisation of the scientific method in the late nineteenth century among natural scientists was manifested in the transformation of the child into a mechanistic object, an instrument for the discovery of medical and scientific truths that simplified the work of scientists. In relation to adults, the mechanistic, natural and instinctive nature of children often seemed to give permission to suspend the complex philosophical and moral questions related to experimentation with human subjects. The most obvious manifestation of this reduction *ad infantiam* was none other than the recurrent denial of infant pain. While Darwin and Preyer did not subscribe to this belief, their attention to children as a sign of human evolution – rather than as self-sufficient objects of knowledge – and the understanding of crying as a *natural* expression paved the way for later treatment of children as incapable of authentic suffering. Together with the extreme experimental caution that treated infant expressions of suffering through the sceptical interpretation of reflex actions, the chapter has presented two major conditions for the consolidation of infant pain denial in scientific practice during the twentieth century, further sustained by the arrival of behaviourism and the increasing emphasis on brain and nervous system development, both covered in Chapter 2.

122 See Biagoli and Galison, *The Disunity of Science*, 1–37.

While the scientific method transformed the child into a scientific and mechanistic object, paediatricians saw children from the perspective of disease and treated pain communication as the main access to the roots of the medical problem. In contrast to scientists and psychologists – who saw the child as a fledgling adult – children's doctors recognised the existence of a language of pain specific to childhood and thus stressed the great distance between children and their being understood as mere men and women in miniature. While the main arguments surrounding adult gestural languages centred on their transparency and how much they revealed about moral character and inner feelings, doubts about a 'natural language' that anyone could read were not enough to deter the effort to find such a language in the field of paediatrics. Thus, one could argue that the rights of children in the paediatric world were not based on the right to be treated as future adults, but they were a form of insulation: the children's hospital physically institutionalised and constructed the right to be a child and to exist in a space separated from the adult world. Additionally, we cannot forget that healthy children were considered a national asset, and their health was the health of the country.[123] In the Great Ormond Street Hospital photographs, the sick child became a discursive category, an object of institutional efforts to return children both to health and to the values of innocence and goodness belonging to the Romantic conception of childhood. However, photography did more than record the sick body: the very act of taking pictures, and the performances of courage and play that were enacted during the photographic sessions, also shaped the children's experiences of pain and relief.

The debate about childhood pain provides more information about the cultural dominance of certain ideals of childhood than about the lack of unity in the sciences. Debates within paediatrics, physiology and evolutionary and behavioural psychology drew upon and reinforced two approaches to childhood that had formed the Western view of childhood. On the one hand, childhood was considered as a road towards adulthood, a fundamental phase in the development of a complete human being. On the other hand, childhood was respected for its autonomy, often seen in idealised or Romantic terms. The ambivalence between childhood as a refuge of personal identity and as a testimony of past civilisations marked by the scars of heredity generated strong tensions in the nineteenth century. Filtered through the problem of childhood pain, this ambivalence makes itself felt in our present frames of reference.

[123] For example, see: Harris, *The Health of the Schoolchild*; Dwork, *War Is Good for Babies*; Anna Davin, 'Imperialism and motherhood', *History Workshop Journal*, 5 (1978), 9–65; G. R. Searle, *The Quest for National Efficiency* (Basil Blackwell, Oxford, 1971); and Harry Hendrick, 'Child labour, medical capital, and the school medical service, c.1890–1918', in Cooter (ed.), *In the Name of the Child*, 45–71.

2 Infant Pain Denial

At the start of the twentieth century, new disciplines in the study of children started to emerge. This did not, however, represent the start of what Ellen Key[1] has described as the 'century of the child', in which humanity realised its spiritual essence through the care of its children. It was, rather, a period in which children were progressively objectivised and turned into subjects of study and rational organisation. As child development as a field of inquiry started to take off, scientific observation categorised children's development in progressive stages within the context of a universal ideal. As Chapter 1 suggested, a new view of the dynamic nature of human development had emerged in the nineteenth century as a result of evolutionary theories.[2]

This chapter continues the exploration of the debates about the emotional expression of children's suffering between scientists and psychologists, on the one hand, and paediatricians, on the other. To a great extent, it uses the same sources and methodologies as Chapter 1. Indeed, the inspiration drawn from Bourke's revisionist work in *The Story of Pain* continues, although the conclusions reached here are significantly different: in fact, infant pain denial appears as only one form among many figurations of children's pain. The scope is expanded further with the inclusion of the child study movement in addition to paediatrics, which was already considered in Chapter 1.[3]

A key development that emerged from the debate around infant pain was precisely the gradual consolidation of its denial. As the nineteenth century gave way to the twentieth, scientific disciplines became clearly separated from each other in both theory and practice. As Claudia Castañeda has pointed out, much of the writing about the figure of the child in the nineteenth century came from the work of 'gentlemen scientists' who worked across the boundaries of biology, anthropology and other emerging disciplines. In contrast, she noted,

[1] Key, *Century of the Child*.

[2] Wertheimer, 'Evolution of the concept of development', 13–26.

[3] Another author who has devoted time to this topic, in the framework of the child study movement, is Sally Shuttleworth, although her study does not extend into the twentieth century. See Shuttleworth, *Mind of the Child*, especially chapters 14 and 15.

twentieth-century scientific discourses drew a very different map of knowledge-making and practice, and scientific knowledge was divided into increasingly specialist subdisciplines, which often provided rival interpretations and perspectives.[4]

In this chapter, I focus on figurations of the child in pain from the 1890s until the Second World War in three scientific disciplines: the child study movement, behavioural psychology and paediatrics. Each discipline approached the question of the child in pain – and the concept of infant pain denial – in a different way. But there was also some overlap between the disciplines and a certain amount of cross-fertilisation. The child study movement, which drew on Darwinism and anthropological theory (in particular 'recapitulation theory'), argued that children embodied the primitive past of the species and could thereby reveal the processes that formed adult capacities.[5] The child study movement presented pain as a reflex action in infants and as a sensation that children learned through experience, which was tied to the evolutionary process and to the emergence of self-consciousness. In contrast, the advocates of behavioural psychology adopted a mechanistic approach and were sceptical about the value of children's expressions of pain. In particular, expressions of pain by newborn children were seen as mechanical reflex responses to stimuli – a perspective that led to the scientific hypothesis that infants did not feel pain.[6] Meanwhile, as the discipline of paediatrics became increasingly scientific, it was influenced by mechanistic and developmental theories. In the early days of paediatrics, figures such as Charles West had compared the figure of the paediatrician to that of the explorer, investigating an uncharted terrain.[7] However, children's medicine now became likened to veterinary science, and children's development was seen in relation to that of animals. In this 'scientised' context, there was no longer room for subjective signs of pain or for the testimony of mothers about their children's suffering. There were also significant debates within paediatrics about the use of anaesthesia when surgeries were performed on infants.[8]

Both the child study movement and behavioural psychology enquiries were largely based in the United States and linked to the United Kingdom and the

[4] Castañeda, *Figurations*, chapter 2.

[5] On child study and the colonisation of childhood, see Varga, 'Look – normal' and Gaile Sloan Cannella, *Childhood and Postcolonization: Power, Education, and Contemporary Practice* (Routledge, New York, 2004).

[6] On infant pain denial and behaviourism, see Rodkey and Riddell, 'The infancy of infant pain research', 338–50.

[7] See Chapter 1.

[8] For a discussion on the sentience of embryos, see Bourke, *Story of Pain*, 218. See also, Boddice, *Knowing Pain*, 95–96.

wider transnational English-language scientific culture. This chapter analyses the discourse of the child study movement and behavioural psychology – together with their techniques, methods and materials – to illustrate the role played by these disciplines in the scientific colonisation of childhood. It argues that, in terms of discourse, child development became structured according to the concepts of rational achievement that gained dominance over other views of the child and childhood. The chapter also examines the role played by pain in understanding human development and how Eurocentric ideas about 'white' development meant that developmental differences were seen as pathologies.[9]

By moving away from strictly scientific discourses to analyse the child in pain in the field of paediatrics – including debates about surgery and anaesthesia in the context of medical practice – this chapter argues for the simultaneous existence of rival and sometimes contradictory versions of the figure of the child in pain in different places – even within the same discipline. In fact, the archival work for this study shows that there were somewhat contradictory factors driving the disciplinary trends that were reconstructed in the form of a unifying history. Thus, while the distance between medical theory and medical practice seems to have had important consequences in terms of differing epistemic considerations of pain – which was an *abstract* instrument of knowledge for the former and a *factual* symptom for the latter – it is also true that, during the first half of the twentieth century, the mechanistic view of childhood and scepticism about infant pain shaped paediatric and clinical practice, as surgery on infants was routinely carried out with minimal or no anaesthesia even as late as the 1980s.[10]

This chapter seeks to give a historical explanation of how scepticism about infant pain became more common among paediatricians by analysing the experimental research on infant pain that was carried out in the early twentieth century and which played a significant role in the development of infant pain denial. Three interrelated causes encouraged the denial of infant pain, each corresponding to a different disciplinary perspective: the Darwinian view that the child was a lower being (child study movement), a perspective grounded in mechanistic behaviourism (behavioural psychology) and experimental caution (paediatrics and anaesthesia).

Pleasure and Pain in the Child Study Movement

The beginning of anthropologist Alexander Francis Chamberlain's book *The Child: A Study in the Evolution of Man*, published at the turn of the twentieth

[9] For a discussion on the scientific comparison of non-white adults with the period of white childhood, see: Bill Ashcroft, *On Post-Colonial Futures: Transformations of Colonial Culture* (Continuum, London, 2001); Castañeda, *Figurations*, chapter 1.

[10] Rodkey and Riddell, 'The infancy of infant pain research', 345.

century, features an image of a four-year-old white child.[11] The photograph shows the child, wearing a smock, from above the waist, and the only visible parts of his body are his face and his hands, which are folded in his lap. With a wide-open gaze, he looks slightly upwards towards the left. For Chamberlain, this boy embodied everything that was normal. The photograph was an image of a boy who 'might stand for the child type in its most genial form and expression'.[12] Around the turn of the century, child-study scientists such as Chamberlain sought to interpret the essence of childhood development, establishing what was 'normal' and what was 'deviant'.[13] In this fin-de-siècle projection, the child was both atavistic and prophetic, and it became the bearer of all future hope. Chamberlain's text expresses the intense interest in the figure of the child that was a characteristic of the 1890s. In this image, one can see the child as playing three roles: the key to unlocking understanding of the self, the door to a long-lost past and a guarantee of a better future.[14]

The science of child study, which was loosely based on evolutionary assumptions, developed quickly in the United States and in Europe. In the United Kingdom, the movement's pioneer was the psychologist James Sully (1842–1923), whose work contributed significantly to the initial conceptualisation of the 'maladjusted child'.[15] Sully's interest in the psychology of children emerged both from his own experience of mental breakdown as a young man and from a philosophical background, rather than from formal medical training. Originally trained as a nonconformist minister, Sully studied at the German universities of Göttingen and Humboldt, where he encountered the work of the psychologist Wilhelm Wundt (1832–1920).[16] In 1871, Sully returned to England and sought a career in writing journal articles on philosophy. His first published piece about children – 'Mental development in children' in *Mind* in 1880 – drew heavily on the diary observations of Darwin and Preyer.[17] Following his own breakdown, Sully believed that the early recognition of the signs of mental fatigue could prevent susceptible individuals from

[11] Alexander Francis Chamberlain, *The Child: A Study in the Evolution of Man* (Walter Scott Ltd., London, 1900), frontispiece.

[12] Chamberlain, *The Child*, frontispiece. [13] Varga, 'Look – normal', 140.

[14] See Sally Shuttleworth, 'Childhood, severed heads, and the uncanny: Freudian precursors (Critical essay)', *Victorian Studies*, 58 (2015), 84–110.

[15] The scientific study of child behaviour in Britain originated from the work of Sir Francis Galton (1822–1911) who, in 1883, introduced the term 'eugenic', defined as 'the science of improving stock'. Francis Galton, *Inquiries into the Human Faculty and Its Development* (Macmillan, London, 1883), 25. For details on Galton's life and work, see Dorothy Middleton, *Sir Francis Galton, 1822–1911* (Eugenics Society, London, 1982).

[16] Considered by historians to be the 'founder of modern psychology', Wundt opened his laboratory in Leipzig in 1879. It subsequently became the model for psychological methodology throughout the world. For more details on the work of Wilhelm Wundt, see Thomas Leahey, *A History of Psychology* (Routledge, London, 2015), 249–60.

[17] Rodkey and Riddell, 'The infancy of infant pain research', 344.

becoming 'psychic invalids' in later life. His work was thus framed within the context of a preventive approach, and he was also one of the first researchers to shift the focus of attention for the welfare of children's physical and mental health onto parents, arguing that scientific observation of children was the duty of responsible parents.

Sully, who reviewed Preyer's Die Seele des Kindes (later translated as The Mind of the Child) for Mind in 1882, published *Studies of Childhood* in 1895, a text that established child study as a disciplinary field. Sully's interest in the child is primarily evolutionary:

> The first years of a child, with their imperfect verbal expression, their crude fanciful ideas, their seizures by rage and terror, their absorption in the present moment, acquire a new and antiquarian interest. They mirror for us, in a diminished distorted reflection no doubt, the probable condition of primitive man, the intellectual and moral resemblances between the lowest existing races of mankind and children are numerous and close.[18]

Based on the Lamarckian premise of inheritable abilities, the quotation states the theory of recapitulation, by virtue of which individual development proceeds through the evolutionary phases of one's own species until reaching its current developmental level.[19] Children were thus observed to discover 'the beginning of things, the way in which human life begins to take its characteristic forms'.[20] The observation of children's behaviour can be seen as an extension of interest in natural history. Following Herbert Spencer and G. H. Lewes, Sully rejected the idea that the infant started out at the level of a mollusc, as had been claimed by George Romanes. Rather, he equated the infant with primitive man, entering the world with additional 'ancestral dowering' in such a way that he began life at a level that was higher than 'the race's starting point'.[21] This view offers a progressive vision of human progress, to which the key is held by the infant.[22]

Sully, in common with other contemporary scientists who studied childhood, took a strong interest in the relationship between thought, language and self-consciousness. While Romanes had suggested that it was self-consciousness rather than language that made human life distinct from that of animals, Sully took the view that thought and self-consciousness could precede language. He argued that even before 'the age of speech' children could be observed thinking.[23] Considering 'pre-linguistic babblings', Sully states:

> As everybody knows, long before the child begins to speak in the conventional sense he produces sounds. These are at first cries and wanting in the definiteness of true articulate

[18] James Sully, *Studies of Childhood* (D. Appleton and Company, New York, 1896), 8–9.
[19] Varga, 'Look – normal', 141.
[20] Sully, *Studies of Childhood*, 4.
[21] Sully, *Studies of Childhood*, 9.
[22] Shuttleworth, *Mind of the Child*, 281.
[23] Sully, *Studies of Childhood*, 4.

sounds. Such cries are expressive, that is, utterances of changing conditions of feeling, pain and pleasure, and are also instinctive, springing out of certain congenital nervous arrangements by which feeling acts upon the muscular organs.[24]

For Sully, this crying 'gradually differentiates itself into a rich variety of expressions for hunger, cold, pain, joy and so forth, of which it is safe to say that the majority of nurses and mothers have at best but a very imperfect knowledge'.[25] Following Preyer, Sully interpreted pleasure and pain as basic instincts in the child and as the primary motivations for action, writing, 'The earliest idea of self seems to be obtained by the child through an examination by the senses of touch and sight of his own body.' It is through 'self-graspings, self-strikings, self-bitings, aided by the very varied, and often extremely disagreeable operations of the nurse and others on the surface of their bodies, they probably reach during the first year the idea that their body is different from all other things, is "me" in the sense that it is the living seat of pain and pleasure'.[26] Pain was presented as a sensation the child learned through experience and which was tied to the evolutionary process and the emergence of self-consciousness.

Sully's interpretation of pleasure and pain as basic instincts in the child, as well as the comparison of the infant with the animal, was common at the end of the nineteenth century and the beginning of the twentieth century, and it had its origin in Darwinism as part of a wider project for explaining behaviour in adaptive terms. The persuasiveness of the core assumption that gaining pleasure and avoiding pain were primary motivations for action expanded, perhaps unconsciously, among diarists such as the American psychologist Milicent Washburn Shinn, whose book *The Biography of a Baby* was published in 1900.[27] While journal entries did offer descriptions of changes in behaviours, the diarists' preferences were individual and idiosyncratic, which allows for very little comparative analysis. Unlike Preyer, whose son's skin sensitivity was 'surprisingly great', Shinn maintained that her baby 'had no experience of skin pain in her early days, and being kept at an equable temperature probably received no definite sensations either of heat or of cold'.[28] Shinn went on to argue that pain was a sensation learned through experience and tied to the evolutionary process of self-consciousness.

The child study movement also took up the question of the relationship between the child and the animal.[29] Louis Robinson, one of the early British

[24] Sully, *Studies of Childhood*, 4. [25] Sully, *Studies of Childhood*, 4.
[26] Sully, *Studies of Childhood*, 4.
[27] On Shinn see von Oertzen, 'Science in the cradle', 175–95.
[28] Milicent Shinn, *The Biography of a Baby* (Houghton Mifflin, Boston, 1900), 47.
[29] For a discussion on the relationship between the child and the monkey in the child study movement see Shuttleworth, *Mind of the Child*, chapter 14.

followers of Kussmaul, performed experiments on babies in an attempt to show the relationship between monkeys and infants. In 'Darwinism in the nursery' (1891), Robinson claimed that opening the nursery to science could help fill the vast gap between embryology and anthropology. He argued that 'the average mother, in spite of many unquestioned merits, is about as competent to take an unprejudiced view of the facts bearing on the natural history of her infant as a West African negro would do to carry out an investigation of the anatomy and physiology of a fetish'.[30] Robinson attempted to prove the arboreal ancestry of humans by testing whether babies had sufficient strength of grip to hang from a bar.[31] Robinson's article 'Reflex action' in D. H. Tuke's *Dictionary of Psychological Medicine* (1892)[32] includes images of babies clinging onto a branch in a way that encouraged readers to imagine them as monkeys swinging through the trees. According to Robinson, the hanging babies' posture and the 'disproportionately large development of the arms compared with the legs, give the photographs a striking resemblance to a well-known picture of the celebrated chimpanzee "Sally" at the Zoological Gardens'.[33]

Sully was not the only advocate of child study at this time. In the United States, psychologist G. Stanley Hall (1844–1924) played a major role in establishing psychological approaches to child development. The biological theories about recapitulation were initially posited in terms of the development of foetal anatomy. However, Hall extended the concept and applied recapitulation theory to the study of consciousness and human behaviour from infancy until early adulthood. A student of psychologists William James and Wilhelm Wundt, Hall published a seminal work in 1893 introducing the concept of childhood as a specific and emotionally complex stage of life, when individuals were particularly vulnerable and malleable.[34] He created a science of 'pedagogy', aimed at making large-scale empirical studies of children and their development.[35] In later work, he categorised specific stages of childhood, introducing the term 'adolescence' in 1904 as a stage of development with particular problems that could not be considered either adult or strictly childlike.[36]

30 Louis Robinson, 'Darwinism in the nursery', *Nineteenth Century*, 30 (1891), 832.

31 Robinson, 'Darwinism', 832.

32 Louis Robinson, 'Reflex action (physiological)', in D. H. Tuke (ed.), *A Dictionary of Psychological Medicine*, 2 vols. (Churchill, London, 1892), 1074–76. The drawing is on page 1076.

33 Robinson, 'Darwinism', 838.

34 G. Stanley Hall, *The Contents of Children's Minds on Entering Education* (E. L. Kellogg & Co., New York, 1893).

35 In 1891, Hall founded the journal *Pedagogical Seminary*, which he used as a tool both for publicising his theories and for collecting data, with issues containing surveys that could be filled in by parents and teachers and returned to his laboratory.

36 Hall, *Adolescence*.

Hall spent a year in Germany studying physiological psychology.[37] Strongly influenced by Ernst Haeckel's recapitulation theory, he had a deep interest in evolutionary psychology and child development. As in the work of Shinn, the study of the child and the adolescent was always conducted within the structural framework of biological and cultural evolution. Although there was strong opposition to recapitulation theory within psychology – because it was not able to explain development – Hall popularised the concept among teachers and parents.[38] Applying Haeckel's theory, Hall made the bold claim that children's play was an 'expression of earlier activities of the race' – something that was a necessary in order that civilised behaviour could later emerge. He also argued – somewhat more fancifully and showing the rather haphazard way in which observations were used to support theory – that early childhood play with sand and water was a replication of humankind's emergence from its aquatic origins.[39] Hall coupled recapitulation theory to Romantic conceptions of the child. His faith in recapitulation as the key to human development seems hard to reconcile with twentieth-century demands for scientific procedures based on systematic observation, behavioural records and quantitative analysis.

Back in the United States, Hall sought to apply what he had learnt in Europe to study children's thought processes, interests and capacities, in the belief that this would lead him to discover a genetic – or 'racial' – basis for development. In 1894, he had set up a child-study department within the US National Education Association. Often seen as the 'father' of child study, he published the first systematic study of the infantile mind carried out in North America, *Aspects of Child Life and Education*, in 1907. Hall's sources included white adults, who provided memories of their childhood; white teachers, who described the white children in their schools; and white children. Although at the time, data sources were described as surveys and questionnaires, information was actually provided in the form of written reports based on anecdotes.[40] Parents and teachers were told how to collect data and instructed to consider their own childhoods and the childhoods of others in relation to a list of characteristics, to which they were invited to add their own variations.

[37] For a discussion on the emergence of what became known as physiological psychology see Kurt Danziger, 'Mid-nineteenth-century British psycho-physiology: a neglected chapter in the history of psychology' and Lorraine J. Daston, 'The theory of will versus the science of mind', both in *The Problematic Science: Psychology in Nineteenth-Century Thought*, William R. Woodward and Mitchell G. Ash (eds.) (Praeger, New York, 1982).

[38] Varga, 'Look – normal', 143.

[39] Varga, 'Look – normal', 143.

[40] Varga, 'Look – normal', 142.

There was enthusiastic participation in Hall's extensive research, and between 1894 and 1896, he sent out thirty-one separate surveys, each one involving 800 correspondents.[41] The more than 120 themes studied in *Aspects of Child Life and Education* were divided into various general groups, such as 'Relations to Nature', which included such topics as children's experience of light and dark, and the 'development of the sense of self'. Closely connected with this, Hall discussed the studies of the 'fundamental affectivities of the child' such as pleasure and pain, including crying and laughing. Hall understood pleasure and pain as the child's fundamental and primary affectivities. He believed that physical self-consciousness started with the child's recognition of its own hand and then the foot, but that 'psychic self-consciousness is commonly only of pain, either internal, as of stomach ache, or peripheral, as of cuts, bruises'.[42] Hall also discussed pain in the section devoted to children's curiosity and interest, where he claimed that there were many cases of 'children deliberately exposing themselves to pain to satisfy a desire for knowledge'. While Hall acknowledges children's capacity to feel both pain and pleasure, some lines later he adds, 'though probably with the same lack of actual realization of pain as in the case of experiments on animals'. Thus, one child who 'had previously experienced an attack of colic' deliberately ate 'green grapes' to see if it were true that they would make her sick, but the 'mere memory of pain was not sufficiently vivid to check her desire for experiment'.[43]

In a similar way, Hall recounted, 'another child on being told that iron on a very cold day would burn her tongue deliberately tried it; and a boy of nine exposed himself to whooping cough to see how it felt'. A five-year-old girl, seeing her mother cry while she was peeling onions, said, 'Mamma, the onions must hurt you. Give me an onion and let me find out where the hurt is.'[44] Hall's conclusion is clear: many cases that at first seem to suggest callousness in children in relation to the sufferings of others in fact concern children's inability to appreciate the situation because they lacked experience of 'physical or mental suffering'. While 'most children have, of course, temporary experiences of pain', children have short memories 'and pain, unless exceptionally sharp or prolonged, is quickly forgotten'. Therefore 'the average healthy child has very slight appreciation of illness or suffering, and exhibitions of sympathy

41 Varga, 'Look – normal', 142.

42 G. Stanley Hall, *Aspects of Child Life and Education* (D. Appleton and Company, New York, 1921), 30.

43 Hall, *Aspects of Child Life and Education*, 94.

44 Hall, *Aspects of Child Life and Education*, 94.

are largely imitative'.[45] Hall argues that a habitually cruel child is an abnormality and will almost certainly have other signs of cruelty. However, in all the cases cited above, the child's underlying motive is curiosity, a desire for knowledge, rather than cruelty.

Similar sentiments are found in the writings of the anthropologist Alexander Francis Chamberlain, Hall's pupil, who argued that there was an instinctive sense of self-preservation in children 'as if they felt the fragility of their existence and clung to it with all their strength[:] this is true physiologically and psychologically'.[46] According to Chamberlain, the lack of sensitivity to pains, blows and wounds during the early years of life was often surprising: 'not localising pain very readily until two or three years of age, they seem to resemble the savages in their resistance to their physical pain and their desperate clinging to life.'[47] Chamberlain's text also expresses the belief that less-evolved cultures had a greater resistance to pain. In the scientific context of child study, the mapping of children was necessary so that the rational adult mind could come to understand childhood. It was assumed that such mapping would be done by members of the white bourgeoisie, which would thereby enable the understanding of that which Sully termed 'the race-mind'[48] – in other words, the history of the mental processes of the white 'race'. The work of Sully, Hall and Chamberlain illustrates the centrality at the turn of the nineteenth century of scientific attempts to understand the child mind and children's development, which involved a range of disciplines and forms of practice.[49]

Stanley Hall had a profound effect on American psychology, particularly child psychology and adolescent development, and many of his students went on to lead the new discipline of child psychology. Among the most notable was Arnold Gesell (1880–1961), who fully adopted Hall's view of recapitulation theory and invented the term 'maturation' to describe the integration of physical and social growth that Hall had defended. Gesell, director of the Clinic of Child Development and professor of child hygiene at the University of Yale, focused on children with developmental problems. He believed that to understand abnormality, it was first necessary to understand normal child development. His studies started with infants and preschool children and later extended to children aged from five to ten, and then to those aged up to sixteen.

45 Hall, *Aspects of Child Life and Education*, 105. 46 Chamberlain, *The Child*, 337.
47 Chamberlain, *The Child*, 338. 48 Sully, *Studies of Childhood*, 8.
49 For a discussion of Sully, Hall and Chamberlain in relation to the mind of the child see Shuttleworth, *Mind of the Child*, 267–90.

Gesell and his co-investigators largely invented the observation techniques and methodologies that soon became the standard means for identifying the normal child's innate (or natural) characteristics and for distinguishing between the normal and the deviant. As these technologies and methodologies were implemented, they had the effect of standardising and objectifying the child's subjective life (nurture) to create a supervisory manipulation that would prevent deviant development.

In 1925, Gesell published his initial observations, a six-year 'systematic survey of the ordinary and normal behavior of infancy and normal childhood',[50] which provided what Hall had been unable to come up with: the construction of normative developmental schedules that set down children's physical, mental, emotional and social abilities, and which he used to measure and classify childhood.[51] In 1934, in *Infant Behavior, Its Genesis and Growth*, Gesell studied the normal development of the infant. In the section devoted to perceptual and adaptive behaviour, he discussed infants' sentience. After stating that 'the sensory life of the prenate is no longer a completely closed book', he said that extensive observations of prematurely born infants had demonstrated a wide range of forms and degrees of receptivity. So, although sensitivity to light and changes of temperature 'is probably present during the latter half of the gestation period', sensitivity to pain 'is more in doubt'. Gesell's work helped to crystallise the idea of child pain as a reflex action, 'prompt but immature', even though he affirmed that sensitivity to painful stimuli definitely increases in the first week after birth.[52]

The Influence of Behaviourism

At the end of the nineteenth century, an accumulation of factors contributed to a mechanistic vision of childhood, which in turn explains how the experimentation with childhood pain in the twentieth century was naturalised: the clinical and academic interest in the functioning of reflex actions and the nervous system, the development of the scientific method, together with the Darwinist vision of the infant as an inferior primitive being and the child as an adult in training. Since evolutionary psychology was coming to be the dominant

[50] Arnold Gesell, *The Mental Growth of the Pre-school Child* (The Macmillan Company, New York, 1925), 3.
[51] Varga, 'Look – normal', 142–44.
[52] Arnold Gesell, *Infant Behavior: Its Genesis and Growth* (McGraw-Hill Book Company, New York, 1934), 281.

paradigm, behaviourism applied to clinical practice both Darwinian theories and anatomical and histological data from the fields of embryology and physiology, thereby reinforcing the idea that babies and children were relatively insensitive to pain.[53] Behaviourism was one of the scientific schools that focused most intently on children, paying specific attention to the importance of pain. Although it soon lost traction to developmental psychology as the leading theory for framing pain, the influence of behaviourism is eye-catching: its methodological assumptions led to the widespread belief that infants' expression of pain cannot be connected to the experience of pain, thereby giving rise to the more established scientific hypothesis that denied that infants felt pain.

The experiments on sensitivity and childhood pain made their appearance in the history of behavioural psychology with the work of Margaret Gray Blanton (1887–1973), a specialist in the field of speech pathology. Blanton performed a series of experiments at Johns Hopkins University in Baltimore under the supervision of the psychologist John Broadus Watson (1878–1958). Watson, who was especially interested in studying the classical behaviourist model of stimulus–response and its applicability to the prediction and control of human behaviour, focused on what he considered the three fundamental human emotions – love, hate and fear. The experiments of his disciple, however, focused on the study of pain. The investigation of pain fitted particularly well with the values of behaviourist psychology, given that expressions of pain could be interpreted as a mere mechanical response to stimuli. Blanton analysed the reactions of a group of babies to harmful stimuli, such as the extraction of blood and pricks on the wrist while sleeping. The babies reacted with defensive attitudes to the experiments: extracting blood produced exaggerated crying, while pricking the babies with pins while they slept caused half of the sample to move their hands and forearms, and the rough rubbing of the back of their heads to remove vernix caseosa provoked the children to move their hands vigorously, to attempt to crawl away, and to cry angrily. Nonetheless, Blanton resists concluding that the medical procedure was the cause of the crying, arguing that, as expressions proper to infantile behaviour, no actual feeling could be firmly inferred from such reactions.[54] Finally she concluded, 'the reflex and instinctive equipment of the child at birth is more complex and advanced than has hitherto been thought'.[55]

The increasing sophistication of behaviourist experiments led to a more exact control of the experimental situation. This resulted in the replacement of

[53] Rodkey and Riddell, 'The infancy of infant pain research', 344.

[54] Margaret Gray Blanton, 'The behavior of the human infant in the first 30 days of life', *Psychological Review*, 24 (1917), 472.

[55] Blanton, 'Behavior of the human infant', 474.

the earlier harmful stimuli with electrical discharges, which removed the variability in the pressure of a pin. This approach was continued in experiments at the Lying-In Hospital and Northwestern University in Chicago under Mandel and Irene Sherman.[56] Nearly all newborns reacted on the first day after their birth and the researchers concluded that they tended to react more to lesser stimulation between the first and the twelfth day. Their conclusion was that this finding suggested that children were not more sensitive in the moments immediately after birth, but rather that their sensitivity increased gradually.[57] Like Blanton, the Shermans noted that the babies attempted to escape and moved in a defensive way, including hitting against the object to get away from it, but they doubted whether conclusions about pain in babies could be drawn from their own experiment: 'Perhaps the responses of infants to pain stimuli cannot be called "pain" responses, as their psychological nature is unknown'.[58]

The Shermans' experiments were published in *The Journal of Comparative Psychology* and in *Comparative Psychology Monographs* alongside the results of similar experiments that used discharges in animals and registered the resulting 'reflexes', pointing to the dominant mechanistic vision of babies, together with the dominance of the analogy between children and animals.[59] Like beasts, babies constituted perfect passive objects for experiments that were carried out from a reductionist behaviourist perspective, given that the investigators were looking for reflexes and not consciousness. Having interpreted their results as proving the existence of the 'decorticate infant', the widespread impact of the Shermans' research paved the way for routine experimentation on babies' pain thresholds, with no requirement for a specific ethical justification.[60]

The Shermans' presentation of the 'decorticate infant' somehow anticipated the fate of behaviourism, which lost its dominance in psychological thinking to a new focus on research about pain in babies: brain development. The research by Myrtle McGraw (1899–1988) at the beginning of the 1940s at the University of Columbia and in the Babies' Hospital in New York was particularly influential. According to Victor Bergenn, during the previous decade, the opinions of Gesell and the behaviourist John Watson were dominant in the field of the psychology of infant development. Watson insisted that training could influence development only when the nervous system of an infant had

[56] Mandel Sherman and Irene Sherman, 'Sensori-motor responses in infants', *Journal of Comparative Psychology*, 5 (1925), 53–68; Mandel Sherman and Irene Sherman, 'Infant behavior', *Comparative Psychology Monographs*, 12 (1936), 1–107.

[57] Sherman and Sherman, 'Infant behavior', 8.

[58] Sherman and Sherman, 'Infant behavior', 38.

[59] Rodkey and Riddell, 'The infancy of infant pain research', 345.

[60] Rodkey and Riddell, 'The infancy of infant pain research', 345.

reached the appropriate stage of growth. Both Gessel and Watson stressed developmental norms and applied standardised scales and texts. It was in this context that McGraw became involved in the direction of the Normal Child Development Study at the Babies' Hospital in New York City. She worked with neurologist Frederick Tilney and neuro-embryologist George Coghill and drew on a variety of approaches as she sought to understand the process of growth itself, rather than the specific norms associated with growth.

It was McGraw's research with the Woods twins that made her work popular, but she also performed an ambitious study using pin pricks to reveal the process by which nerves mature.[61] The researcher evaluated the reactions of children to pain provoked by pricking the head, the trunk and the hands and feet during the taking of blood samples.[62] She made a total of 2,008 observations, evaluating seventy-five children aged between a few minutes of life and four years. Her discoveries were that the youngest patients (those up to several days old) either did not react to pain or demonstrated a dispersed reaction, while there was a more localised reaction in older children. McGraw believed that, in the newborns, there was a high pain threshold in relation to external stimuli, as they were not capable of identifying or localising the external source of pain. She also reported that some neonates did not show any response to being pricked by pins and indicated that the typical response 'consists of diffuse bodily movements accompanied by crying, and possibly a local reflex'.[63] Reacting to the pinpricks, the babies cried and tried to remove their arms and legs. Despite this observation, McGraw confidently concluded that they possessed a very limited sensitivity to pain. In her view, a child's first week or ten days was a period of 'hypaesthesia' (a diminished capacity for physical sensation, especially of the skin).[64] The 'local reflex' referred to by McGraw refers to the widely accepted medical view at the time that reactions were of a merely mechanical nature and therefore had no mental or emotional significance. 'Even when there is sensitivity is it reasonable to assume that neural mediation does not extend above the level of the thalamus', she wrote in the article's discussion section.[65]

[61] Psychologist Myrtle McGraw gained prominence through her extensive research on the twins Jimmy and Johnny Woods. Less well known is that McGraw also conducted tests on the twins' pain responses using the blunted tip of a pin on various parts of their bodies, including their legs, forearms, trunks and cheeks. Myrtle B. McGraw, *A Study of Johnny and Jimmy* (Appleton Century Crofts, New York, 1935).

[62] Myrtle B. McGraw, 'Neural maturation as exemplified in the changing reaction of the infant to pin prick', in Myrtle B. McGraw (ed.), *The Neuromuscular Maturation of the Human Infant* (Hafner, New York, 1969), 42–47.

[63] McGraw, 'Neural maturation', 39–40.

[64] McGraw, 'Neural maturation', 40.

[65] McGraw, 'Neural maturation', 42.

The 'Scientisation' of Paediatrics

Following the trend inaugurated by Charles West, doctors at the beginning of the twentieth century continued exploring how to determine the symptoms of children's illness, and interpreters such as David Forsyth, a doctor at the Evelina Hospital for Sick Children in London, still described pain as one of the many symptoms of disease, stressing that 'none can rival it in diagnostic value'.[66] Like many other authors who have commented on the diagnoses of children's illnesses, Forsyth was very much concerned with the difficulty that children had in communicating an object as elusive as pain. He reminded his readers that:

> at the age when children have no power of verbal expression, it is not always easy to recognise its presence, character, or intensity, still less to localise it or trace its distribution. This comes not only from the infant's inability to speak, but also from his own ignorance of the site of his pain.[67]

These problems were far from being exclusive to babies, and doctors also lacked confidence in the testimony of older children: although a child might be able to speak, he 'is quite incompetent to describe symptoms or to locate pain with trustworthy accuracy', affirmed Forsyth.[68] Another doctor who specialised in paediatrics and who was a pioneer in the study of children in institutions, the American Henry Dwight Chapin, argued in 1911 that the different parts of the child's face betrayed the localisation of pain in certain parts of the body. The upper part of the face would point to pains or illnesses of the head; the alteration of the middle part of the face would be related to chest pains, and the lower part of the face would be an expression of pain in the abdominal organs.[69] The obstetrician Pierre Budin warned mothers how to 'detect disease at its first appearance, and thus insure for her child timely medical assistance'.[70] Like Holt, Budin argued that the mother could carry out a diagnosis of the child by observing its expressions. If the eyebrows were contracted, it indicated that the child had a headache. This gesture was often considered to be the first exterior sign that something was wrong and, Budin affirmed, always occurred 'at the very onset of disease'.[71] If this sign were not identified by the mother and the illness followed its course, 'the eyes will become fixed and staring'. Later would come the grinding of teeth, movements of feet and

[66] David Forsyth, *Children in Health and Disease: A Study of Child-Life* (John Murray, London, 1909), 18.

[67] Forsyth, *Children in Health*, 20.

[68] Forsyth, *Children in Health*, 20.

[69] Henry Chapin, *Diseases of Infants and Children* (W. Wood and Co., New York, 1911), 58.

[70] Pierre Budin, *The Nursling: The Feeding and Hygiene of Premature & Full-Term Infants* (Caxton Publishing Company, London, 1907), 165.

[71] Budin, *The Nursling*, 13.

hands and – of course – crying. If the lips were separated in a way that the doctor could see the child's teeth or gums, the pain was localised in the belly, while the expansion of the nasal cavities implied chest pain.[72]

In 1913, the English doctor Archibald Garrod put forward once more the idea that love and sympathy were indispensable conditions for the satisfactory conduct of medical practice. In this narrative, Garrod hailed the qualities that the doctor who was dedicated to this period of life should have, commenting: 'The young child cannot tell us what he feels, and the seat of pain in an infant has often to be inferred from its actions . . . the youth of the patient calls for the exercise of special qualities in the medical attendant, and no man can be a good children's doctor who has not a real love of children.'[73] As written, Garrod's narrative can be understood as a continuation of the discourse that Charles West and other paediatricians had started fifty years earlier. However, in the 1920s, medical discourse started to change.

At about that time, the mechanistic vision of the child started to permeate paediatric practice, which had by now achieved recognition by the medical profession.[74] While in West's time the absence of a direct account of the patient and the consequent insistence on the fundamental importance of the doctor's physical examination led to the identification of the paediatrician with the figure of the explorer, now children's medicine started to be compared with veterinary practice.[75] The Scottish paediatrician Robert Hutchison used the analogy to rule out any attempt at constructing patient histories:

> With what are called 'subjective symptoms' in children you are not in any way troubled, because there are none. Paediatrics is like veterinary work in this, that the patient is unable to give you an account of his sufferings, and you are thrown back entirely on your own observation, which, of course, makes the necessity for careful examination all the greater.[76]

Some years later, Edmund Cautley recommended not looking at children directly in the eyes when carrying out a diagnosis, because 'like animals, [they] intensely dislike being stared at'.[77] Like Hutchison, Cautley compared practising on children with practising on animals, 'for in each case we are dependent on the observation of onlookers, and on physical examination, and

[72] Budin, *The Nursling*, 13.

[73] Archibald Garrod, in Archibald E. Garrod, Frederick F. Batten, and Hugh Thursfield (eds.), *Diseases of Children* by various authors (Edward Arnold, London, 1913), 1.

[74] Institutionalisation was crystallised in 1928 with the formal constitution of a professional body of child-health specialists, the British Paediatric Association, followed two years later by the foundation of the American Academy of Pediatrics.

[75] Jonathan Gillis, 'Taking a medical history in childhood illness: representations of parents in pediatric texts since 1850', *Bulletin of the History of Medicine*, 79 (2005), 429.

[76] Robert Hutchison, *Lectures on Diseases of Children* (Edward Arnold, London, 1904), 4–5.

[77] Edmund Cautley, *The Diseases of Infants and Children* (Paul B. Hoeber, New York, 1912), 3.

are neither assisted nor deceived by subjective symptoms'.[78] If, as happened with the metaphor of the explorer, the analogy with the veterinarian strengthened the need for the doctor to develop a specialist capacity for carrying out a direct clinical evaluation of the child patient, at the same time it connected with late nineteenth-century observations about the animal characteristics of younger children, which were considered to be a 'recapitulation' of the evolution of the species.[79]

In paediatric treatises written at this time, the perception of the child had changed. There is an increasing accordance with the scientific method and ideas coming from the experimental sciences, including behaviourism. In his *Introduction to Child Study*, William Blackley Drummond outlined the way different branches of science had approached the child: 'The philologist, for instance, turns to baby linguistics in the expectation of gaining a better understanding of the origin of human speech. The anthropologist, unable to discover a living specimen of primitive man, turns to the child as his nearest representative. The archaeologist finds valuable material in the child's attempts to draw.'[80] Some lines later, the Scottish doctor comments how, unlike anthropologists, philologists and physiologists, the main interest of most students of children lay in the impact of 'of child-study upon the direct welfare of the children themselves'.[81]

Drummond's text reflects the change that was now being forged in the field of paediatrics. The doctor argues that the first stage of an individual's development is characterised by a 'sensation' stage, 'in which the various sense organs are acted on by the outside world, and responsive movements are noticed more or less definitely of pleasure or pain'. From his point of view, the expressive movements of the 'babies' indicated initially only pleasure or pain; thus 'the smiling, laughing, and crowing accompanied by movements of the limbs', were early signals of pleasure, while the downwards contraction of the corners of the mouth and the frowning of the brows indicated the appearance of tears.[82] Even though Drummond recognised the child's capacity to experience pain, he referred to Preyer's investigation, introducing these sensations in the section dedicated to 'reflex movements'. His reference to Preyer is particularly relevant when talking of the 'child's first cry on entering the world', and he agreed with the physiologist that the child's first cry had a reflex origin, 'a much more reasonable vision than that of Kant when he spoke of it as the cry of indignation or anger, or of the common notion, according to which it is the result of pain'.[83] Within the framework of paediatrics as an institutionalised

[78] Cautley, *Diseases of Infants*, 4. [79] Gillis, 'Not just small adults', 946.
[80] William Drummond, *An Introduction to Child Study* (Edward Arnold, London, 1907), 4.
[81] Drummond, *An Introduction to Child Study*, 5.
[82] William Drummond, *The Child: His Nature and Nurture* (Dent, London, 1902), 76.
[83] Drummond, *The Child*, 73.

practice, paediatricians started to apply the theory of childhood development to their work, equating the infant and infantile development with animal development, at the same time as they introduced and established the standards of biological normality for life stages.[84] Thus, although many of the treatises of the period still started with a section dedicated to the examination of children, there was no longer room for the subjective signs of pain or the mother's account.

Even though Cautley started his treatise by referring to the words of the Romantic poet William Wordsworth – commenting 'The child is the father of the man, but is by no means a miniature adult' – he emphasised the importance of understanding childhood illness with the aim of developing an 'appreciation of the problems of life and pathology necessary for those whose work is mainly among adults'.[85] Children are not adults in miniature, but have their own identity, which will be given to them, above all, through growth. This orientation appears explicitly in other paediatric texts of the period, such as those of George Frederic Still (1868–1941), the first full-time child health specialist in the United Kingdom and the first Professor of Child Health at King's College, London. Still did not start his treatise with a section dedicated to the diagnosis of childhood illnesses and titled his first chapter 'Medical aspects of growth and development'. These treatises by Cautley and Still incorporated new understandings generated from the field of child physiology that allowed knowledge of the normal functions for each sub-stage of children's lives, and studies of the medical data corresponding to the evolution of the child in the different stages of life, through anthropometric measures covering the period from neonatal until puberty. Thus, the sections dedicated to diagnosis are no longer centred on pain and its signs but on weight – considered by many to be a more sensitive index of the health of an infant – the size of the head, dentition and mental development.[86]

Infant Pain Denial and the Use of Anaesthesia

In 1920, treatises such as that of the Austrian doctor August Ritter von Reuss, director of the neonatal department at the University Women's Clinic of Vienna, started to present the theory that babies had a lesser sensibility to pain because of the immaturity of their nervous systems, commenting:

84 Sydney Buckman, 'Babies and monkeys', *The Nineteenth Century*, 36 (1984), 727–43; W. Kidd, 'The prehensile power of the hands of the human infant', *The Lancet*, 150 (1897), 1010.

85 Cautley, *Diseases of Infants*, 1.

86 George Frederic Still, *Common Disorders and Diseases of Childhood* (Henry Frowde, London, 1910); A. E. Garrod, in Garrod et al. (eds.), *Diseases of Children; By Various Authors*; Wilfred J. Pearson and W. G. Wyllie, *Recent Advances in Diseases of Children* (P. Blakiston's Son & Co. Inc, Philadelphia, PA, 1935).

> Children under three weeks old remained comparatively quiet when stimulated by currents so strong as to be almost unendurable by adults; it is difficult to decide how far this is due to incomplete development of the peripheral nerve tracts or to backwardness of the central pain receptors.[87]

Surprisingly, this specialist did not deny that babies showed obvious signs of suffering when subjected to 'stimulation of the skin, such as smack'. Moreover, the infant responded to these stimuli 'with loud screams, thus showing that it is sensitive to pain'. Nevertheless, Ritter von Reuss continued,

> it is generally accepted that while the reflex excitability for local tactile stimulation in the new-born is even greater than at a later period, the perception of pain is considerably less; that the time of reaction is longer than the pain, such as in operations, has on the whole not nearly so great an intensity and duration as in the older child.[88]

The dominant view in psychology and physiology that infants and children had a reduced sensitivity to pain was reinforced within paediatrics by a fear about the use of opiates on young children, which justified the minimal use of anaesthesia in children's surgery. In 1938, when describing a surgical procedure in a child, Max Thorek, founder of the International College of Surgeons, wrote: 'anaesthesia is often not required. In many cases, a sponge soaked in the mixture of water and sugar is sufficient to calm a child'.[89] A few years later, the English medic Gordon Jackson Rees published a paper on paediatric anaesthesia that explored complications such as how infants of less than six months tended to become hypothermic in response to anaesthesia, while older infants, in contrast, tended towards hyperthermia. Of the two conditions, it was easier to manage hypothermia, and sometimes hyperthermia could lead to convulsions and even death, with the use of ether anaesthesia and atropine premedication increasing that risk. Rees wrote:

> The respiratory deficiencies of the infant during early life and the hazards of hyperthermia in older children suggest that controlled ventilation during the maintenance of anaesthesia has special advantages. It should be regarded as an essential part of the technique for prolonged operations, and is highly desirable for shorter procedures. Anaesthesia can be maintained at very light levels with nitrous oxide-oxygen and a relaxant drug, with the result that recovery is rapid. There are, therefore, cogent practical and theoretical reasons for maintaining anaesthesia with controlled ventilation, a relaxant drug, nitrous oxide and oxygen.[90]

87 August Ritter von Reuss, *The Diseases of the Newborn* (John Bale, Sons & Danielsson Ltd., London, 1920), 73.

88 Ritter von Reuss, *Diseases of the Newborn*, 77.

89 Max Thorek, *Modern Surgical Technique*, vol. III (Lippincott, Montreal, 1938), 20–21.

90 Jackson Rees, 'Anaesthesia in the newborn', *British Medical Journal* (23 December 1950) 1419–22, cited in *Oxford Textbook of Paediatric Pain* (Oxford University Press, Oxford, 2013), 12.

But this view was strongly opposed by others, such as Charles Robson, an anaesthetist at the Hospital for Sick Children in Toronto – who may have been the first paediatric anaesthesiologist – who responded:

> First, it has been stated that infants under seven days of age do not require anesthetics for operations – that their association tracts for pain are not fully established and that minor operations may be carried out without any damaging effects on the infant. Personally, I do not believe this and it is simply vivisection to operate on a conscious screaming wriggling infant without using a general or local anesthetic.[91]

Robson's practice was to use open-drop ether, cyclopropane, and tracheal intubation to provide infant anaesthesia.[92]

Robson's views were probably not those of the majority. Early textbooks on paediatric anaesthesia provide little discussion of pain, even in relation to newborns.[93] For instance, there is only one substantive comment in Digby Leigh's and M. K Belton's Pediatric Anesthesia, which became a reference text in many countries:

> Newborn infants are not as sensitive to pain and some degree of analgesia is present without anesthetic. Most infants, however, do have some pain sensation even at birth and one cannot rely on the old adage that there is no pain sensation for the first three weeks of life. It is nearer the truth to say that sensitivity to pain is decreased. Since there is some basic analgesia, very low concentrations of anesthetic agent will produce complete analgesia.[94]

In 1950, J. L. Henderson's article 'The relief of pain in childhood' still argued that children appeared to 'tolerate pain better than adults'.[95] A decade later, David M. Levy argued that as neonates lacked memories, it was not possible to compare their pain with that experienced by adults.[96]

In 1952, French neurologist André Thomas issued a warning about the function of the myelin sheath, based on studies in animals that had shown how non-myelinated fibres could be excited. In 1957, Ernest Jones encapsulated the theory that in order for pain to be felt the capacity to remember it needed to be in place and that in order to feel pain sensations there first needed to be a mature nervous system. He argued that while an individual subject might recognise pain mentally he could not reconstruct it and that repeated

[91] Charles Robson, 'Anesthesia in children', *Anesthesia and Analgesia*, 4 (1925), 235–40.

[92] C. M. Mai and M. Yaster, 'Pediatric anesthesia: a historical perspective', *American Society of Anesthesiologists*, 75 (2011), 10–13.

[93] Bonnie J. Stevens, Gareth Hathway and William T. Zempsky (eds.), *Oxford Textbook of Pediatric Pain*, 2nd ed., Oxford Textbook (Oxford Academic, Oxford, 2021; online ed., 1 June 2021), 5.

[94] M. D. Leigh and M. K. Belton, Pediatric Anesthesia (Macmillan, New York, 1948), 30.

[95] J. L. Henderson, 'The relief of pain in childhood', in Sir Heneage Ogilvie and William A. R. Thomson (eds.), *Pain and Its Problems* (Eyre and Spottiswoode, London, 1950), 171–72.

[96] David M. Levy, 'The infant's earliest memory of inoculation: a contribution to public health procedures', *Journal of Genetic Psychology*, 96 (1960), 3–46.

pain sensations did not provide resistance.[97] Harold Merskey suggested that children had an immature perception of pain and acquired this ability as they grew older.[98] He argued that even if small children were able to feel pain, their reaction to it involved a weaker expression than that of adults. Merskey was a member of the panel that proposed the first definition of pain adopted by the International Association for the Study of Pain (IASP) as 'an unpleasant sensory or emotional experience associated with actual or potential tissue damage or described in terms of such damage. Noteworthy, pain is always subjective. Everybody learns it through experiences related to injuries in early life'.[99]

Conclusion

This chapter has shown how scientific disciplines – and paediatrics in particular – changed between the latter part of the nineteenth century and the first half of the twentieth century. Scientific understanding of pain and childhood became the domain of increasingly specialist – and often competing – disciplines, each of which had its own perspective on pain in childhood. Thus, the child study movement, heavily influenced by Darwinism and recapitulation theory, envisioned the child as an entity that embodied the species' primitive past and held that pain was a mere reflex action in infants and a sensation that children learned as they grew. The mechanistic vision of behaviourism dismissed children's expressions of pain, particularly those of infants, which were seen as reflex responses to stimuli. While paediatrics in the nineteenth century was often not considered as a branch of science, this changed in the twentieth century. However, far from consolidating the factual consideration of pain, the 'scientisation' of paediatrics led to the influence of mechanistic and developmental theories, and eventually to the rejection of 'subjective' testimony as a methodological approach to children. On the one hand, paediatrics started to conceive pain in a more theoretical perspective; on the other hand, practice was based on the underlying analogy between animals and children, and between veterinarians and paediatricians. The increasingly mechanistic vision and the dismissal of 'subjectivity' and mothers' accounts of children's pain led to the growing importance of observation (by professionals rather than parents, and by doctors rather than nurses). But some of the observational practices – notably those of Hall and Gesell – were hardly as scientifically rigorous as they were presented at the time. They owed much to Romantic conceptions of the child and to the theory of recapitulation, and they used the child as a symbol of the development of the human species. They were also informed by racial and class prejudices and emerged at a time of increasing industrial

[97] Ernest Jones, 'Pain', *International Journal of Psychoanalysis*, 38 (1957), 255.
[98] Harold Merskey, 'On the development of pain', *Headache*, 10 (1970), 116–23.
[99] H. Merskey et al., 'Pain in terms: a list with definitions and notes on usage', *Pain*, 6 (1979), 249.

institutionalisation. Although they had different theoretical perspectives, all three disciplines – child study, behavioural psychology and paediatrics – came to embrace the idea that infants did not feel pain or had considerably less sensitivity to pain than older children and adults.

The debate about infant pain denial encapsulates two important issues in both the history of pain and the history of childhood. First, that of the *politics of pain*, an idea defended by several important writers.[100] Lucy Bending's argument that the appropriation of physical pain by different interpretations opens the door to potential abuse by the authorities means that pain is not only subject to cultural conditioning but also susceptible to being represented or distorted by those power groups.[101] The infant pain research this chapter has explored can be seen as a paradigm for the ways in which pain can be manipulated and defined by those in power. Whenever the communicative power of language is weakened or linguistic communication disappears, Elaine Scarry's thesis – that the inexpressibility of personal pain makes someone more vulnerable to being exploited, oppressed or tortured by those who have power – resonates.[102] Connected to the politics of pain is the power of representation. Here, the 'normal' example takes the place of the species, and the species the place of the specific individual, who disappears. This leads to metaphorical representations where the child takes the place of the savage and vice versa, where the normal replaces the abnormal, and so on. This kind of representation allows the creation of taxonomies and theories about development.

The second issue concerns the child's status as a developing body and the significance of pain in the scientific construction of the development process. In the twentieth century, the child came to embody a normative developmental process. The experience of pain was an important aspect in marking the distinct phases of development, both in the child study movement and in behaviourism. In the nineteenth century, scientific figurations had used the form of the child body to generate hierarchies based on race, gender, sexuality and class. But in the twentieth century, there was a change as the child's body was seen more in terms of its human potential. Nonetheless, in both nineteenth- and twentieth-century science, the child was essentially valued as a future adult.

[100] Elaine Scarry insists that power can ignore the pain of those that do not have the capacity to express themselves, leading to a greater vulnerability to all kinds of physical abuse (Scarry, *Body in Pain*). Martin Pernick presents an account of the selection of human typology that needed or even deserved anaesthesia when it was making its entrance into habitual medical practice in the United States at the end of the 1840s and the beginning of the 1850s (Pernick, *A Calculus of Suffering*). On the politics of pain see Bourke, *Story of Pain*; Wailoo, *Pain: A Political History*. See also Mary Poovey, *Uneven Developments: The Ideological Work of Gender in Mid-Victorian England* (Chicago University Press, Chicago, 1988), chapter 2.

[101] Bending, *Representation of Bodily Pain*, 1–11.

[102] Scarry, *Body in Pain*, 27.

3 Articulating Mental Pain

In October 1875, the British doctor William H. Spurgin described one of his patients, a ten-year-old girl whom he named 'S.T.' The girl's parents called the physician in September 1874 after the child complained of 'severe pain at the epigastrium'.[1] According to her parents, who provided Spurgin with details of their child's story, S.T. had always been healthy until three months before the doctor was sent for, when she started suffering 'of the same pain once or twice a week', a pain that progressively worsened. Spurgin reported that, on his first visit, S.T. was 'a rosy healthy-looking child', but the increasing pain meant that she 'soon became sallow', developed an 'abdominal aspect' and 'became quite unable to walk', and then had convulsions and screaming fits.[2] Eventually, the child 'appeared in the greatest agony and misery in spite of all treatment'. S.T.'s symptoms and her lack of response to treatment led Spurgin to diagnose hysteria. Even though there was confusion about the symptoms of hysteria, nineteenth-century alienists agreed that the most unusual manifestations of hysteria always involved the continuous experience of chronic pain. S.T. was one of many children and young people in the second half of the nineteenth century who suffered from mental health disorders and ended up being cared for by doctors or confined in state institutions. Her case provides insights into the overlapping ways in which the mental disorders of childhood were understood in relation to pain, which is the subject of this chapter.[3]

[1] Spurgin, 'Case of hysteria', 555. [2] Spurgin, 'Case of hysteria', 555.

[3] The historiography of children's insanity has grown considerably since Sally Shuttleworth's 2010 publication *The Mind of the Child*, but historians have paid little attention to the broader topic of children's pain in post-Darwinian psychiatry. For a discussion of child insanity, see: Shuttleworth, *Mind of the Child*; Sally Shuttleworth, 'The psychology of childhood in Victorian literature and medicine', in Helen Small and Trudi Tate (eds.), *Literature, Science, Psychoanalysis, 1830–1970: Essays in Honour of Gillian Beer* (Oxford University Press, Oxford, 2003), 86–101; Steven Taylor, *Child Insanity in England, 1845–1907* (Palgrave Macmillan, London, 2016); Steven Taylor, '"All his ways are those of an idiot": the admission, treatment and social reaction to two idiot children of Northampton Pauper Lunatic Asylum, 1877–1883', *Family & Community History*, 15 (2012), 35; K. Gingell, 'The forgotten children:

In *The Body in Pain*, Elaine Scarry makes a clear distinction between physical and psychological pain, arguing that psychological pain is present in almost all forms of literature, but that physical pain has received scant attention.[4] This chapter argues, however, that during certain historical periods, this kind of stark distinction between mental and bodily pain is not supported by the evidence.[5] To make this argument, the analysis returns to the second half of the nineteenth century, when boundaries between psychiatry, psychology, neurology and neighbouring medical and scientific disciplines were still blurred. The analysis thus focuses on the overlapping ways in which the mental disorders of childhood were understood in relation to pain and, in some cases, the absence of pain. By arguing that mental illness and insanity often became known precisely through the physical manifestation of a pained body, this chapter supports the view voiced by, among others, Rob Boddice and Louise Hide, whose work explores the complex cultural connections between the body in pain and the disordered mind.[6]

The main methodological challenge in researching this chapter was the identification of references and ideas connected to pain in the context of children's insanity. While the previous two chapters explored the expression of children's pain and infant pain denial – notions directly mentioned by both theorists and practitioners – the interest in pain in the context of the authors and topics covered in this chapter is more indirect. For this reason, the following pages explore different mental conditions in search of ties with childhood and suffering, instead of pointing directly at statements, principles and practices directly related to that central topic.

To explore the intersection of children's mental illness and pain at the end of the nineteenth century from the perspective of the practising psychiatrists of the time, this chapter presents different mental diseases that represent distinct ways of framing the complex interactions between the child's mind, body and pain. The varied representations of pain that emerge straddle a range of scientific judgements and underlying theories. The first section marks the

children admitted to a county asylum between 1854 and 1900', *Psychiatric Bulletin*, 25 (2001), 432–34.

4 Scarry, *Body in Pain*, 11.

5 Sarah Chaney makes a similar point in the context of pain and self-mutilation in later nineteenth-century psychiatry. See Sarah Chaney, 'Anaesthetic bodies and the absence of feeling: pain and self-mutilation in later nineteenth-century psychiatry', *19: Interdisciplinary Studies in the Long Nineteenth Century*, 15 (2012), 1–19.

6 Rob Boddice, 'Hysteria or Tetanus? Ambivalent embodiments and the authenticity of pain', in Dolores Martin Moruno and Beatriz Pichel (eds.), *Emotional Bodies: Studies on the Historical Performativity of Emotions* (University of Illinois Press, Urbana-Champaign, 2019), 19–35; Morris, *Culture of Pain*, 103–24; Louise Hide, 'Making sense of pain: delusions, syphilis and somatic pain in London County Council asylums, c. 1900', *19: Interdisciplinary Studies in the Long Nineteenth Century*, 15 (2012), 1–20.

central year of 1860 as the date when the concept of the 'child mind' was introduced by the psychiatrist Sir James Crichton-Browne, who strongly advocated the extension of the notion of insanity to children. It then goes on to cover 'night terrors', a new category of disease strongly linked to hallucinations and painful attacks, which rapidly gained popularity among theorists of mental illness despite the lack of documented cases. Night terrors were often attributed to pain – typically intestinal disorders. First presented in Charles West's *Lectures on the Diseases of Infancy and Childhood*, the night-terrors category was further elaborated by Crichton-Browne, among others.[7] The importance of night terrors is that it is the first example of a form of mental illness considered to be suffered exclusively by children. Crichton-Browne believed night terrors to be a passing form of 'pantophobia' that was common in infancy and childhood, and both night terrors and daydreams came to be seen as part of a continuum that led directly to mental illness, a view that shaped the late nineteenth-century development of child psychiatry.[8]

The second section covers melancholia – also defined as 'mental pain' and as a form of 'affective insanity' – and explores the Darwinist, physiological research programme that presumed that this form of mental illness resulted from an irritated brain.[9] This new concept of melancholia and the distinction between emotional and intellectual maladies relied on ideas about non-intellectual insanity that had emerged in the early nineteenth century, such as 'moral insanity' – introduced by James Cowles Prichard in his 1835 book *Treatise on Insanity and Other Disorders Affecting the Mind* – where the moral faculties and emotions were considered disordered.[10] The next section analyses hysteria, an umbrella or catch-all notion that included a multitude of bodily manifestations with the only common trait being that of manifest pain, often of an emotional nature. It shows how hysteria was used to explain all kinds of conditions – including religious ecstasy and sexual deviance (beyond

[7] West, *Lectures*, 188.

[8] James Crichton-Browne, 'Psychical diseases of early life', *Journal of Mental Science*, 6 (1860), 312–13.

[9] Åsa Jansson's book *From Melancholia to Depression: Disordered Mood in Nineteenth-Century Psychiatry* (Palgrave Macmillan, Cham, 2021) has been very useful for an understanding of children's melancholia in relation to Victorian physicians diagnoses of adults. See also, Åsa Jansson, 'Mood disorders and the brain: depression, melancholia, and the historiography of psychiatry', *Medical History*, 55 (2011), 398; Åsa Jansson, 'From statistics to diagnostics: medical certificates, melancholia, and suicidal propensities in Victorian psychiatry', *Journal of Social History*, 46 (2013), 716–31.

[10] For a discussion of moral insanity see German Berrios, *The History of Mental Symptoms: Descriptive Psychopathology since the Nineteenth Century* (Cambridge University Press, Cambridge, 1995). German Berrios, 'Mood disorders: clinical section', in German E. Berrios and Roy Porter (eds.), *A History of Clinical Psychiatry: The Origin and History of Psychiatric Disorders* (Athlone Press, London, 1995); German Berrios, 'Classic Text No. 37: J.C. Prichard and the concept of moral insanity', *History of Psychiatry*, 10 (1999), 111–26.

the scope of the current study) – and how although it was initially applied particularly to adult women, it was later extended to children. The final section explores children who enjoy inflicting pain on others. For the leading British alienist Henry Maudsley, such behaviour indicated 'homicidal monomania'. This chapter focuses on the British context from the 1860s until the end of the nineteenth century, a period during which diagnostic categories passed from being fluid to becoming clearly defined diseases with – for its time – a notably consistent symptomology.

These various conditions each involved different figurations of pain. So, while physical pain was considered the cause of hallucinations and irrational fears in the case of night terrors, with both melancholia and hysteria, pain was seen in affective and emotional terms. In the case of hysteria, pain became the unifying symptom and articulating notion that allowed the construction of a range of bodies in emotional pain.

The Victorian system for classifying mental disorders placed a plethora of conditions within two main categories: idiocy and insanity. Children and young people who would today be diagnosed as having learning disabilities often found themselves labelled 'idiots', 'imbeciles' or 'feebleminded'.[11] And the label 'insanity' was applied to any disorder or mental illness in which the mind did not conform to normal activities and patterns, and which resulted in socially unacceptable behaviours. This chapter focuses on insanity, showing how neurologists, psychiatrists and paediatricians understood pain of non-organic origin.

Researching this chapter involved an extensive literature search for historical publications on children's insanity and pain, and I began with two historical reviews of the development of child psychiatry: Alexander von Gontard's article 'The development of child psychiatry in 19th century Britain' (1988) and M. Neve's and T. Turner's *History of Child and Adolescent Psychiatry* (2002).[12] Von Gontard's article stands out for its thorough research, based mainly on the writings of nineteenth-century medical practitioners, as well as its description and analysis of the early development of

[11] For a discussion on disability, see: Anne Borsay and Pamela Dale (eds.), *Disabled Children: Contested Caring, 1850–1979* (Pickering & Chatto, London, 2012); Pamela Dale and Joseph Melling, *Mental Illness and Learning Disability since 1850: Finding a Place for Mental Disorder in the United Kingdom* (Routledge, London, 2006); Stephen Humphries and Pamela Gordon, *Out of Sight: The Experience of Disability, 1900–1950* (Northcote House, Plymouth, 1992); Mary Clare Martin, 'Disabled children and domestic living spaces in Britain, 1800–1900', in M. S. Romero, E. A. Garcia and G. A. Jimenez (eds.), *Children, Spaces and Identity: Childhood in the Past Monograph Series* (Oxbow Books, Oxford, 2015), 136–54.

[12] Alexander von Gontard, 'The development of child psychiatry in 19th century Britain', *Journal of Child Psychology and Psychiatry*, 29 (1988), 569–88. M. Neve and T. Turner, 'History of child and adolescent psychiatry', in M. Rutter and E. Taylor (eds.), *Child and Adolescent Psychiatry* (Blackwell, Oxford, 2002).

child psychiatry in Britain. This chapter focuses on works published by British alienists and paediatricians, as well as the European and American texts they cite, from 1860 to 1900, the period in which the first studies of child psychiatry appeared. These texts, written in a discursive and scholastic style, seem likely to have been aimed at elite physicians rather than the public. Although nearly all these texts are dedicated to adult conditions, the sections on childhood reveal a great deal about medical perceptions and treatment of children.

The Mind of the Child

Despite widespread agreement on the nature of imbecility and idiocy, defining insanity proved a difficult task for late nineteenth-century alienists and some British clinicians questioned whether children could be insane.[13] Even physicians who specialised in children – such as Fletcher Beach and John Langdon Down – found few cases that appeared to be obvious examples of insanity. 'Acute insanity arising before the age of puberty is rarely met with in asylum practice; and there are, so far as I am aware, very few such cases recorded,' wrote M. B. Ray, an assistant medical officer at the West Riding Asylum, in 1896.[14]

As Sally Shuttleworth has pointed out, during the first half of the nineteenth century, there had been considerable reluctance to accept the idea that children could be afflicted by the same mental illnesses that affected adults, and the reported cases tended to point towards poor parenting or teaching rather than being related to the child mind itself.[15] Notwithstanding worries about 'degeneration' and inherited insanity, in the 1850s the medical consensus was that children could be imbeciles or 'idiots' but not insane.[16] Thus Jean Étienne Dominique Esquirol argued: 'it is only at puberty, during the earliest menstrual efforts, or during, and after a too rapid growth, that we begin to notice certain cases of mental alienation. [. . .] Mental alienation might, therefore, be divided, relative to ages, into imbecility for childhood, mania and monomania for youth, lypemania or melancholy for consistent age, and into dementia for advanced life'.[17] But the picture begins to change after 1860, with the advance of psychiatry and the emergence of the view that children were in fact *more* vulnerable to certain forms of insanity than adults were.

[13] Shuttleworth, *Mind of the Child*, 21.

[14] M. B. Ray, 'A case of acute melancholia occurring in a child', *The Quarterly Medical Journal: A Quarterly Review of the Medical Sciences for Yorkshire and Adjoining Counties*, 5 (October 1896–July 1897), 242.

[15] Shuttleworth, *Mind of the Child*, 21.

[16] Von Gontard, 'Development of child psychiatry', 569–88.

[17] Jean Étienne Dominique Esquirol, *Mental Maladies: A Treatise on Insanity* (Lea and Blanchard, Philadelphia, PA, 1845), 34.

Crichton-Browne[18] warned in 1860 that attention needed to be paid to children's language because 'those incoherent speeches, or odd remarks, which are attributed to childish unmeaning babbling and folly, may sometimes be in reality the result of delusions, illusions and hallucination'.[19]

Crichton-Browne's 1860 essay 'Psychical diseases of early life' had a major impact on the emerging discipline of child psychiatry, arguing that 'monomania or delusional insanity, we believe to be more common during infancy and childhood than at any other period of life'.[20] Citing recent research on heredity and idiocy, Crichton-Brown argued that 'almost every form of mental disease which may attack the adult, may also attack the infant and the child'.[21] His approach, derived from Esquirol's theories about monomania, listed childhood mental disorders including melancholia, mania, kleptomania, homicidal mania, pantophobia, moral insanity and night terrors.[22]

But, at the time of publishing this influential essay, Crichton-Browne was far from being an experienced physician. He was a twenty-year-old student and would not qualify as a doctor for another year. While drawing on established medical paradigms, his essay also anticipates the work of late nineteenth- and early twentieth-century psychiatrists in its concern for sexuality and suicide. He takes a dim view of the common childhood activity of daydreaming, arguing that such imaginative projections – 'castle building' – are a 'pernicious practice' and that 'much mental derangement in mature life, we believe, is attributable to these reveries indulged in during childhood'.[23]

Soon after the publication of Crichton-Browne's essay, the eminent psychiatrist John Conolly called for a greater understanding of the child mind, writing in 1862: 'In innumerable respects society and manners and modes of thinking have undergone great changes since the beginning of this century, but in no respect more strikingly than in the greater attention paid to the minds of children of every class.'[24] Crichton-Browne and Conolly were not alone. As Sally Shuttleworth has argued in *The Mind of the Child*, although it was not until the end of the nineteenth century that the two fields of child psychology and child psychiatry started to consolidate, as early as the middle of the century, 'the inner workings of the child mind [were] opened up to

[18] Crichton-Browne's life has been extensively examined in a comprehensive and well-documented study conducted by historian Michael Neve and psychiatrist Trevor Turner. Neve and Turner, 'History of child and adolescent psychiatry'.

[19] Crichton-Browne, 'Psychical diseases', 287.

[20] William Ll. Parry-Jones, 'The history of child and adolescent psychiatry: its present-day relevance', *Journal of Child Psychology and Psychiatry*, 1 (1989), 3–11.

[21] Crichton-Browne, 'Psychical diseases', 320. [22] Shuttleworth, *Mind of the Child*, 38.

[23] Crichton-Browne, 'Psychical diseases', 303.

[24] John Conolly, 'Recollections of the varieties of insanity', *Medical Times and Gazette*, 1 (1862), 235.

medical interrogation and intervention'.[25] There was no specialist science in childhood mental conditions, and the studies were carried out by specialists in adult illnesses.

Perhaps the most dramatic claim in this 1860 essay is that insanity could occur 'in utero'.[26] This idea opened the door to an increasing focus on hereditary transmission, a trend that was aided and abetted by the development of evolutionary psychology and psychiatry following the publication of Darwin's *On the Origin of Species* in 1859. From having previously been seen as incapable of suffering from most mental disorders, the child was now deemed vulnerable to the full array of adult conditions. For Crichton-Browne: 'From the end of the first dentition, up to puberty, we may state, as a general principle, that there is a liability to every psychical disease from which the adult may suffer, together with certain conditions peculiar to that stage of life.'[27] At the same time, there was a wider cultural concern about the child mind. Research into children's mental capacity played a role in the introduction of compulsory education in the UK, and by the end of the century specialised care was being offered to children deemed abnormal or mentally deficient.[28]

From 1860 onwards, medical professionals debated not only whether children could be insane but also at what stage could insanity be present. Many tried to distinguish between the sane and the insane mind. Scottish physician William Ireland observed: 'Sanity is generally regarded as a natural and healthy growth of a man's character, and insanity as something diseased or abnormal.'[29] A mind afflicted by insanity was seen as deviating from the characteristics of a normal childhood, corrupting children's natural innocence and manipulating their natural tendencies. There was also much debate about the developmental stage after which children could become insane. Considering the question 'How soon can a child go mad?', Henry Maudsley argued 'obviously not before it has got some mind to go wrong, and then only in proportion to the quantity and quality of mind which it has'.[30]

Crichton-Browne was not alone in his claims, although his tone may have been fiercer and more provocative. As shown in Chapter 1, Charles West had called for more attention to be paid to the unique nature of the physical constitution of children and their pathologies. In his textbook on children's

[25] Shuttleworth, *Mind of the Child*, 42. [26] Shuttleworth, *Mind of the Child*, 37.

[27] Crichton-Browne, 'Psychical diseases', 286.

[28] Eleanor Betts, 'From Juvenile Delinquent to boy murderer: understanding children who killed, 1816–1908' (Unpublished PhD thesis, Queen Mary University, 2016), 152.

[29] William Ireland, *The Mental Affections of Children: Idiocy, Imbecility and Insanity* (J & A Churchill, London, 1898), 272.

[30] Henry Maudsley, *The Pathology of Mind: A Study of Its Distempers, Deformities and Disorders*, 2nd ed. (Macmillan and Co., London, 1895), 364.

diseases and in a subsequent publication titled 'On the mental Peculiarities and Mental Disorders of Childhood' published in The Medical Times and Gazette, West suggested that similar consideration should be given to children's minds and claimed that the advances in the study of adult illnesses, which had enabled the move from studying symptoms – 'diseases' – to studying the individuality of the patient – the 'diseased' – had no equivalent in studies of children's ailments.[31] According to West, medical practitioners who did not take into account the 'mental and moral peculiarities of childhood' in the development of childhood illness would never be able to make a secure diagnosis. Just as happened 'in the grown person', factors such as anxiety and grief were actual factors 'in conducting the patient to death, or in bringing his recovery'. It was thus fundamental to study the child 'from its mental as well as from its physical side' to understand 'how in its immaturity the mind reacts on the body as well as the body on the mind'.[32]

In the third, expanded, edition of his *Lectures on the Diseases of Infancy and Childhood* (1854), West enlarged the chapter on mental health, including new material about children's imagination, dreams and nightmares, and various mental pathologies.[33] In this edition, West confronted child insanity more directly. He notes that 'perversion of the intellect or of the moral faculties, as distinguished from mere feebleness of mind, is met with in childhood as well as in adult age, and deserves to be regarded and to be treated as insanity no less in the one case than in the other'.[34]

By pointing out the role of anxiety and mental unrest in sick children and introducing the topic of mental disorders into a text on the physical ailments of children, West became a key figure in the development of child psychiatry.[35] Noting the role of anxiety and mental unrest in sick children, he challenged the assumption that children, not having yet attained a state of reason, were incapable of losing it and therefore of becoming insane. As Sally Shuttleworth has argued, this perspective led to the definition of mental disorder as a kind of 'heightened state of childhood', a change in the understanding of the child mind, which opened the door to the idea that the causes of insanity might be

[31] Charles West, 'On the mental peculiarities and mental disorders of childhood', *Medical Times and Gazette*, 1 (1860), 133–37.

[32] West, 'On the mental peculiarities', 133.

[33] For a discussion of West's work in relation to the mind of the child, see Shuttleworth, *Mind of the Child*, chapter 2, and Boehm, *Charles Dickens*, chapter 3.

[34] West, *Lectures*, 188.

[35] As Janet Oppenheim has argued in her discussion on nervous children, the growth of child psychology was only one aspect of the gradual development of paediatrics as a reputable branch of medicine during the nineteenth century. See Janet Oppenheim, *'Shattered Nerves': Doctors, Patients, and Depression in Victorian England* (Oxford University Press, Oxford, 1991), 234.

related to a child's freedom from adult mental constraint.[36] The following section analyses the disease defined by West as 'night terrors' and its relation to pain, taking this as a characteristic example of the new disciplinary categorisation of incipient child psychiatry.

Night Terrors, Pain and Hallucinations

To illustrate children's vulnerability to monomania or delusional insanity, Crichton-Browne referred to children with visions of ghosts and to the diagnostic category of 'night terrors' recently unveiled by Charles West.[37] Despite the Romantic interest in dreams, nightmares and apparitions, West's text was the first nineteenth-century medical textbook to consider children's night terrors as a specific category.[38] In the 1848 edition of the *Lectures*, West had presented the idea of an apparently psychological disorder originating from a somatic source in digestive dysfunction. West's lecture about night terrors begins with a graphic description of a child afflicted by this phenomenon. While sleeping one night, a little boy of eleven months awoke 'with a sudden start, and a scream so violent that all the people in the house heard it'.[39] After he was removed from his bed, he continued to cry loudly for a while and then, little by little, he calmed down and 'fell asleep again, sweating profusely'. After an interval – sometimes half an hour, sometimes as much as two hours – he would wake up again in the same sudden way and with the same violent scream. And then, after a few minutes, he would again 'sink into slumber'.[40] Six days later, the attacks returned more vehemently and increased in frequency, with 'as many as seven or eight having occurred in the course of a single night'. The child also suffered similar attacks when he was sleeping during the daytime. His parents recalled that before the first attack the child had suffered for ten days with mild diarrhoea, 'with dark and slimy evacuations'.[41] Despite the apparent gravity of the illness, the child was cheerful, sucked well, did not vomit and did not present fever. The only physical symptomology present was a swollen and tender abdomen, swollen gums and a furry tongue. The boy's doctor, West, diagnosed the condition as a case of *night terrors* dependent upon intestinal disorder.

This account is one of various cases used to illustrate the new diagnostic category. Both in the second edition of the *Lectures* and in his essay 'On the

[36] Shuttleworth, *Mind of the Child*, 50.

[37] From this point on, night terrors became a standard entry in medical manuals, usually citing West. See, for example, T. H. Tanner, *A Practical Treatise on the Diseases of Infancy and Childhood* (Henry Renshaw, London, 1858), 276–79.

[38] Sally Shuttleworth, 'Night terrors: medical and literary representations of childhood fear', in Anne-Julia Zwierlein (ed.), *Unmapped Countries: Biological Visions in Nineteenth Century Literature and Culture* (Anthem Nineteenth-Century Series) (Anthem Press, London, 2005), 198.

[39] West, *Lectures*, 188.
[40] West, *Lectures*, 188.
[41] West, *Lectures*, 188.

Mental peculiarities and mental disorders of childhood', West expanded his understanding of the aetiology of night terrors, highlighting the connection with organic injuries and adding experiences of intense physiological pain – especially following surgery – to other factors such as intestinal worms and digestive problems. West also saw a relationship between bodily pain and the persecutory delusions and hallucinations children experienced.[42]

Although West admitted the paucity of relevant works to cite in support of his arguments, his comments on the connection between pain and hallucinations follow the emerging tradition in psychiatry that attempted to find a somatic location for conditions – such as melancholia, neuralgia and hallucinations – with no obvious organic origin. Historians have generally agreed that, after the middle of the nineteenth century, a new generation of medically trained alienists placed a greater emphasis on somatic explanations of insanity.[43] These accounts involved both biological heredity and the rather vaguely defined concept of 'nervous impulses', principles that were used in the classification of children's insanity. Such late nineteenth-century definitions of insanity can be seen as part of a wider mindset – manifested both in scientific and popular literature – that placed a twin emphasis on volition and self-control on the one hand, and the biology of the brain on the other.

This new generation of medical experts was convinced that insanity had a physical cause – whether a brain injury or some other kind of organic lesion – that could be brought to light by sophisticated medical practices. Thus, G. Fielding Blandford wrote in *Insanity and Its Treatment* (1871): 'Disorder of the mind means disorder of the brain, and [. . .] the latter is an organ liable to disease and disturbance, like other organs of the body, to be investigated by the same method and subject to the same laws.'[44] The psychiatrist Henry Maudsley dismissed psychological enquiries into insanity as metaphysical and unscientific musings.[45] British and continental psychiatrists generally agreed that considerably more research was needed to establish the physical location of insanity. Maudsley, though, suggested that, until hard evidence

[42] See Hide, 'Making sense of pain'.

[43] Andrew Scull, *The Most Solitary of Afflictions: Madness and Society in Britain, 1700–1900* (Yale University Press, New Haven, CT, 1993); L. S. Jacyna, 'Somatic theories of mind and the interests of medicine in Britain, 1850–1879', *Medical History*, 26 (1982), 233–58; Michael J. Clark, 'The data of alienism': evolutionary neurology, physiological psychology, and the reconstruction of British Psychiatric Theory, c.1850–c.1900' (Unpublished PhD thesis, University of Oxford, 1982).

[44] George Fielding Blandford, *Insanity and Its Treatment: Lectures on the Treatment, Medical and Legal, of Insane Patients* (Oliver and Boyd, Edinburgh, 1871), 6.

[45] See Henry Maudsley, *The Physiology and Pathology of the Mind* (Macmillan, London, 1867); Henry Maudsley, 'The genesis of mind', *Journal of Mental Science*, 7 (1862), 461–94. For the broader implications of such attitudes, see L. S. Jacyna, 'The physiology of mind, the unity of nature, and the moral order in Victorian thought', *The British Journal for the History of Science*, 14 (1981), 118.

became available, diagnoses should be made on the basis of the compendium of nervous symptoms. More than any other figure, he shifted the focus of British psychiatry from the metaphysical to the physical, arguing that the psychological symptoms of insanity were not especially significant and amounted to epiphenomena. Maudsley was convinced that organic causes would one day be found that corresponded with the various symptoms that were the basis of classification. Within this medical cosmology, insanity in children could be viewed as 'evidence' of anatomical lesions (in the brain), of pathological instinct or of a functional disorder.

Within the wider literature about insanity, there has been much debate about the extent to which the insane should be treated in institutions or at home.[46] However, historians agree about the marginality of discussion about child insanity – which, when it took place, was generally within the context of adult insanity – even though children's hallucinations and other mental disturbances were recognised. In the Victorian period, children and adults were sent to the same county asylums and had similar experiences of confinement.[47] However, the emergence of the concept of night terrors challenged both the theory and the practice of approaching children and adults in similar terms regarding diagnosis and treatment. Night terrors were widely discussed in publications by alienists who dealt with insanity, but the concept had emerged from the study of diseases in children, which suggests that medical professionals had begun to see childhood insanity as a valid area warranting attention. Another factor to consider is that children were being diagnosed and treated for mental illnesses not only within British asylums but also in the new hospitals that specialised in children's ailments. Child patients who showed signs of insanity were treated in hospitals such as Great Ormond Street Hospital, Evelina Hospital and Glasgow Children's Hospital, and their conditions were usually categorised as disorders of the nervous system.[48] It would be wrong to

[46] P. Bartlett and D. Wright (eds.), *Outside the Walls of the Asylum: The History of Care in the Community 1750–2000* (Athlone, London, 1999); D. Mellett, *The Prerogative of Asylumdom: Social, Cultural and Administrative Aspects of the Institutional Treatment of the Insane in Nineteenth Century Britain* (Garland, New York, 1982); Amy Rebok Rosenthal, 'Insanity, family and community in Late-Victorian Britain', in Borsay and Dale (eds.), *Disabled Children*, 29–42; Andrew Scull, *Museums of Madness: The Social Organization of Insanity in Nineteenth Century England* (Penguin Books, London, 1979); J. K. Walton, 'Casting out and bringing back in Victorian England: pauper lunatics, 1840–70', in W. F. Bynum, R. Porter and M. Shepherd (eds.), *The Anatomy of Madness: Essays in the History of Psychiatry*, vol. 2 (Tavistock, London, 1985), 132–46.

[47] Steven Taylor, 'Insanity, philanthropy and emigration: dealing with insane children in late-nineteenth-century North-West England', *History of Psychiatry*, 25 (2014), 224–25.

[48] W. H. Dickinson, on the staff of Great Ormond Street Hospital from 1869–82, was the first to keep separate volumes of case notes for particular groups of conditions. His volume for 'Nervous Diseases' (so large that it was rebound in three parts) is very broad in its definition by today's standards, ranging from what today would be neurosurgery cases to what would now

conclude that the absence of published material about children's medical conditions in the years following West's text implies that children were not treated in hospital wards. Hospital case notes make repeated references to conditions such as night terrors, hysteria, melancholia and monomania. Practical interest in children's insanity may, in fact, have been stronger and more widespread than might be suggested by the lack of consideration within contemporary theoretical discussions.

The diagnosis of 'night terrors' applied specifically to children became very popular, although the amount of disagreement between physicians is striking. If for West the nocturnal terrors had their origin in a digestive condition or a cerebral condition, for Crichton-Browne they were 'usually associated with, perhaps dependent upon, cardiac disease', while authors such as Maudsley attempted more complex physiological explanations in the mechanism of the nervous system.[49] In any case, it seems that West's lectures gave medical and scientific respectability to the popular perception of the mentally disturbed child.[50] The fact that West's account is repeated in nearly all the publications about night terrors implies that few Victorian medical professionals – not even those who, like Maudsley and Crichton-Browne, started to specialise in the care of children and young people – were involved in cases that could be identified clearly as insanity. Often, the clinical cases used to support the existence of insanity in childhood did not come from the actual medical practice of these alienists but rather from earlier publications or cases of colleagues that had been recorded in articles or medical treatises.

An interesting example is offered by Daniel Tuke, an English physician and writer who made a detailed entry about the terrors in his *Dictionary of Psychological Medicine* (1892). Tuke uses a narrative structure like that of West, showing how information was exchanged between the various medical disciplines and their different knowledge bases,[51] and his medical compendium includes accounts of child psychiatry, with contributions from Thomas Clouston on 'Developmental Insanities and Psychoses' and H. B. Donkin on

be called psychiatric cases. GOS/10/26, Dr W. H. Dickinson's casenotes (1869–82), Great Ormond Street Archives.

49 Crichton-Browne, 'Psychical diseases', 312.

50 Shuttleworth, *Mind of the Child*, 51; Boehm, *Charles Dickens*, 123–24.

51 'An hour or two after onset of sleep, the child affected suddenly screams out and wakes in a great fright, not at first recognising its surroundings or nurse. The child often has difficulty in getting to sleep again, the fright passing off gradually. As a rule, there is no recurrence the same night, but there usually is on succeeding nights.' Tuke, *Dictionary*, 857. Tuke and Bucknill's *Manual of Psychological Medicine* was the major standard British textbook at the time, J. C. Bucknill and D. H. Tuke, *A Manual of Psychological Medicine: The History, Nosology, Description, Statistics, Diagnosis, Pathology, and Treatment of Insanity* (Blanchard & Lea, Philadelphia, PA, 1858).

hysteria.[52] Clouston's contribution to the publication included a systematic study of 'night terrors'.[53] The Scottish psychiatrist, who was the superintendent of several asylums and a celebrated lecturer on mental diseases, framed this phenomenon within his theory about the occurrence and form of insanity related to developmental stages. The view that insane children and young people were subject to similar theoretical and practical considerations regarding diagnosis, treatment and confinement as insane adults faced opposition from a contrasting viewpoint that emphasised the unique nature of child insanity. Authors such as Clouston identified differentiated developmental phases. Thus, according to Clouston, it was during the process of teething when children of a 'neurotic heredity and an unstable quality of brain' were 'especially subject to convulsions, that being the prevailing neurosis under four years of age'.[54] The two main ways in which 'brain instability' manifested itself in early childhood, argued Clouston, were 'convulsions and delirium', both of which were transitory and nearly always without any nervous effects once the initial attack was over. The condition known as 'pavor nocturnus' or 'night-terrors' fell into the second category, being 'a form of transitory child delirium that rarely occurs except during sleep'.[55] Clouston found two causes for this phenomenon. First, the night terrors that belonged to early childhood were already symptoms of an excess of imagination: 'anything that rouses into premature activity the imagination of nervous children in whom the fancy is already very active may be followed at night by night-terrors', especially 'if there is undigested food in the stomach'.[56] Second, the appearance of night terrors was common 'after surgical injuries or during severe and painful inflammations'.[57] As often happens with hallucinations and delusions, regardless of their cause, the night terrors supposedly induced by pain were often frightening and involved persecution and condemnation.

James Taylor also supported the theory that 'bodily pain' was an 'excitant' of the hallucinations proper to night terrors, and that it could determine their character. Taylor referred to a case of night terrors described by a Dr Colman, in which a child 'woke up screaming that some one was in the room hurting his finger. Although recognising his parents, he continued to see this phantom and in a second similar attack he said his finger was not only hurt but bleeding, and

52 Clouston, Developmental Insanities and Psychoses, 357–71; Donkin, Hysteria. 618–27 in D. H. Tuke, *A Manual of Psychological Medicine: The History, Nosology, Description, Statistics, Diagnosis, Pathology, and Treatment of Insanity* (Blanchard & Lea, Philadelphia, PA, 1858), volume 1.

53 Clouston, Developmental Insanities, in Tuke, Dictionary, 358.

54 Clouston, Developmental Insanities, in Tuke, Dictionary, 358.

55 Clouston, Developmental Insanities, in Tuke, Dictionary, 358.

56 Clouston, Developmental Insanities, in Tuke, Dictionary, 358.

57 Clouston, Developmental Insanities, in Tuke, Dictionary, 358.

pointed to imaginary spots of blood on the sheets'.[58] 'Intestinal disturbance is the most commonly alleged cause of night terror,' concluded the doctor.[59] Likewise, for Henry Maudsley, the appearance of night terrors went hand in hand with a morphological condition. Adopting the reflex action model and an evolutionary approach, Maudsley attempted a classification of child development in a series of neural centres: from the tertiary, which transmits reflex actions from the moment of birth with no associated sensations, to the primary or ideational, which allows the appearance of adult forms of insanity. Maudsley hoped that this approach to classification would lead to the revelation of associated lesions in the brain or nerves and thereby advance the medical-scientific side of psychology because diagnosis would be grounded in physiological research. In this model, the night terrors and other seemingly natural hallucinations suffered by infants and small children were often the result of a brain injury or the presence of a 'morbid deposit' in the brain.[60]

Hallucinations thus arose as the major aspect of insanity in night terrors, which might otherwise have been classified as a merely physiological disease. In his 1860 essay, Crichton-Browne cited West in support of the connection between night terrors, hallucinations and bodily pain, arguing that delusions in childhood could have the consequence of mental derangement in adult life. On top of West's description of night terrors, Crichton-Browne claimed that 'many cases of infantile insanity owe their origin to fear'.[61] Thus night terrors and daydreams are viewed as belonging to a continuum that leads directly to mental illness, a view that would become very influential in the early years of child psychiatry. Crichton-Browne relates the case of 'a boy, who, during infancy, was subject to night terrors, and who, at the age of twelve, and for many succeeding years, was frequently attacked by pantophobia. The attacks were always introduced by palpitation and characterised by the most intense, yet unaccountable, dread, by temporary loss of identity, and by trembling over the whole body.'[62] The alienist concluded by urging parents to be unceasingly alert to signs of similar states in their children – such as daydreaming and those conditions related to an 'excess' of imagination – as Crichton-Browne felt confident that, if detected at an early stage, they could still be remedied by rest and a nourishing diet.[63]

Although brain injury and pain were often seen as the causes of the hallucinations of night terrors, they also impacted the patient's emotional state. Maudsley criticised the way that adults were ignorant of children's suffering,

[58] James Taylor, *Paralysis and Other Diseases of the Nervous System in Childhood and Early Life* (J & A Churchill, London, 1905), 304.

[59] Taylor, *Paralysis and Other Diseases*, 304.

[60] Maudsley, *Physiology and Pathology*, 370.

[61] Crichton-Browne, 'Psychical diseases', 313.

[62] Crichton-Browne, 'Psychical diseases', 312–13.

[63] James Crichton-Browne, 'On dreamy mental states', *Stray Leaves from a Physician's Portfolio* (Hodder and Stoughton, London, 1927), 7–9.

writing in 1895: 'It is difficult for grown-up persons, unless perchance helped by a hateful memory of their own terrors in childhood, to realise the terrible agonies of fright and anguish which seize some nervous children when they are alone in the dark.'[64] Addressing 'Disorders of sleep' and 'The fears of neurotic children', Leonard Guthrie, a senior physician at Paddington Green Children's Hospital in London, described 'a peculiarly horrible dream' that he himself had experienced repeatedly since childhood.[65] Guthrie expands the category of night terrors to include similar experiences during the day, dream hallucinations and 'educational night terrors'. Like West, Guthrie sees these problems as arising from impressions acting on a child brain that was morbidly excitable. Attempting to explain the apparently inexplicable, writers often sought an external cause – such as the 'corrupting' influence of the working-class nurse and her terrifying stories on children in bourgeois nurseries – or adopted an evolutionary perspective that emphasised the influence of inherited memories and thereby located the origin of a child's night terrors in the distant reaches of prehistory. Here, the somatisation of an internal injury is replaced by an environmental, acquired factor. Although clearly different, both explanations maintained the boundaries of childhood purity and innocence.

Melancholia and Mental Pain

In an 1883 lecture, the Scottish physician Thomas Clouston defined melancholia as 'mental pain, emotional depression, and sense of ill-being, usually more intense than in melancholy, with loss of self-control, or insane delusions, or uncontrollable impulses towards suicide, with no proper capacity left to follow ordinary avocations, with some of the ordinary interests of life destroyed, and generally with marked bodily symptoms'.[66] At that time, melancholia was one of the most standard diagnoses of mental suffering, with a coherent symptomology and an explanatory biological model.[67] Although the term melancholia had been used since antiquity to describe a form of illness or madness, the mid nineteenth century biomedical model of melancholia was completely new and conceptually different. In this new context, melancholy was seen as a form of 'affective insanity' – a mental illness whose main symptom was a disordered mood and which could take place without any kind of intellectual delusion[68] – or as 'an emotional disorder with

[64] Maudsley, *Pathology of Mind*, 370.

[65] Leonard Guthrie, *Functional Nervous Disorders in Childhood* (Henry Frowde and Oxford University Press, London, 1907), 40–41.

[66] Thomas S. Clouston, *Clinical Lectures on Mental Diseases* (J & A Churchill, London, 1883), 37.

[67] Jansson, *From Melancholia to Depression*, 6.

[68] Jansson, *From Melancholia to Depression*, 6.

neurophysiological basis'.[69] Writing in 1867, Maudsley suggested that 'sympathetic' or 'reflexive' morbid bodily activity that caused repeated 'irritation' of the brain would gradually distort the 'tone' of this organ and eventually lead to 'disordered emotion'.[70]

Based on the Darwinian understanding of the mind, emotion was seen as a process that took place within the human nervous system.[71] Wilhelm Griesinger in Germany and Thomas Laycock in the UK developed the idea of 'reflex' to include operations of the mind.[72] According to Laycock, a mere idea was capable of triggering a morbid emotional reaction, which produced an involuntary muscular movement (claiming, for example, that hydrophobia could arise from the mere mention of water). For Griesinger, ideas could excite both motor action and emotional reactions, and the brain could produce fresh impressions and ideas in reaction to both internal and external stimuli. Interactions between these stored impressions and ideas could provoke 'irritation' to the brain and lead to morbid reactions.[73]

This physiological model was adopted by many late nineteenth-century psychiatrists, including Maudsley, who claimed that the 'equilibrium between the individual and his surroundings' could 'be disturbed by a subjective modification, or an internal commotion, as well as by an unwonted impression from without'.[74] With the brain already morbidly affected, new impressions could cause painful emotions, and Maudsley's radical suggestion was that pathological emotionality could occur without any intellectual disturbance. He rejected 'the present artificial classification [of insanity], which is not really in conformity with nature'.[75] In its place, he put forward the two general categories of *affective* and *ideational* insanity, thereby establishing the possibility of a pathological mood that did not involve any derangement of the intellect.

As with hysteria, some medical professionals were reluctant to diagnose children with melancholia. Others – including Crichton-Browne and Maudsley – were convinced that the 'insanities of early life' could include melancholia.[76] Maudsley described a range of melancholic disorders, led by 'pure, abstract indefinite

69 Jansson, 'Mood disorders and the brain', 398.

70 Maudsley, *Physiology and Pathology*, 139.

71 Jansson, 'From statistics to diagnostics'.

72 Wilhelm Griesinger, 'Ueber psychische Reflexactionen: Mit einem Blick auf das Wesen der psychischen Krankheiten', reprinted in *Gesammelte Abhandlungen, Ersters Band: Psychiatrische Abhandlungen* (E. J. Bonset, Amsterdam and Berlin, 1968 [1843]), in Jansson, 'Mood disorders and the brain', 396. Thomas Laycock, 'On the reflex function of the brain', *British and Foreign Medical Review*, 19 (1845), 298–311.

73 Griesinger, *Die Pathologie*, 24–25; 35–36 in Åsa Jansson, 'The creation of "disordered emotion": melancholia as biomedical disease, c.1840–1900' (Unpublished PhD thesis, Queen Mary University of London, 2014)., 78.

74 Maudsley, *Physiology and Pathology*, 129, 134–35.

75 Maudsley, *Physiology and Pathology*, 137, 322.

76 Crichton-Browne, 'Psychical diseases', 312–13.

depression' and religious melancholy, with hypochondriasis and some other disorders rarer before puberty ('as their existence implies subjectivity of thought'), and 'simple melancholia [. . .] a mere exaggeration of that feeling of depression to which we are all at times liable, [that] may, in youth, as in mature life, exist without at all involving the intellectual faculties'.[77]

This new concept of melancholia and the distinction between emotional and intellectual maladies are also related to ideas about non-intellectual insanity that emerged in the early nineteenth century, such as 'moral insanity', introduced by James Cowles Prichard in his 1835 book *Treatise on Insanity and Other Disorders Affecting the Mind*, whereby the moral faculties and emotions were considered capable of being disordered.[78] According to Prichard, 'this form of mental disease has been said above to consist of a morbid perversion of the feelings, affections, habits, without any hallucination or erroneous conviction impressed upon the understanding; it sometimes co-exists with an apparently unimpaired state of the intellectual faculties'.[79] He considered children as natural sufferers of moral insanity: since it was assumed that the emotions developed in childhood before the capacity for reasoning, it was only a short step to arguing that forms of insanity affecting only the emotions could exist in childhood. Maudsley, who also used the term 'affective insanity', described this condition as 'a form of disease which undoubtedly occurs in early life, and which, indeed, is more readily acknowledged when it is met with in such young children than when it is met with in the adult'.[80] To Maudsley, depressive symptoms amounted to 'a constitutional defect of nervous element whereby an emotional or sensational reaction of a painful kind follows all impressions; the nervous or cyclical tone is radically infected with some vice of constitution so that every impression is painful'.[81] For Maudsley, all impressions (whether positive or negative) received by a morbidly sensitive brain would produce feelings of displeasure.

Maudsley described the various forms of childhood melancholic states and attempted to correlate the type of melancholia with the child's developmental level at the time the illness first manifested. Thus, in infants in whom feeling manifested 'before thought in the order of mental development', melancholy was a 'primitive language of cries, grunts, exclamations, tones of sounds, gestures and features'.[82] Children aged four or five might have 'fits of moaning, melancholy and apprehensive fears', while the symptoms among

[77] Crichton-Browne, 'Psychical diseases', 312–13.

[78] J. C. Prichard, *A Treatise on Insanity and Other Disorders Affecting the Mind* (Sherwood, Gilbert and Piper, London, 1835), 14.

[79] Prichard, *A Treatise on Insanity and Other Disorders*, 14.

[80] Maudsley, *Physiology and Pathology*, 328.

[81] Maudsley, *Physiology and Pathology*, 328.

[82] Maudsley, *Physiology and Pathology*, 329.

older children might be more like those of typical adult melancholy, perhaps including suicidal ideation.[83]

Throughout the Victorian period, descriptions of melancholia often relied on 'symptoms' deduced from observing patients' general demeanour. 'The child suffering from melancholia,' maintained William Ireland, 'gives up his play, neglects his lessons, avoids his companions, shows little affection for his parents, seeks to be alone, and in general loses interest in everything, and is in a depressed state of mind.'[84] Such children manifested deviance from conventional perceptions of 'normal' juvenile behaviour. Maudsley described such children as 'capricious and wilful in behaviour, perplexing and distressing parents by perverse whims, outbreaks of temper, rude speeches, and sullen defiance of authority'.[85] Thus, while other conditions, such as hysteria, involved intense and frantic behaviour, melancholia was characterised by listlessness, a general lack of interest and depression.[86] Crichton-Browne argued that melancholic children 'are given up to "black despair"'.[87] Understood as one of the types of delirium proper to childhood, for Clouston the diagnosis of 'excited melancholia' also involved a subjective symptomology: the child 'talks excitedly, screams, hears terrible voices, sees frightful sights, clings to its nurse or hides under the bedclothes, stares wildly through dilated pupils at its visual hallucinations'.[88] According to this psychiatrist, 'painful hallucinations' and a depressed emotional state were the main psychological characteristics of this delirium. Hence, while melancholia was mainly listed as an emotional disease, the links to cognition and the faculties of representation could also sometimes appear.

Attention was also given to children's size, physiognomy and bodily functions, as physicians continued to use antiquated terms such as the melancholic 'constitution' and 'temperament'[89] well beyond 1850, and such terminology came to be used within the Darwinian physiological framework. Darwin himself suggested that emotional expressions could begin as conscious acts that became wholly preconscious and automated reflex actions through repetition, continuing because of the force of habit. He quotes 'Dr Maudsley' on the subject: '[R]eflex movements which commonly effect a useful end may, under changed circumstances of disease, do great mischief, becoming even the occasion of violent suffering and of a most painful death.'[90] He argued that if initially 'exciting' painful emotions might lead to impulsive bodily movement and actions, they could later manifest as a 'depressing' state. Melancholia

[83] Maudsley, *Physiology and Pathology*, 329. [84] Ireland, *Mental Affections*, 294.
[85] Maudsley, *Pathology of Mind*, 393. [86] Jannson, *From Melancholia to Depression*, 185.
[87] Crichton-Browne, 'Psychical diseases', 63.
[88] Thomas Clouston, 'Developmental insanity', in Tuke, *Dictionary*, 358.
[89] See, for example, William Bevan Lewis, *Text-Book of Mental Diseases* (Charles Griffin and Company, London, 1899), 115–16; Tuke, *Dictionary*, 220.
[90] Darwin, *Expression of Emotions*, 48.

appears here not only as the result of an unbalanced internal life but also as the final stage of a convulsive struggle to escape pain.

A direct connection developed in the mid- to late-nineteenth century between melancholia, depression and mental pain. This relationship had several uses. It played a crucial role in standardising the portrayal of melancholia in medical literature, contributing to the transformation of psychological medicine into a recognised modern scientific field and a specialised branch of medicine.[91] Practitioners observed symptoms of melancholia through the lens of physiology using biomedical language, which gave prominence to 'depression' and 'mental pain'. These terms were also reconceptualised within a modern scientific framework.[92]

The notion of 'mental pain' has a long and eclectic history. While it seems that late-nineteenth-century British medical psychologists decoded mental pain as analogous to physical pain, within physiological psychology it had an ambiguous status, as something both literal and metaphorical. Terms such as 'irritation', 'tone' and 'pain' were used to explain both cerebral and psychological processes. 'If a child ever shows depression or mental pain', argued Clouston, 'then there is certainly something wrong, some organ is disordered, the child is being poisoned by bad food or bad air, or some irritation is going on in its bodily processes'.[93] In other words, both mental pain and depression were associated with somatic or physiological problems.

The main problem with trying to record and diagnose the pain of emotional life was that it manifested mainly through language. So, as well as observing a patient's bodily state, demeanour and behaviour, medical psychologists increasingly started to base their diagnoses on the content of conversations with patients, along with reports from family members, friends and workhouse officials. Physicians emphasised the importance of comprehensive patient histories, in part to reveal possible 'hereditary predispositions' to insanity if there were other cases of madness in the family.[94]

[91] Jannson, *From Melancholia to Depression*, 11.

[92] For a discussion on 'emotion' as a physiological and thus biological process, see: Ruth Leys, *From Sympathy to Reflex: Marshall Hall and His Opponents* (Garland Pub., New York, 1990); Roger Smith, *Inhibition: History and Meaning in the Sciences of Mind and Brain* (Free Association Books, London, 1992); Georges Canguilhem, 'The concept of reflex', in *A Vital Rationalist: Selected Writings from Georges Canguilhem*, ed. François Delaporte (Zone Books, New York, 1994), 179-202; Edwin Clarke and L. S. Jacyna, *Nineteenth-Century Origins of Neuroscientific Concepts* (University of California Press, Berkeley, 1987); Robert M. Young, *Mind, Brain, and Adaptation in the Nineteenth Century: Cerebral Localization and Its Biological Context from Gall to Ferrier* (Oxford University Press, New York, 1990); Jean Starobinski, *Action and Reaction: The Life and Adventures of a Couple* (Zone Books, New York, 2003) and (trans. Judith P. Serafini-Saul), 'The word reaction: from physics to psychiatry', *Psychological Medicine*, 7(3) (1977), 373–86.

[93] Clouston, Developmental Insanities, in Tuke, *Dictionary*, 370.

[94] This approach was strongly influenced by Darwinian-based eugenic theories and, in Britain, reinforced through the work of prominent medical professionals, most notably the psychiatrist

In their study of the medical history of insane children and young people, British practitioners emphasised circumstances and events that might have played a role in their patients' diagnosis. They considered that sometimes a specific incident that provoked an intense emotional response could have a direct effect on a patient's mental health – for instance, a tragedy, fear, religious fervour, 'excessive' study or family problems. The emotional stress provoked by the death of a family member was a common feature. M. B. Ray wrote in the *Journal of Mental Science* in 1898 of the case of J.W., a fifteen-year-old boy with a diagnosis of mania.[95] The boy was thin, poorly nourished and otherwise in ill health, and his mental state involved excitement, restlessness and incoherent chatter.[96] After assessing this case, Ray determined that the boy's mother's death a few months earlier was the cause of the boy's illness.[97] Sometimes the traumatic trigger for mental illness came from the domestic environment. Alexandre Brière de Boismont, for instance, described the case of M, a boy who from a very young age was 'a witness of and actor in domestic scenes which reacted only too strongly upon an excitable organization'.[98] Soon he became melancholic, and at twelve years of age 'was heard to say he should be glad to die'. With this disposition, claimed Boismont, 'it was not surprising that he attempted suicide at sixteen years of age'.[99]

Probably the most manifest and extreme indication of children's melancholia was the suicide attempt, which some contemporary medical authors chose to conceptualise as a deliberate act of self-harm.[100] 'Whilst speaking of melancholia, we must devote a few words to the consideration of suicide in early life', argued Crichton-Browne: 'Even in infancy and childhood, when

Henry Maudsley (1835–1918). On eugenics see, for example, Bashford and Levine (eds.), *The Oxford Handbook of the History of Eugenics*. For further reviews of the field, see: Thomson, *The Problem of Mental Deficiency*; Bowler, *The Mendelian Revolution*; Searle, *Eugenics and Politics*; Mazumdar, *Eugenics, Human Genetics and Human Failings*; Soloway, *Demography and Degeneration*; Turda, 'Recent scholarship on race and eugenics'; Dikötter, 'Race culture'; Nye, 'The rise and fall of the eugenics empire'.

95 M. B. Ray, 'Case of acute mania occurring in a boy', *Journal of Mental Science*, 44 (1898), 320.

96 Ray, 'Case of acute mania', 321. 97 Ray, 'Case of acute mania', 320.

98 Alexandre Brière de Boismont, 'On the insanity of early life', *Journal of Psychiatric Medicine*, 10 (1875), 630.

99 Boismont, 'On the insanity of early life', 630.

100 On child suicide, see: Sally Shuttleworth, 'Jude the Obscure and child suicide', in Shuttleworth, *Mind of the Child*; Shuttleworth, 'The psychology of childhood', 86; and Betts, 'From Juvenile Delinquent'. For a scholarly discussion of suicide in Victorian society, see: Olive Anderson, *Suicide in Victorian and Edwardian England* (Clarendon Press, Oxford, 1987); Barbara T. Gates, *Victorian Suicide: Mad Crimes and Sad Histories* (Princeton University Press, Princeton, NJ, 1988); and Howard I. Kushner, 'Suicide, gender and the fear of modernity in nineteenth-century medical and social thought', *Journal of Social History*, 26 (1993), 461–90. On self-harm see Sarah Chaney, *Psyche on the Skin: A History of Self-Harm* (Reaktion Books, London, 2017).

cares and sorrows are comparatively unknown, and when sensations and feelings, pleasurable or painful, are transient and evanescent, we frequently meet with deliberate acts of self-destruction.'[101] Thus, in his Report of the Devon Asylum for 1856, a Dr Bucknill relates the case of a twelve-year-old child, who had attempted suicide by drowning and strangulation. After arriving at the asylum, he 'cried incessantly, "I wish to die, I wish to die"' and engaged in acts of self-harm: 'He struck his head against the wall and tried to suffocate himself by pressing his fist against his throat.'[102]

Hysteria

Children's hysteria – a condition which Charles West did not discuss in his texts on the mental peculiarities of childhood – has not been studied in detail. Recent historiography on adult hysteria has argued that, very often, the illness was a vehicle for the expression of emotional pain that found no other form of medical recognition.[103] While the evidence collected in the archival research of this study may not suffice to determine the extent to which this performative notion of hysteria – which implies a complex collaboration between the medical community and patients in the enactment of the hysterical body – also applies to children, it might start to lay the foundations for a better understanding of the interplay between child emotional suffering and the normative way in which the patient with hysteria was expected to behave. In discussing the notion of the performative character of hysteria, the recognition of an almost infectious quality to hysteria in children – among whom symptoms were imitated – is an important factor. According to the physician and alienist John Conolly, in addition to their weak nervous constitution, 'the proneness to imitation which is observable in all persons in early life' helped to spread hysterical symptoms among children. He noted, 'this is particularly seen in schools, which have sometimes furnished remarkable cases of squinting, stammering, and awkward motions, solely occasioned by imitation'.[104] Conolly's point was not that children were engaging in conscious mimicry, but rather that hysterical convulsions could become infectious among an impressionable audience. Complex learning and imitative processes were often involved in the development of hysterical symptoms.

[101] Crichton-Browne, 'Psychical diseases', 316.
[102] Boismont, 'On the insanity of early life', 625.
[103] See Boddice, 'Hysteria or Tetanus?'; Morris, *Culture of Pain*, 103–24.
[104] John Forbes (ed.), *The Cyclopaedia of Practical Medicine: Comprising Treatises on the Nature and Treatment of Disease, Materia Medica and Therapeutics, Medical Jurisprudence*, vol. 1 (Sherwood, Gilbert, and Piper, and Baldwin and Craddock, London, 1833–35), 578.

While nineteenth-century texts about childhood insanity devote less attention to hysteria than to other conditions, they do recognise the existence of hysterical disturbances in children.[105] In fact, it seems that hysteria may have been far more frequent than other conditions that received greater attention from theorists. Even though 'night terrors' occupied a central position in Charles West's writings within the emerging field of paediatrics, it is striking that there are records of only three children admitted to the Great Ormond Street Hospital suffering from this pathology between 1880 and 1900.[106] In contrast, hysteria occupies a central place in the case notes of doctors who at the end of the nineteenth century were working on nervous conditions in the new hospitals including Great Ormond Street.[107] It seems likely that, despite the neglect and even dismissal of this concept by contemporary theoretical literature, there was considerable practical interest in it.

Medical writers explained the phenomenon relying on the contemporary belief that children, like adult women, lacked an adequately developed will. According to this theory, the higher centres of children's immature brains could not completely control the lower ones, while the unstable nature of children's nerves – with their tendency to spontaneous discharges – also served to encourage the unpredictable symptoms of hysteria. J. Michell Clarke, physician and pathologist at the Bristol General Hospital and lecturer on practical physiology at the Bristol Medical School, argued that 'the greater frequency of the affection in childhood' was to be expected because children's nervous systems had 'not acquired that degree of stability which frequent repetition of the movement ensures in the adult'. According to this view, 'the paths for nervous impulses are not so definitely marked out, and there is less resistance to irradiation of impulses along other channels than in the adult'.[108]

As with melancholia, physicians addressed hysterical conditions through the symptoms observed in their child patients and the accounts given by parents or other relatives. The first signals were always physical, and the disease was construed on a physiological basis. However, the clinical paradigm of the bodily location of disease proved problematic when pain flared up in the apparent absence of manifest external lesions, as in cases of hysteria. During the nineteenth century and part of the twentieth century, hysteria was perceived

105 See Oppenheim, *Shattered Nerves*, 237.

106 Harriet Busby, GOS/9/1/4, 1879–83 General Admissions Register, Great Ormond Street Archives; William Wanstell, GOS/9/1/12, 1906 Admissions Register, Great Ormond Street Archives; Doris Ford, GOS/9/1/14, 1908 Admissions register, Great Ormond Street Archives.

107 The Historical Admission Records Project (HHARP), has 200 records of children diagnosed with hysteria from 1859 to 1897. See The Historic Hospital Admissions Records Project (HHARP) database (Great Ormond Street Hospital for Children/University of Kingston).

108 Michell Clarke, 'Clinical observations on hysteria', *The Lancet*, 141 (20 May 1893), 1185–89.

as a disorder of nervous organization. Physicians focused on physical symptoms, provided physical treatments and avoided dealing with the mind.[109] With hysteria, they highlighted the physical, emotional and intellectual aspects of the condition, which was defined in a way that was now free from the previous gynaecological aetiology and – at least in principle and certainly in relation to childhood hysteria – gender non-specific.[110] Clarke argued that at this period of life, the 'ratio of hysterics to the sexes is about equal' but after the age of twelve, 'the paths of the two sexes widely diverge, and the educational factor comes into full force'.[111]

As in the case of adult hysteria, the presence of pain or symptoms that did not appear to be related to a structural lesion constituted one of the constant manifestations of hysteria.[112] Charles West describes the case of Sophia Banquett, a 'delicate' nine-year-old girl who 'was taken with great pain in the Chest and Head, and also had pains in the limbs'.[113] Apart from pain in the limbs and joints, the little girl had been experiencing violent fits, during which 'she has broken several of her teeth' and 'has lately been several times found asleep at odd times; and has been noticed to stand and stare, and to leave off talking in the middle of a sentence'.[114] Although her pains were 'said to be rheumatic', after she was admitted to the Great Ormond Street Hospital, Dr Charles West diagnosed Sophia with hysteria and malingering. Like the early French psychiatrist Étienne-Jean Georget (1795–1828), who argued that the continuous experience of chronic pain invariably resulted from the more extreme manifestations of hysteria, late nineteenth-century texts that referred to hysteria in children also maintained that, while hysterical behaviour could be characterised by convulsive movements or nervous attacks, its symptomology was manifested above all in a constant and intractable pain. William H. Spurgin, for instance, considered 'severe pain at the epigastrium' as one

[109] Sander L. Gilman, Helen King, Roy Porter, G. S. Rousseau and Elaine Showalter (eds.), *Hysteria Beyond Freud* (University of California Press, Berkeley, 1993). The pre-Freudian physiological focus in studies of hysteria and related disorders has been documented by, among others, Lilian R. Furst, *Before Freud: Hysteria and Hypnosis in Later Nineteenth-Century Psychiatric Cases* (Bucknell University Press, Lewisburg, 2008).

[110] On hysteria and gender, see Mark Micale, *Hysterical Men: The Hidden History of Male Nervous Illness* (Harvard University Press, Cambridge, MA, 2008); see also Elaine Showalter's classic, *The Female Malady: Women, Madness and English Culture, 1830–1980* (Virago, London, 1987).

[111] Clarke, 'Clinical observations', 1185–89.

[112] On pain and hysteria see: Moscoso, *Pain*, 172–81; Morris, *Culture of Pain*, 103–24; Boddice, 'Hysteria or Tetanus?'

[113] GOS/10/12 of Dr Charles West's notes series, Great Ormond Street Archives, Great Ormond Street Archives.

[114] GOS/10/12 of Dr Charles West's notes series, Great Ormond Street Archives, Great Ormond Street Archives.

of the constant manifestations of hysteria.[115] In the case of the ten-year-old girl patient S.T., with which this chapter began, it was precisely this symptom that led the parents to summon the physician, who examined the child, prescribed various treatments that proved ineffective and then decided upon a diagnosis of hysteria because she 'appeared in the greatest agony and misery in spite of all treatment'.[116]

As with night terrors, hysteria was also often considered to result from recent accidents or previous injuries. An 1885 issue of the *Journal of Mental Science* describes the case of A.W., a twelve-year-old boy who was diagnosed and treated for hysteria after receiving a hard blow to the head in the schoolyard. Michell Clarke described the case of a boy aged fourteen whose illness began after he fell from a chair, 'striking his back'.[117] Another case described by Clarke featured a girl whose 'illness began after a fall on the back, which caused much pain, and since the inability to stand or walk had compelled her to remain in bed except for a day or so for the past three months'.[118] Some of these cases were labelled as hysterical paraplegia and all started after a fall or blow followed by pain, but with no sign of organic disease.

British alienists had some measure of success in mapping hysteria onto the body. Like Charcot, they encountered hysterogenic points, palpitations, patches of cutaneous hyperaesthesia and hysterical cough.[119] Clarke narrates the case of a twelve-year-old child where 'each spasm of "cough" consisted of a loud noise, repeated spasmodically four or five times with expiration, and partly of an articulatory noise made in the throat, harsh, rasping or sawing in character, and so loud as to be heard over the whole house'.[120] The absence of response to pain stimuli, as well as the absence of pain itself, was one of the most conclusive symptoms in diagnoses of hysteria. 'Patches of cutaneous hyperaesthesia are not uncommon in hysteria', argued Clarke, 'and the patients are generally aware of their existence'. In a study of ten children with hysteria, he described the case of a 'general condition of moderate hyperaesthesia of

115 Spurgin, 'Case of hysteria', 555. 116 Spurgin, 'Case of hysteria', 555.

117 Clarke, 'Clinical observations', 1186. 118 Clarke, 'Clinical observations', 1186.

119 The classic lines of enquiry about hysteria, and the ways it was gendered, centre on figures such as Charcot and Freud. The bodily effects of the emotionally traumatised were, through medical universalisation, ultimately directed away from mainstream medicine toward psychoanalysis. How hysteria was conceptualised varied between countries. As Edward Shorter notes, 'the underlying incidence of the disorder may well be constant across the ages but its form changeable, in accordance with [. . .] cultural influences.' See Edward Shorter, 'Paralysis: the rise and fall of a "hysterical" symptom', *Journal of Social History*, 19 (1986), 549. See also Nicholas P. Spanos and Jack Gottlieb, 'Demonic possession, mesmerism, and hysteria: a social psychological perspective on their historical interrelations', *Journal of Abnormal Psychology*, 88 (1979), 540–41.

120 Clarke, 'Clinical observations', 1187.

the whole cutaneous surface', and in another, 'there was hyperaesthesia over the whole anterior surface of the trunk'.[121]

As in their study of the medical history of children with melancholia, when looking at hysteria, British practitioners emphasised the circumstances and events that might have played a role in their patients' diagnosis. For instance, in a 'Case of Marked Hysteria in a Boy of Eleven Years', Savage describes a child who was healthy until 4 January 1885, when he attended the 'funeral of a little sister who died as the result of an accident'.[122] The following day he did not play, 'gave up all his ordinary habits, became dull, his appetite failed, and his bowels became confined'.[123] Savage suggests that the child was deluded about his 'motions' because 'he did not pass anything; but it was found out that he threw one motion out of the window'. Although refusing to eat with his family, the child 'would steal food or eat it on the sly'. When admitted to hospital on 23 April, 'he was crouched into a ball, his face tied up in a handkerchief, and both his legs drawn up under his buttocks, and both his feet turned inwards, so that he stood – when forced to stand – on his outer malleoli'.[124]

The cases of children's hysteria discussed in the late nineteenth century can be reread from another perspective – the suffering of the child in question. Take the case of nine-year-old Rebecca Novis, the daughter of the pharmacist at the Islington Workhouse, who was admitted in 1871 with the diagnosis of 'hysteria', having spent several weeks as a 'voluntary mute', unwilling or unable to speak or walk and spending long periods in a passive state with closed eyes, although able to use gestures to answer questions.[125] Two weeks before her hospitalisation, she refused to open her eyes, spent her days quietly crying – which was interrupted only for meals – and trembled constantly. Upon examination, she concealed her eyes behind her left arm and displayed difficulty in smiling, despite the doctor's persistent efforts. In the case of Rebecca Novis, the physician William Howship Dickinson, assistant physician at the Great Ormond Street, applied a robust treatment that included speech and activity provocation by pinching and attempting to prise open her eyelids, together with warm baths and galvanic stimulation.[126] She eventually became more active and was sent home, briefly relapsed, was readmitted and then discharged when she improved. She was one of the first Great Ormond Street patients to be photographed and one of the images in the case notes was later adapted for use in fundraising literature. Or the case of Emma Allwood, who

[121] Clarke, 'Clinical observations', 1187.

[122] George Savage, 'Case of marked hysteria in a boy of eleven years', *The Journal of Mental Science*, 31 (1885), 201.

[123] Savage, 'Case of marked hysteria', 202.

[124] Savage, 'Case of marked hysteria', 202.

[125] GOS/10/26, Dr W. H. Dickinson's casenotes, Great Ormond Street Archives.

[126] GOS/10/26, Dr W. H. Dickinson's casenotes, Great Ormond Street Archives.

had suffered headaches for several years and then developed pain in the back and had fits in which she cried, laughed, fainted, screamed and jumped up and down. Dickinson's case notes tell of how 'the fits are gradually leaving her, but she has pain in the back, drags her legs after her, especially the left (walking badly during the last fortnight)' and how throughout the day – unless asleep or particularly interested in something – she let out a 'peculiar sobbing noise or slight scream'.[127]

Despite – or perhaps because of – the elusiveness of hysteria, physicians talked of the difference between 'true' and 'false' hysteria. For instance, an 1885 article in the *Journal of Mental Science* noted that a doctor who treated the case of a twelve-year-old boy ('A.W.') who had lost the capacity to speak considered three possible diagnoses: '[T]he diagnosis', the author reported, 'lay between malingering, hysteria, or grave cerebral disease'.[128] In this particular case, malingering – that is, feigning illness – was eventually ruled out, and the presence of a severe pain in the head led the doctor to diagnose that the boy was suffering from hysteria. In the spring of 1866, ten-year-old Eliza Holden was admitted to the hospital complaining of pain over the spine. A month before admission she began to have pains in the chest and down the left side, could not sleep at night and these pains continued. Two weeks later, she began to twitch her arms. She complained of great paroxysmal pain over the spine. When the pain come on, it was so strong that she 'cried out'.[129] The medical examination 'detected nothing', and based on the symptoms – twitching muscles and odd pains – the child was diagnosed with hysteria. In the case notes, the child's physician Dr West notes that 'Her behaviour while in the hospital was not of a child who wishes to deceive',[130] thus acknowledging the possibility of malingering but recognising this child's symptoms as real. She recovered after being put on a meat diet and made to help in the ward. However, hysteria and children's insanity certainly got caught up in contemporary debate about the concept of malingering, which was claimed to be reaching 'a high level of perfection' by the start of the twentieth century.[131] Cases such as this constantly reiterated the elusive nature of hysteria and other types of insanity. In fact, the categories of mania, melancholia, hysteria and moral insanity were not entirely separate. For instance, Maudsley and some other British practitioners considered hysteria to be a manifestation of moral insanity.[132] Identifying and categorising mental disorders in their patients required medical professionals to exercise their keenest skills of observation.

[127] GOS/9/1/2, 1864–72 Admissions Register, Great Ormond Street Archives.
[128] P. Smith, 'Case of hysteria in a boy', *Journal of Mental Science*, 31 (October 1885), 370.
[129] GOS/9/1/2, 1864–72 Admissions Register, Great Ormond Street Archives.
[130] GOS/9/1/2, 1864–72 Admissions Register, Great Ormond Street Archives.
[131] Editorial, 'Malingery', *The Lancet*, 165 (1905), 45–46.
[132] Maudsley, *Pathology of Mind*, 397.

The Harmful Child, or Moral Disease as the Cause of External Pain

Even though in the cases of insane children the pain suffered by the patient served to unravel the diagnosis, alienists such as Maudsley considered that a central factor in determining if a child was suffering from insanity was whether patients seemed to take delight in inflicting pain and physical injury both on themselves and on other children.[133] Maudsley saw homicidal monomania as particularly noteworthy in childhood, describing a 'destructive impulse which sometimes reaches such an extreme degree in the madness of childhood [and which] is afforded by the instance of homicidal impulse'.[134] The idea that there was a specific form of insanity that involved the impulse to kill emerged in France at the beginning of the nineteenth century, as illustrated by Jean Étienne Dominique Esquirol's *Mental Maladies: A Treatise on Insanity* (1845), which includes an account of 'homicidal monomania' in two young female patients. In one case, a seven-year-old girl wished to kill her mother; in the other, a girl had an irrational desire to kill her stepmother. In the latter case, there had apparently been no mistreatment of the child by the stepmother, yet the girl spoke calmly and with certainty about her homicidal plans.[135]

In the second half of the nineteenth century, the press started to apply a new discourse of otherness to children found guilty of killing, as new ideas of child development emerged. In the late nineteenth century, medical professionals increasingly recognised adolescence as a specific phase between childhood and adulthood – between the ages of twelve and twenty – that involved physical and emotional changes taking place rapidly. In this context, rebelliousness and misbehaviour were seen as natural for youths, and many late-nineteenth-century child psychologists believed that one effect of adolescence was to increase the likelihood of criminal behaviour.[136] Thus, Stanley Hall argued in 1904 that 'adolescence is the best key to the nature of crime. It is essentially antisocial, selfishness, refusing to submit to the laws of altruism'.[137] Furthermore, 'all boys develop a great increased propensity to fight at puberty', so their bloody noses and black eyes were to be seen as part of the process of development by which a boy became a man.[138] Child development, puberty and adolescence were also used to explain violent acts against animals. According to the psychologist James Sully, children's natural curiosity often led them to be cruel to animals and that it was from inflicting such injuries that

[133] On self-harm in Victorian times see Chaney, *Psyche on the Skin*. Also, the same author's 'Anaesthetic bodies and the absence of feeling'. On Maudsley and homicidal insanity see, Betts, 'From Juvenile Delinquent', 153.

[134] Maudsley, *Physiology and Pathology*, 283.

[135] Esquirol, *Mental Maladies*, 371.

[136] Betts, 'From Juvenile Delinquent', 272.

[137] Hall, *Adolescence*, 405.

[138] Hall, *Adolescence*, 356.

children learned about the consequences of causing pain.[139] The psychologist Eugene William Bohannon argued that cruelty was inherent in childhood and youth. While these actions were more typical of adolescence, there were also cases involving younger children. Thus, a six-year-old girl '[p]icked up a little chicken and wrung off its head, then broke its legs'.[140] She also 'delights to be "mother," when playing with children, so she can beat them'. Another six-year-old '[p]unishes dogs and cats in any way she can'.[141]

'Homicidal monomania' was the most common category of insanity used by late nineteenth-century alienists to account for violent children and children who killed. An 1848 article in the *Journal of Psychological Medicine and Mental Pathology* defined it as a 'peculiar condition of a man in which, without derangement of the intellect, he is hurried away by an irresistible inclination, driven, *impelled* by a blind instinct that cannot be accounted for'.[142] Diagnosing a case of homicidal monomania in an eighteen-year-old boy, Henry Maudsley wrote that the boy 'said that he had felt "an impulse to kill someone"'. After examining the boy's family for evidence of hereditary illness, Maudsley discovered that 'his mother had been twice in a lunatic asylum, having been desponding, and having attempted suicide; his brother was of weak intellect [and] the person to whom he was apprenticed and others gave evidence that he was always strange and not like other boys'.[143]

Esquirol also subscribed to the idea that homicidal monomania could manifest in young children and that accidents at birth or in early childhood – as well as any hereditary tendency – could play a role. It was a child falling on his or her head that was the most-often cited reason for homicidal monomania in children.[144] According to Esquirol, 'a child of three years of age, falls upon his head. He complains from that time of headaches. At puberty, the pain in the head increases, and mania manifests itself'.[145] At the murder trial of thirteen-year-old Robert Coombes in 1895, expert medical witnesses testified that the accused's history of debilitating headaches – which followed falling on his head when aged three, as well as cerebral damage from the forceps used during his birth – meant that he was insane when he killed his mother.[146] Both medical professionals and criminologists believed that certain forms of insanity could cause criminality, and saw murders carried out by children as evidence to prove their

[139] Shuttleworth, *Mind of the Child*, 283.
[140] E. W. Bohannon, 'A study of peculiar and exceptional children', The Pedagogical Seminary: An International Record of Educational Literature, Institutions and Progress, 4 (1896), 26.
[141] Bohannon, 'A study of peculiar', 26.
[142] Anon, 'Homicidal insanity', *Journal of Psychological Medicine and Mental Pathology*, 1 (1848), 330.
[143] Henry Maudsley, Responsability in Mental Disease (D. Appleton, New York, 1899) 169.
[144] Betts, 'From Juvenile Delinquent', 235. [145] Esquirol, *Mental Maladies*, 51.
[146] 'Robert Allen Coombes', *OBP*, 9 September 1895, cited in Betts, 'From Juvenile Delinquent', 154.

case. A *Daily News* article said that 'Robert, the murderer, is certainly insane. It is a matter of an accident of birth complicated by heredity'.[147]

In his article 'On the insanity of early life', Brière de Boismont also discussed the cases of children who took pleasure in inflicting pain, a condition that he described as 'mental derangement'. Thus, he describes the case of an 'extremely difficult to manage' six-year-old boy who, once admitted to the asylum, would threaten the doctors: 'As soon as I am at liberty, I will set fire to the house, and if I can find a pointed knife, I will stab you to the heart; I should rejoice to see your blood flow, and to kill you.'[148]

Some medical accounts of homicidal mania suggested a link between mental illness and poverty. Maudsley, for example, claimed a direct connection between socioeconomic conditions and the emergence of this particular form of insanity in children. 'Unequal to the social ways and regular work of their fellows', he argued, 'they drift apart into idle brooding and sauntering, and, when they belong to the lowest classes, gravitate vagrantly into workhouse or gaol. From time to time one of this class commits arson, rape or even homicide.'[149] An unsigned 1870 article in the *British Medical Journal* proclaimed: 'It is only fair to conclude that, with an increased number of such persons [pauper lunatics] at liberty, drawn from a less safe class, we should have a much richer harvest of murders, acts of violence, and legal transgressions, committed by lunatics.'[150] John Langdon Down also highlighted the possible links between mental illness, poverty and crime, noting that children and young people from families with financial resources often escaped the fate of their poorer peers. He cited a specific case of a boy from a well-off family who was diagnosed with moral insanity and became a thief: 'Had he been a member of a lower stratum of society he would have become a jail-bird. Great pains were taken to prevent his getting into the hands of the police.'[151]

Conclusion

As previously noted, in *The Body in Pain*, Elaine Scarry argued that psychological pain is present in almost all forms of literature, but physical pain has received very limited attention.[152] By looking at the overlapping ways in

[147] 'The Plaistow Murder', *Daily News*, 18 September 1895, cited in Eleanor Betts, 'From Juvenile Delinquent to boy murderer', 155.

[148] Boismont, 'On the insanity of early life', 623.

[149] Maudsley, *Pathology of Mind*, 380.

[150] Anon, 'Lunatics at home', *British Medical Journal* (28 May 1870), 552, in Rosenthal, 'Insanity, family and community in late-Victorian Britain', 33.

[151] John Langdon Down, *On Some of the Mental Affections of Childhood and Youth: Being the Lettsomian Lectures Delivered before the Medical Society of London in 1887, Together with Other Papers* (J & A Churchill, London, 1887), 57.

[152] Scarry, *Body in Pain*, 11.

which the mental disorders of childhood were understood in relation to pain, this chapter has argued that it is not always possible to clearly distinguish the suffering of the body from that of the mind. Studying children's mental disorders as seen by psychiatrists in late nineteenth-century England provides a helpful way to examine the intersection of notions of body and mind and contemporary ideas about pain. When we examine the various forms of insanity that were diagnosed in children, it becomes clear that separating physical and emotional pain is impossible. This poses wider questions about how late-nineteenth-century psychological medicine considered the relationship between the body and the mind.

The concept of night terrors was significant as it was the first example of a diagnosis of a mental illness suffered exclusively by children and not by adults. Night terrors sometimes involved delusions that were misperceptions of bodily sensations, thus providing insights into patients' subjective experiences. Many medical accounts of night terrors attributed their cause to physical pain, such as intestinal disorders. Thus, this diagnosis – whose popularity was never backed up by experimental evidence – highlights the close connection between physical and psychological pain, which were difficult to separate and whose boundaries were rather vague.

The mental suffering of melancholia was also considered, by researchers following a Darwinist tradition, to have somatic origins, resulting from an irritated brain. Melancholia – a term that dates back to antiquity – was reconceptualised in the nineteenth century as a form of 'affective insanity', a mental disorder devoid of intellectual delusions, primarily characterised by mood disturbances. This new notion of melancholia was also linked to the emergence of ideas of other forms of insanity where it was the moral faculties or the emotions, rather than mental or intellectual capacity, that were considered disordered. Children were considered to be particularly prone to both 'moral' and 'affective' insanity. As in the case of adult hysteria, the presence and the absence of pain or symptoms that did not appear to be related to structural lesions constituted one of the constant manifestations of hysteria. However, while the diagnosis of hysteria in adults was almost exclusively applied to women, in children gender did not play much of a role.

The question of the desire among some children to inflict physical pain upon others or upon themselves was also explored extensively during the late nineteenth century. These tendencies were considered to be among the main symptoms of mania and homicidal monomania. Discussion of children who inflict harm on other children or on animals played an important role in the emergence of ideas about developmental phases and to the concept of adolescence.

Thus, pain played multiple roles in discussions about mental illness in the second half of the nineteenth century and there was such an intertwining of physical, emotional and psychological pain that it was impossible to separate clearly the somatic and the mental. There were assumptions that disordered mental states in children had physical origins – whether in the intestines, from old injuries, or in the 'nerves' – even if these could not be proven experimentally. In cases where patients complained of physical pains that had no obvious organic cause, the umbrella term of 'hysteria' was often applied, as with the case of S.T. with which this chapter began. At the same time, mental illness also started to be seen as an expression of emotional pain for which there was not yet a frame of reference. As the century drew to a close, Josef Breuer and Sigmund Freud published their studies of hysteria, which would lay the foundations for the creation of such a framework. In the twentieth century, through the influence of psychoanalysis, the debates about pain and the respective roles of body and mind would take a new direction.

4 The Nervous Child

In 1906, an eleven-year-old girl was taken to the medical practice of Dr Thomas D. Savill. After examining her symptoms, the British physician excluded any kind of structural injury. While the child had previously been affectionate and in no way troublesome, some weeks earlier, she had started to experience 'attacks of crying and depression, two or three times a day'. As well as these symptoms, 'her sleep was broken and disturbed by bad dreams, and she wandered downstairs to her parents almost every night on account of the gloom and sadness of her thoughts'.[1] Her appetite was poor, and she suffered from a chronic pain in her stomach. According to Savill, the symptoms presented by the child were not related to any injury or visible morphological change, nor were they related to intellectual retardation. On the basis of the combination of symptoms, the child was diagnosed as suffering from 'neurasthenia'.[2] According to this view, the patient wrongly believed that her pain was located in the stomach when, in fact, it originated in the nervous system as a whole.

Thirty years later, the British pioneer of child psychology and psychotherapy Margaret Lowenfeld discussed the same type of chronic pain in her article 'A new approach to the problem of psychoneurosis in childhood' (1931). Her conclusions could not have been more different from Savill's. The latter argued that the child's symptoms were located in the body and in the general physical condition of the nervous system. His diagnosis presented the somatic location of the nerves as the site of several conditions with no obvious organic origin – including insomnia, lethargy, depression, headache and bodily aches and pains. Lowenfeld, on the contrary, claimed that symptoms such as 'vomiting, diarrhoea, constipation, skin eruptions' were merely 'the physical side of a mass of fused experiences containing physical as well as mental experiences'.[3]

1 Thomas Dixon Savill, *Clinical Lectures on Neurasthenia* (Henry J. Glaisher, London, 1899), 131.

2 Savill, *Clinical Lectures*, 131.

3 Margaret F. Lowenfeld, 'A new approach to the problem of psychoneurosis in children' (Paper read to the Medical Section of the British Psychological Society on 25 March 1931), *British Journal of Medical Psychology* (November 1931), 3.

Lowenfeld embraced psychotherapy and its redefinition of nervous states in mental rather than somatic terms. In attempting to collapse the distinction between physical and emotional pain, Lowenfeld's article anticipates the debates within psychoanalysis about psychogenic pain[4] – or physiological pain of an emotional nature – that would take place in Britain in the following decades.

This chapter continues to trace the issues analysed in Chapter 3 as they unfolded in the first half of the twentieth century under the light of two emerging disciplines: the new psychology and psychoanalysis. The chapter explores the polarised model of children's pain in the context of British children's studies, in which similar symptoms were identified and treated according to different theoretical frameworks: the clinical tradition – which still strove for the somatic articulation of maladies – and the emerging field of psychoanalysis. As seen in the first chapter, the Cartesian mechanical tradition held that pain was a strictly physical phenomenon. However, historians of science and pain, especially those who have looked at chronic pain, have argued that the connection between physical injury and harmful experience 'was called into question during the second half of the twentieth century'.[5] As David Biro has documented, by the second half of the twentieth century, researchers had observed devastating injuries where pain was absent and excruciating pain with minor or no injuries whatsoever. Together with this evidence, neurologists began to accept that many psychological factors – such as emotions, memories, attitudes and expectations – could act as major modifiers of the experience of pain.[6] This chapter builds on that body of knowledge to argue that, long before the second half of the twentieth century, some interpreters believed that affective states imagined as injuries to the mind could trigger pain that resembled physical injuries.

The relationship between body and mind has been widely discussed in the recent historiography of childhood. Historians who have studied the development of child-centred interventions in the interwar period have generally agreed that the transformation of physiological disorders into psychological conditions can be explained by the fundamental shift in medical paradigms that took place in the early twentieth century, with a move from a 'hygienist' focus on the bodies of children and their physical health to an emphasis on their minds and emotions.[7] Given that British medicine was relatively conservative,

[4] Psychogenic pain is non-organic pain associated with psychological factors. See, G. Engel, '"Psychogenic" pain and the pain-prone patient', *American Journal of Medicine*, 26 (1959), 899–918.

[5] David Biro, 'Psychological pain: metaphor or reality?', in Rob Boddice (ed.), *Pain and Emotion in Modern History* (Palgrave, London, 2014), 53.

[6] Biro, 'Psychological pain', 53.

[7] For a discussion on the shift from children's bodies to children's minds, see: Steedman, *Strange Dislocations*; Carolyn Steedman, *Childhood, Culture, and Class in Britain: Margaret McMillan,*

it may be unsurprising that here the move from bodies to minds was often a slower and more tentative process that might be suggested by the term 'paradigm shift'. In this chapter, I examine this emergence closely and show how the acceptance of psychotherapy – and, with it, the perspective of nervous states more in mental rather than somatic terms – did not take place overnight.[8] The central claim of this chapter is that during the first half of the twentieth century there was continuing debate over the medical status of children's somatic pain: neurologists and some paediatricians argued that pain without physical injury was to be located in the nervous system,[9] while other physicians and psychologists asserted that these so-called nervous conditions should be explained in mental rather than somatic terms.[10]

Much of the nineteenth-century literature on nervous disorders refers to harmful symptoms unrelated to structural injuries.[11] Nonetheless, medical experts and scientists of the time, working under the principle of clinical causality, believed that behind all these pains there *was* some kind of injury, whether a dysfunction, nervous irritation or psychological trauma.[12] The general historiographical consensus is that during the twentieth century 'nervous pain' gradually disappeared from medical and popular literature due to a fundamental change in medical paradigms. In line with historians who have suggested that this transition was a tentative and prolonged process[13] and with Javier Moscoso's argument that, in the early twentieth century, both neurology and psychiatry expanded the notion of the nervous pain by putting forward the idea of the existence of unconscious cognitive activity and psychological

1860–1931 (Virago Press, London, 1990); Carolyn Steedman, 'Bodies, figures and physiology: Margaret McMillan and the late nineteenth century remaking of working class childhood', in Roger Cooter (ed.), *In the Name of the Child: Health and Welfare, 1880–1940* (Routledge, London, 1992); Cathy Urwin and Elaine Sharland, 'From bodies to minds in childcare literature: advice to parents in Inter-War Britain', in Cooter, *In the Name of the Child*, 44; Harry Hendrick, 'Children's emotional well-being and mental health in early post-Second World War Britain: the case of unrestricted hospital visiting', in Gijswijt-Hofstra and Marland (eds.), *Cultures of Child Health*, 215; Harry Hendrick, *Child Welfare: England 1872–1989* (Routledge, London, 1994); Shapira, *The War Inside*, 1–23.

8 A similar argument has been made by Mathew Thomson in the context of adult neurasthenia. See Mathew Thomson, 'Neurasthenia in Britain: an overview', in Marijke Gijswijt-Hofstra and Roy Porter (eds.), *Cultures of Neurasthenia from Beard to the First World War* (Rodopi, Amsterdam, 2001), 79.

9 For example, David Morris, 'An invisible history of pain: early 19th-century Britain and America', *Clinical Journal of Pain*, 14 (1998), 191–96.

10 For example, Noémi Tousignant, 'Pain and the pursuit of objectivity: pain-measuring technologies in the United States *c*. 1890–1975' (Unpublished PhD thesis, McGill University, 2006); Marcia Meldrum, 'A capsule history of pain management', *Journal of the American Medical Association*, 290 (2003), 2470–75.

11 See Chapter 3.

12 Andrew Hodgkiss, *From Lesion to Metaphor: Chronic Pain in British, French and German Medical Writings, 1800–1914* (Rodopi, Amsterdam, 2000).

13 Thomson, 'Neurasthenia in Britain', 79.

trauma,[14] this chapter's account of children's nervous pain in British medical practice assumes that its history ran parallel to that of unconscious pain.[15]

This chapter is organised around two themes. First, nervous pain, a concept that emerged in the nineteenth century as medical professionals sought to explain pain that appeared to have no morphological cause. It explores the use of the term 'neurasthenia',[16] the battle between accounts that emphasised heredity and those that highlighted the environment, and the differences between the perspectives of neurologists, psychologists and paediatricians. This section considers the work of experts such as George Frederic Still, Gilbert Ballet, Thomas Dixon Savill, Leonard Guthrie and Archibald Garrod.

The second part focuses on unconscious pain and addresses the major shift that took place at the beginning of the twentieth century, with the decline of ideas about the nervous system as the location of certain illnesses and the growth of new ideas that focused on mental rather than somatic problems.[17] My argument is that, in practice, the change in perspective was more complex than suggested by the straightforward, linear 'from bodies to minds' narrative. For instance, the chapter reveals how the concept of neurasthenia – or nervousness – survived well into the interwar period and how it seemed to be given a new life in the area of children's health. Thus, the figure of the 'nervous child' is studied along with the influence of Freud and psychoanalysis together with that of the 'New Psychology' and the child guidance clinics.[18]

[14] Moscoso, *Pain*, 172–90.

[15] See, for instance, Hector Charles Cameron, *The Nervous Child* (Geoffrey Cumberlege/Oxford University Press, London, 1946).

[16] The idea of neurasthenia was introduced by George Miller Beard as a diagnostic category based on the notion of 'nerve fatigue' and came to encompass a wide range of symptoms, including headaches, insomnia, anxiety, depression, neurosis, hysteria and mania. In his foundational essay, Beard defined neurasthenia as an entirely somatic disorder, subject to physiological inquiry, but caused by the close relationship of body and mind, being brought about by 'bereavement, business and family cares, parturition and abortion, sexual excesses, the abuse of stimulants and narcotics, and civilized starvation'. See George Miller Beard, 'Neurasthenia, or nervous exhaustion', *Boston Medical and Surgical Journal*, 3 (1869), 47. For details on Beard's work in the context of nineteenth-century psychiatry, see Trevor Turner, 'The early 1900s and before', in Hugh Freeman (ed.), *A Century of Psychiatry: Vol I* (Mosby-Wolfe, London, 1999), 3–29.

[17] The First World War was unique in the means and extent to which it precipitated a transformation of the popular and scientific understandings of the human body and its selfhood. See Stefanos Geroulanos and Todd Meyers, *The Human Body in the Age of Catastrophe: Brittleness, Integration, Science, and the Great War* (University of Chicago Press, Chicago, 2018).

[18] Various studies have examined the use of the term 'nervous' in medical approaches, particularly towards women, during this period. See, for example, Showalter, *The Female Malady*. However, the concept also played a leading role in framing approaches to children, influencing medical theories that focused on the development of children's brains and which linked the state of a child's mind to physiology. See Michael Roper, 'From the shell-shocked soldier to the nervous child: psychoanalysis in the aftermath of the First World War', *Psychoanalysis and History*, 18 (2016), 39–69.

The claims of such authors as Nelleke Bakker and Mathew Thomson that the terminology of 'nervousness' was gradually replaced by 'neurosis' are tested and expanded to the field of child studies in Britain; however, instead of focusing on Thomson's differentiation between elite and general practitioners, the chapter is organised around interdisciplinary comparisons. This second part of the chapter considers the work of Hector Cameron, Hugh Crichton-Miller, Anna Freud, Melanie Klein, Donald Winnicott, Millais Culpin and Margaret Lowenfeld.

This chapter explores the published texts of British neurologists, paediatricians and psychologists from 1900 to 1939. It explores how different concepts proved attractive to distinct professional groups at different times. According to the neurologists – and in strict observance of the anatomo-clinical tradition – the nervous system was considered to be the 'seat of disease' for different types of pain without a lesion. As a result, such pains fell under the purview of this medical discipline. The emergence of new knowledge led to a reframing of the ways in which this knowledge was structured. As they sought to identify causal factors, neurologists came to study children as well as adults. At the same time, paediatricians extended their focus on children to embrace psychogenic pain, to allow for labelling beyond their previous diagnostic models.[19]

In addition to scientific sources previously analysed in the published works, this chapter draws on an extensive literature search for medical and paediatric publications on children's nervous pain that began with the Institute of Child Health (University College, London) Library Historical Collections on the History of Paediatrics and included the Archives of Disease in Childhood, BMJ Journals, *The Lancet* and the *British Medical Journal*. To uncover psychological theories and observations of children's pain, I have focused on the published texts of British psychologists and psychoanalysts who conducted research on 'nervous' children. In particular, I explore the findings of those professionals who worked in the Children's Clinic for the Treatment Study of Nervous and Difficult Children (above all, its founder Margaret Lowenfeld), the Tavistock Clinic and its founder, Hugh Crichton-Miller, and the Child Guidance Clinic. Thanks to the Wellcome Trust archive and the archives of the Institute of Education, I was able to study other pioneering figures who contributed to the development of psychoanalysis in Britain, such as Melanie Klein, Donald Winnicott and Susan Isaacs.

[19] Nelleke Bakker, 'A harmless disease: children and neurasthenia in the Netherlands', in M. Gijswijt-Hofstra and R. Porter (eds.), *Cultures of Neurasthenia from Beard to the First World War* (Rodopi, Amsterdam, 2001).

Nervous Pain

The language of 'nerves' and an expanding medical culture concerned with 'nerve management' appeared for the first time in the British literature about childhood conditions just after 1900, nearly twenty years after its first mention in relation to adult medicine in Britain.[20] Previously, when medical culture had paid attention to the pathologies observable in children, it did so only in relation to adult physiology.[21] It was not until the beginning of the twentieth century – with the advent of new disciplines such as paediatrics, educational psychology and child psychology – that a theoretical framework for the study of pain and the nervous conditions that belong to childhood developed.[22] Thus the debates that had already taken place in the nineteenth century about hysteria, neurasthenia and the disorders of the imagination[23] flourished once again in the twentieth century within these new disciplines that sought to create a medical dictionary appropriate to the first years of life. At the same time, children with deviant behaviour passed from the domain of morals to that of medicine and became objects of study in paediatrics and psychology.[24] These children were seen not so much in terms of insanity but according to a range of 'nervous' behaviours. While many discussions centred on neurasthenia, hysterical pain and neuralgia, others also included nervous tics, rheumatism (acute and chronic) and the abnormal modification of sensory thresholds.

At the start of the twentieth century, medical practitioners had two versions of the concept of neurasthenia and other nervous disorders: one based on hereditary determinism and the other on environmental factors. There is a fundamental difference between the two perspectives: while heredity was not something that could be treated, external conditions could be altered or altogether removed, which placed an emphasis on prevention and cure by creating a positive environment. The optimism of environmental approaches might have been an influential factor in their success over Bénédict Morel's theory of degeneration. Usually framed within the context of adult physiology, the study of children's nervous illnesses was also centred on this question: Did the deficiencies of neurasthenia stem from a morbid heredity or from the conditions of modern life? Thus, in one of the biggest and most successful

[20] For a discussion on nervous disorders and modernity see Amelia Bonea et al., *Anxious Times: Medicine and Modernity in Nineteenth-Century Britain* (University of Pittsburgh Press, Pittsburgh, PA, 2019).

[21] See Chapter 3.

[22] See, for instance, George Frederic Still, *Common Disorders and Diseases of Childhood* (Henry Frowde, London, 1910).

[23] See Chapter 3.

[24] This issue is discussed in detail in Mathew Thomson, *Psychological Subjects: Identity, Culture and Health in Twentieth-Century Britain* (Oxford University Press, Oxford, 2006), 5–9.

of the volumes about neurasthenia circulating in Britain during the period – *Clinical Lectures on Neurasthenia* – Thomas Dixon Savill framed childhood within the nature–nurture debate, denying heredity as the only or principal cause but recognising the influence of innate predisposition. After claiming that 'heredity does not seem to play so important a part here as it does in cases of hysteria', Savill dedicated various paragraphs to describing the three ways in which heredity could play a role in the development of neurasthenia. First, a tendency to develop nervous illnesses 'may be present as a general neurotic taint in the family'.[25] In the words of this doctor, 'the children of insane parents, for instance, seem especially prone to cerebral neurasthenia'.[26] Second, a greater predisposition existed in the children of alcoholics, even when the parents had not gone on to present nervous symptoms. Third, there were children with a family history of tuberculosis, followed by those whose mothers had presented 'debility [. . .] at the time of pregnancy'.[27]

While recognising innate predisposition as a 'point of entry' or condition of possibility for the onset of nervous imbalance, neurologists did not deny that educational and developmental factors – such as early ill-treatment or school pressure – could turn a nervous child into a serious case of neurasthenia.[28] Neurasthenia as a diagnosis was closely linked to the growing interest in mental as well as physical hygiene in schools. From the beginning of the twentieth century, 'over-pressure' and resulting nervousness was recognised as one of the main risks for the appearance of the illness. Thus, in *Neurasthenia*, Gilbert Ballet commented that although 'the disease is very rare in childhood and old age', there was a type of neurasthenia that was present only in childhood: 'precocious neurasthenia'.[29] Based on the cases that he had been able to study in his practice, this doctor concluded that the child who suffered from this type of neurasthenia was almost always male, 'notably taller than the average, and whose girth of chest and volume of muscles are not proportionate to their height', and whose nervous system 'is endowed with excessive fragility and yields to the slightest shock'.[30] According to Ballet, the aetiology of this variant of neurasthenia was not so much heredity as a problem of 'over-pressure' and especially 'cerebral over-pressure', which he claimed must figure 'in the front rank of the causes of neurasthenia'.[31] For Ballet, the most extreme manifestations of neurasthenia always led to the continuous

25 Savill, *Clinical Lectures*, 59.

26 Savill, *Clinical Lectures*, 59.

27 Savill, *Clinical Lectures*, 59.

28 The topic of over-pressure has been discussed by Sally Shuttleworth in the chapter 'Progress, pressure and precocity', in Shuttleworth, *Mind of the Child*, 131–150. See algo Oppenheim, *Shattered Nerves*, 244–46.

29 Gilbert Ballet (trans. P. Campbell Smith), *Neurasthenia* (Henry Kimpton, London; Alexander Stenhouse, Glasgow, 1908), 9.

30 Ballet, *Neurasthenia*, 10.

31 Ballet, *Neurasthenia*, 9.

experience of chronic pain, whether 'dull pain', a constant 'pain in the forehand and the back of the neck', pain in the stomach, 'pains all over' or painful sensations in the back very similar to those that constitute headache and rachialgia.[32]

In the 1914 book *Treatment of Neurasthenia*, Paris society nerve doctor Paul Hartenberg commented that together with heredity, 'there is another cause which will elicit a response from the nervous system; this is the hyperactivity of brain and spinal cord'.[33] He located the source of this abnormal hyperactivity in the school, its demanding curriculum and in parents' expectations of their children, because the first symptoms coincided with the moment in which these young patients had been obliged to 'put forth an extra effort which often results in the breakdown of predisposed nervous systems'.[34]

Thomas Dixon Savill, who was a physician at the West End Hospital for Diseases of the Nervous System, cited Ballet and argued that there was a specific form of neurasthenia that belonged to childhood, to which he gave the name 'cerebral neurasthenia', which was produced by over-pressure at school. He mentions the case of Agnes C., 'a healthy-looking child', eleven years old, who was brought to the doctor by her parents because during the preceding weeks, she had displayed 'attacks of crying and depression', two or three times a day.[35] Her sleep was unstable and disturbed by frequent nightmares. While her appetite was poor and the girl complained of a constant pain in her stomach, her bowels and other organs were in a perfect state. A degree of improvement had been achieved through the administration of quinine, hydrobromic acid and bromide, but 'fits of depression' followed, alternating with attacks of excitation and 'silliness', according to her mother. The immediate 'cause of her symptoms appeared to have been a too close application to study', concluded the doctor.[36]

With Ballet, Savill considered that one of the most important aspects of these children was the continuous experience of chronic pain. Like Agnes, a significant number of children suffered pain that could not be explained by any morphological lesion. In defining 'functional nervous disorders', Savill states that the term 'functional' – which had often been used as a synonym for 'hysterical' – in fact denoted an 'absence of anatomical or structural changes to account for the symptoms'.[37] Savill's account represents a borderline case within the anatomo-clinical model of health and disease, which was based on the ability to localise individual agents of disease within structures and

[32] Ballet, *Neurasthenia*, 3.
[33] Paul Hartenberg, *Treatment of Neurasthenia* (Joint Committee of Henry Frowde and Hodder & Stoughton, Edinburgh, 1914), 60.
[34] Hartenberg, *Treatment of Neurasthenia*, 169. [35] Savill, *Clinical Lectures*, 36.
[36] Savill, *Clinical Lectures*, 36. [37] Savill, *Clinical Lectures*, 59.

tissues.[38] Since the axiom of tissue pathologies and structural lesions excluded the possibility of conceiving pain without a lesion, physicians and neurologists simply added it, following Savill's example by suggesting that the lesion was located in the nervous system. Diagnoses of neurasthenia were attractive because they provided a somatic location for a wide range of conditions that had no obvious organic cause. Using the analytic framework of the historian and philosopher of science Thomas Kuhn, these diagnoses could be considered ad hoc adjustments in the predominant anatomo-clinical paradigm to realign evidence and theory: in a naïve conception of the experimental method, the existence of non-somatic pain would have rejected the hypothesis that all pain has a location in the body.[39]

The history of these patients showed an overabundance of afflictions, such as nervousness, headaches, disturbed sleep, restlessness, amnesia, agoraphobia, claustrophobia, irritability, inattention and vasomotor symptoms. As with conditions such as night terrors, pain was not a symptom, in Savill's opinion, but the cause of 'irritable weakness of the nervous system'.[40] Just as in the clinical cases of adult neurasthenia studied by Javier Moscoso, child patients arrived with one illness and left with another.[41] Thus, the parents of the fourteen-year-old William F. C. came to Savill complaining that their son had become 'more and more nervous' during the previous weeks and was 'gradually losing his memory'.[42] After examining the child, who had come to his practice complaining of a fierce headache, the doctor concluded that he was, in fact, suffering a neurasthenic condition. According to the physician, the parents' belief that the pain was localised in the joints was wrong, as it stemmed from the nervous system as a whole. This translation did not imply scepticism on the presence of symptoms or discomfort. Quite the contrary, no one was in any doubt that the pain was anything other than real. Although patients did not know the source of their own suffering – and attributed it to the wrong location – Savill and other doctors did not question the discomfort. Symptomatic cures were not ruled out despite their palliative character.

In 1905, Michell Clarke, Professor of Pathology at University College, Bristol (now Bristol University), also saw chronic pain, either of the back or of the head, as one of the most important symptoms of neurasthenia.[43] To this, he added other complaints such as dizziness and vertigo, mental depression,

[38] Daniel Goldberg, 'Pain without lesion: debate among American neurologists, 1850–1900', *19: Interdisciplinary Studies in the Long Nineteenth Century*, 15 (2012), 4–5.
[39] Thomas Kuhn, *The Structure of Scientific Revolutions* (University of Chicago Press, Chicago, 1962).
[40] Savill, *Clinical Lectures*, 59. [41] Moscoso, *Pain*, 172–81.
[42] Savill, *Clinical Lectures*, 37.
[43] J. Michell Clarke, *Hysteria and Neurasthenia* (J. Lane, The Bodley Head, London, 1905).

inability to carry out mental work, various sleep disorders, irritability of temper, weakness and tremor of the limbs, back pains, palpitation and certain forms of dyspepsia. Clarke describes these children, in terms similar to those used by Ballet, as having 'had a spell of exaggerated growth' after which the nervous troubles appeared. They were 'long and lean', suffered from headaches, had sluggish memories, complained of sleeping badly and, when getting up in the morning, were tired and 'as though palsied'.[44] Along with the pressure of school, Clarke mentioned the development of the imagination, desire and masturbation as causes of neurasthenia.

Medical professionals emphasised the importance of avoiding the overstimulation of the nerves, advocating regular activities, relaxation and the avoidance of risks and dangers. If in each classroom and each family there was a potentially nervous child, it would be the treatment of the children that would decide their future, affirmed these experts. Doctors did not believe it was in the power of the parents or of education to free a child with a neurasthenic predisposition from suffering the symptoms, but they could help to control them. In *Treatment of Neurasthenia*, Paul Hartenberg recommended open air and tonics, as well as the need to 'diminish or entirely suppress all work' in the case of schoolchildren or students.[45] If the condition was severe, the child should be 'confined to bed'. If all this did not have an effect, the doctor had as a weapon the preparation of a 'cereal decoction'.[46]

Despite the importance given to the hereditary factor, some experts believed that self-control was a powerful treatment, if not a cure. Michell Clarke recommended eliminating alcohol, tea and coffee from the child's diet combined with bodily as well as mental training.[47] Regular hours as well as the day-to-day control of the emotions could help to prevent the seed of neurasthenia from germinating. Equally, for Gilbert Ballet, the first measure in preventing neurasthenia was to safeguard children who had been born to parents who were neuropathic or arthritic by repressing their hereditary tendencies and trying to strengthen their nervous centres.[48] To achieve this, the doctor insisted on putting into practice, 'methodically and patiently', all the means at the disposal of hygiene. In *Treatment of Neurasthenia by Teaching of Brain Control*, Roger Vittoz suggested that patients who had fewer possibilities of being cured were those who had been ill since childhood and had no

[44] Clarke, *Hysteria and Neurasthenia*, 59. [45] Hartenberg, *Treatment of Neurasthenia*, 172.
[46] Hartenberg, *Treatment of Neurasthenia*, 172.
[47] Clarke, *Hysteria and Neurasthenia*, 7. See also J. Michell Clarke and G. Scott-Williamson, 'A case of obscure fever with pronounced nervous symptoms, apparently due to infection by a *Leptothrix bacillus*', *British Medical Journal*, 2663 (13 January 1912) 67–68.
[48] Ballet, *Neurasthenia*, 163.

'conception whatever of the idea of an effort of will'.[49] Despite the central role given to either heredity or living standards as causes of the disease, these interpretations of childhood neurasthenia left more room for prevention than the notion that adult neurasthenia was caused by the pace and circumstances of modern life.

Ballet emphasised the importance of studying 'moral over pressure' when considering the aetiology of neurasthenia.[50] For this doctor, states of 'sorrow' and 'discomfort' from 'depressing emotions' that included 'vexation', 'disappointments', 'remorse' and 'thwarted affection' were most crucial in causing children to suffer from nervous exhaustion. Ballet's analysis of children's neurasthenia did not completely conform to the original concept of adult neurasthenia as a weakness of the nerves, which arrived in the United Kingdom from the United States in the 1880s. When it was first described, neurasthenia was depicted as a somatic disease provoked by too much strain on the brain and the digestive system, stemming from modern industrial and urban life. However, Ballet's references to social conditions were usually pushed into the background. Publications such as Ballet's represented an optimistic approach that emphasised how a favourable environment could prevent or even cure neurasthenia.

As late as 1920 – a date that is often considered as marking the end of the peak of neurasthenia – neurologist Ivo Geikie Cobb, assistant to the out-patient physician at the Middlesex Hospital, still defined it as generalised 'irritable weakness' of the entire nervous system.[51] Starting out from an article published by Campbell Smith in the *Practitioner* in 1911, Cobb maintained that while the 'early edition of nerve exhaustion' in children – to which he designated the name 'Neurasthenia Minor' – resembled adult neurasthenia, it presented a series of symptoms and characteristics that belonged to this particular period of life.[52] It is interesting that Cobb only outlined this argument, without going on to explain the nature of these differences. His treatise widened the array of symptoms, mentioning afflictions such as hypersensitiveness of the sensorium, the loss of mental and bodily vigour, disturbed sleep, irritability of temper, muscular weakness, restlessness, nervousness and – above all – 'vague pains'.[53] The fact that many of the treatises about adult neurasthenia written at the beginning of the twentieth century referred to a type of neurasthenia characteristic of childhood reflects the influence and growth of arguments that had emerged from the field of paediatrics, which stressed the

[49] Roger Vittoz, *Treatment of Neurasthenia by Teaching of Brain Control* (Longmans, Green, London, 1911), 80.

[50] Ballet, *Neurasthenia*, 163

[51] Ivo Geikie Cobb, *A Manual of Neurasthenia (Nervous Exhaustion)* (Baillière, Tindall and Cox, London, 1920), 88.

[52] Cobb, *A Manual of Neurasthenia*, 29.

[53] Cobb, *A Manual of Neurasthenia*, 29.

importance of studying childhood pathologies as manifestations independent of those that belonged to the adult world.

Paediatrics and Functional Neuroses in Childhood

Despite its apparently limited acceptance, the concept of neurasthenia permeated both the medical and educational discourses about children during the first decades of the twentieth century. By then, paediatricians had already taken interest in children's nervous problems – including illnesses such as hysteria and neuralgia, as well as neurasthenia – as an object of study in their own right. Although treatises about nervous conditions written by neurologists during this period continued to frame the child within debates about adult conditions, paediatrics focused its attention on conditions that specifically belonged to children.[54] Going beyond earlier diagnostic models, a new nomenclature was taking shape. Childhood neurasthenia, which had been mentioned in some of the foundational studies of adult nervous pathologies, was to be diagnosed in the twentieth century by an expanding medical culture that managed and medicalised children's nervous disorders.

At the beginning of the century, medical pathology, psychiatry and psychology all placed an urgent focus on the rigorous study of childhood conditions that did not depend on the adult world. In so doing, these new disciplines also sought to legitimise and consolidate themselves. Manuals about children's nervous disorders written by medical pathologists and paediatricians were published, covering the physical, mental, moral and emotional aspects of the weakness of nerves as well as the effect of parental shortcomings, parental negligence or a bad environment. Although the treatises produced by the new discipline of paediatrics varied in their assumptions and standards, they had one thing in common: paediatricians (along with pathologists) attacked the authority of neurologists in conceptualising and treating mental illnesses and the child's nervous system.[55] The response of paediatricians to neurology – which, at that time, enjoyed a higher academic and professional status – was to emphasise the unique character of childhood conditions and to use this claim as the basis for diagnosis.[56]

An important figure in this process was George Frederic Still (1868–1941), assistant physician for diseases of children at two hospitals in London: King's College Hospital and the Hospital for Sick Children, Great Ormond Street, where he became one of Charles West's successors and a prominent member

[54] For example: Savill, *Clinical Lectures*; Hartenberg, *Treatment of Neurasthenia*.

[55] A very similar process has been described by Nelleke Bakker in the context of the Netherlands. See Bakker, 'A harmless disease'.

[56] Bakker, 'A harmless disease', 311.

of the hospital's second generation.[57] Still inherited West's legacy of the 'nervous child', first mentioned in the 1848 *Lectures on the Diseases of Infancy and Childhood* in the section on 'nervous disorders'.[58] Still's significance lies in a new definition of children's nervous instability that he called 'defect of moral control', published in *The Lancet* in 1902.[59] In this work, which was based on his three Goulstonian Lectures, 'On some abnormal psychical conditions in children', given at the Royal College of Physicians of London, Still discusses the symptoms that neurologists saw as clear indications of neurasthenia and other disorders of the nervous system. Still divided the cases into two groups. The first comprised children with a 'morbid failure in development of moral control'.[60] The second consisted of children with a 'morbid loss of already acquired moral control'.[61] It is worth noting that Still's use of the word 'morbid' implies the morphological/anatomical claim that the disease entity – the defect of moral control – was linked to a pathological condition. As with the medical conditions analysed by neurologists, the prevailing idea of causation in relation to both groups was that there was an organic cause of the children's defect of moral control. Still argued that a 'lack of moral control may be shown in many ways,' with symptoms including 'nervousness', 'passionateness', 'dishonesty' 'spitefulness and cruelty'.[62]

The psychological symptom was related to a morphological condition, which was generally held to be a physical disease affecting the brain during infancy. Still's demonstration in his Goulstonian Lectures of a causal link between damage to the brain and immoral behaviour in children inscribed his theory in the anatomo-clinical conception of local, discrete entities as pathological causes, a view he shared with rival neurologists.[63] What set Still apart

[57] See P. M. Dunn, 'Sir Frederic Still (1868–1941): the father of British paediatrics', *Archives of Disease in Childhood – Fetal Neonatal Edition*, 91(4) (July 2006), 308–10.

[58] West, *Lectures*, 188.

[59] For example, Frederic Still's concept of defect of moral control, which he developed in his Goulstonian Lectures, a series of three lectures to the Royal College of Physicians of London. In 'On some abnormal psychical conditions in children: the Goulstonian Lectures,' *The Lancet*, 1 (1902), 1008–12, Still discusses 'the particular psychical conditions [. . .] which are concerned with an abnormal defect of moral control in children'.

[60] Still, 'On some abnormal', 1010. [61] Still, 'On some abnormal', 1079.

[62] Still used this diagnostic label in his medical practice as well: GOS/10/229-230: Dr Frederic Still casenotes (1913–16), Great Ormond Street Hospital.

[63] Still's demonstration in his Goulstonian lectures of a connection between brain damage and deviant behaviour in children was highly influential in the conceptualisation of maladjustment and, later, of attention deficit hyperactivity disorder (ADHD). Both ADHD's advocates and those who question its validity trace the lineage of this diagnostic category back to these lectures. R. A. Barkley, *Defiant Children: A Clinician's Manual for Assessment and Parent Training* (Guilford Press, New York, 1997); R. A. Barkley, *Attention Deficit Hyperactivity Disorder: A Handbook for Diagnosis and Treatment*, 3rd ed. (Guilford Press, New York, 2006); R. A. Barkley and K. R. Murphy, *Attention Deficit Hyperactivity Disorder: A Clinical Workbook* (Guilford Press, New York, 2006); R. A. Barkley, *ADHD and the Nature of Self-*

from neurologists is the fact that he was the first expert to describe neurosis as a specific children's disease. He thereby anticipated the change that would take place within the literature of nervous disorders.[64] At the time of his 1902 lectures, Still was already campaigning for the establishment of a specialist discipline for childhood conditions. Known as the 'father of British paediatrics', in 1906 he became Britain's first professor of paediatrics (at King's College Hospital), and in 1933, he was elected president of the first international congress on paediatrics.[65]

Still's *Common Disorders and Diseases of Childhood*, a textbook published in 1909, proved successful and was in its fifth edition by 1927. This work has a chapter dedicated to children's nervous disorders, which is important for two reasons.[66] First, it is one of the first studies to deal with nervous conditions from within the new children's science. Second, it anticipates the paradigm shift that was taking place in the field of the study of childhood nervous conditions and which would be consolidated in debates after the First World War. While other treatises of the time continued to use the heading 'peculiarities of the nervous system', Still called this chapter 'Nervous Children', thereby formulating a new figuration of childhood that would be subject to subsequent conceptualisation and articulation over the following decades.[67] According to Still, these children demonstrated too much intelligence to be labelled under the established terminology of idiocy and they were too young to be understood as 'criminal minds'.[68]

In 1909, Still had to open with an apologetic defence of an 'unscientific title': there was 'no technical term which so well expresses the condition which I wish to emphasise here as the homely word "'nervousness"'.[69] Indeed, the new figure of the nervous child would not establish itself within medical theory and practice until the 1920s, with the consolidation of paediatrics and the

Control (Guilford Press, New York, 2005); R. A. Barkley, G. Edwards and A. R. Robin, *Defiant Teens: A Clinician's Manual for Assessment and Family Intervention* (Guilford Press, New York, 1999); S. Goldstein and M. Goldstein, *Managing Attention Deficit Disorders in Children: A Guide for Practitioners* (John Wiley & Sons, New York, 1990); S. Goldstein and M. Goldstein, *Managing Attention and Learning Disorders in Late Adolescence and Adulthood* (Wiley, New York, 1997).

64 Thomas Armstrong, *The Myth of the ADD Child* (Plume Penguin, New York, 1995); P. Breggin, *Talking Back to Ritalin* (Common Courage Press, Monroe, ME, 1998); P. Schrag and D. Divoky, *The Myth of the Hyperactive Child and Other Means of Child Control* (Pantheon, New York, 1975).

65 Dunn, 'Sir Frederic Still', 308–10.

66 Still, Common Disorders, chapter XXXVIII, Nervous Children, 544–555.

67 Still, *Common Disorders*, 544–555.

68 GOS/10/229-230: Dr Frederic Still casenotes (1913–1916), Great Ormond Street archives.

69 Still, *Common Disorders*, 544.

emergence of educational psychology. Paediatric treatises published in the first two decades of the twentieth century placed conditions such as neurasthenia, hysteria, neuralgia and neurosis under the heading of 'functional nervous disorders' rather than 'nervous children'. Thus, one of the first textbooks on the emerging discipline of child psychiatry was *Functional Nervous Disorders in Childhood* (1907) by the British physician Leonard Guthrie, senior physician at Paddington Green Children's Hospital in London.[70] Like Still, Guthrie based his account on considerations quite distinct from those that had been held during the previous century and that were still defended within the field of neurology, illustrating the big changes that were taking place in the paediatric, psychological and psychiatric approaches to childhood. Guthrie reflects on the early Victorian period when the child mind had yet to capture medical attention:

> If children were ill or ailing, the doctor was called upon to prescribe for their diseases, but advice on their management in general was neither sought not welcomed. He was not asked to see a child because it was wayward, but because it was wasting, not because it was dainty, capricious in appetite, refusing food considered good for it, and craving for all that is unwholesome, but because it had pains in its stomach. Advice was not asked for peevish, passionate children, nor for those who were afraid of the dark, and unnaturally timid, absent-minded, or brooding and morose, jealous, spiteful or cruel, nor for mischievous, untruthful, dishonest, or immoral children. All such defects were regarded as moral rather than morbid, and were treated as such.[71]

As in Still's description, this catalogue of traits neatly summarises precisely the areas of children's behaviour that were being claimed by child psychiatry. However, Guthrie and Still were coming from different places. While Still based his ideas on Charles West and the first texts about children's diseases, Guthrie drew on the complex debate among late nineteenth-century psychiatrists and neurologists about the possibility of children's insanity.[72] Throughout the book's twenty-one chapters, the narrative remains faithful to two guiding principles: a clear opposition to the tendency to blame parents for their children's problems and an insistence on the importance of two factors: personality and environment. Following West's recommendations on the empathetic duties of the paediatrician, Guthrie dictated the need to access a true understanding of childhood and the physical and psychological pain every child endures. In line with the factual acceptance of childhood suffering typical of practising paediatricians, Guthrie claimed its potentially permanent effects on the psyche. Unlike neurologists, he did not believe that the functional neuroses of childhood could be explained by the development of the cerebrospinal system during infancy and argued that 'the environment of

[70] Guthrie, *Functional Nervous Disorders*, 4–5.
[71] Guthrie, *Functional Nervous Disorders*, 4–5.
[72] Shuttleworth, *Mind of the Child*, 16.

the neurotic child as well as his personality have always to be considered in relation to his ailments'.[73]

Guthrie's work describes various specific types of deviant behaviour that he observed in children. Although he still suggested a somatic location of these ailments, Guthrie argued that both emotional and somatic factors played a role in the development of neurosis. Thus, in the chapter 'Effects of emotions on health' he argued that, when diagnosing neurotic children, doctors should take into account the potential effect of mental problems on the origin and course of illness: 'The influence of their mental troubles may be as great as, or greater, than our own, in causing and prolonging their complaints.'[74] He quotes George Eliot's novel *The Mill on the Floss* and argues that because health and happiness go hand in hand, 'if a child is miserable, its health, like that of an adult, suffers. The cause of the misery may seem trivial, but its effect upon health may be prolonged through after life'.[75]

It has been argued that the interwar period involved a 'transformation in the understanding of the moral sphere', with a movement from a 'hygienist' focus on the bodies of children and their physical health to an emphasis on their minds and emotions.[76] However, a less linear, more complex and protracted dynamic starts to appear when disciplines other than child rearing and psychology are added to the analysis, as Guthrie's account exemplifies. Together with West and other paediatricians, he had acknowledged the influence of emotions on the development of children's illnesses and nervous disorders, and the radical enmeshment of 'physical' and 'emotional' pain. When discussing the various functional neuroses of childhood, Guthrie considered 'hysteria and neurasthenia are often met together'. Thus, while he defined neurasthenia as 'hyper-sensitiveness of higher centres with proneness to general exhaustion of nervous energy', Guthrie saw mental and physical hysteria as characterised by 'excitability and explosiveness of higher centres, associated with local sensory and motor paralysis, and deficient powers of control of emotional display'.[77] In the words of this physician, neurasthenia probably caused 'more misery and pain than any organic disease'. 'Children may from very early years be neurasthenic in the highest degree', wrote Guthrie, adding that it was therefore important to recognise early symptoms and tendencies towards the disease, to tackle them if possible and thereby save such children from 'the life-long ill health which has been the lot of many endowed with the highest order of intellect and genius'.[78]

[73] Guthrie, *Functional Nervous Disorders*, 17. [74] Guthrie, *Functional Nervous Disorders*, 7.

[75] Sally Shuttleworth has discussed the work of Guthrie in relation to George's Eliot's *The Mill on the Floss* and Charlotte Bronte's *Jane Eyre*. See *Mind of the Child*, 16–17.

[76] Urwin and Sharland, 'From bodies to minds', 44.

[77] Guthrie, *Functional Nervous Disorders*, 15. [78] Guthrie, *Functional Nervous Disorders*, 17.

Guthrie considered that lower abdominal pains, diarrhoea and vomiting – where there was no specific cause – were constant manifestations of nervous children. His list of symptoms included repeated night terrors, headaches and migraine, urticaria (hives) and other forms of *erythema exudatativum*, poor circulation, dead fingers, cold extremities, sweating and cardiac palpitation. Nervous children were also prone to habit spasms (tics), rheumatic chorea, recurrent tonsillitis and cyclic albuminuria. Although they might suffer from epileptiform seizures, cases involving true epilepsy were rare. Neurotic children could even go on to develop all kinds of hysteria or neurasthenia in later life, risked becoming alcoholics or drug-takers, and could be suicidal, homicidal and/or insane.[79]

Guthrie brought together into the single configuration of the nervous or neurotic child all the distinct figures that had been studied by alienists at the end of the nineteenth century – the child with night terrors, the depressed child, the hysterical child and the insane child – and the different conditions studied by neurologists.[80] For Guthrie, pain was not just a symptom but also an important factor in the aetiology of the condition. Even though neurasthenia, hysteria and children's nervousness often resulted from a specific organic origin – either 'traumatism' or an illness of some kind – for doctors such as Guthrie, the 'perpetuation of the mischief' could well be the result of 'domestic mismanagement'.[81] In Guthrie's view, neurotic people were not necessarily neurasthenic, although they were prone to become so. Neurasthenia was the result of the combination of a neurotic temperament and unfavourable conditions and surroundings. Thus, when considering a neurotic child, both environment and personality had to be considered. Guthrie's text shows the shift in approaches to children's abnormal behaviour, moving away from the neurologists' belief in inherent hereditary factors to consider the significance of environmental influences.

Archibald Garrod, writing in 1913, was not 'disposed to agree with the modern doctrine that functional nervous disorders, such as neurasthenia, "psychasthenia" and hysteria, are entirely psychic in origin'.[82] On the contrary, they were nervous manifestations of a 'psycho-somatic' or 'somato-psychic' origin, which had their base in a physical or bodily change, almost always of a harmful nature.[83] The English physician criticised those psychologists who maintained that 'functional nervous disorders in general are affections of the mind, and not of the brain or body' and that the mind 'is not a function of the brain nor the brain the organ of the mind'.[84]

[79] Guthrie, *Functional Nervous Disorders*, 19–20.
[80] See Chapter 3.
[81] Guthrie, *Functional Nervous Disorders*, 17.
[82] Garrod et al., *Diseases of Children*, 666.
[83] Garrod et al., *Diseases of Children*, 666.
[84] Garrod et al., *Diseases of Children*, 666.

As Sarah Hayes has argued, theories about the influence of environmental versus hereditary factors shaped the medical approaches to the mind of the child in the first decades of the twentieth century.[85] The debate can be followed as closely in paediatrics authors as in neurologists. Still, for example, emphasised hereditary factors and considered that the main causes of childhood 'nervousness' included drunkenness by one of the parents at the moment of conception, the intense feelings of the mother during pregnancy and the presence of mental infirmities in the family.[86] Many doctors recognised that bad treatment or school overload could transform a child who presented only a disposition of minor importance into a serious case of nervousness. While Edmund Cautley argued that a neurotic heredity was the predisposing cause of neurasthenia, psychasthenia and hysteria, Guthrie and others accentuated the importance of the child's environment in the development of these conditions.[87] Calmness, order and regularity were prescribed – along with a host of 'hygienist' remedies such as physical exercise and fresh air – as ways to help to cure this condition. The most optimistic popular version highlighted the possibility of treating and decreasing childhood nervousness through the management of a healthy environment and a sound upbringing. The suffering of a nervous constitution in a child could be avoided, Cautley claimed, through a healthy diet. Good education, acceptance of obedience and self-control could help to combat hereditary predisposition and could act as a prophylaxis against weak nerves.[88] While neither parents nor schools could prevent a predisposed child from suffering the symptoms, they could nonetheless help to control them.

Although they took hereditary tendencies into account, doctors such as Cautley believed that a balanced and ordered life far away from strong impressions could counteract the lively imagination of the child and its nervous tendencies. Cautley's optimistic conclusion was that a tranquil and harmonious environment offered the best chance of avoiding the development of the illness in a child born with this temperament and of helping him or her to develop a stable character, despite the innate propensity towards the contrary. While there were potentially nervous children in every school and family, their future would be decided by how they were treated, according to this perspective. Cautley's account shows that before the First World War, medical professionals had a holistic conception of children's nervous illnesses. The emphasis on specific material lesions was combined with a notion of the interplay between emotions and tissues, between illness and subject.

[85] Sarah Hayes, 'Rabbits and rebels: the medicalisation of maladjusted children in mid-twentieth century Britain', in Mark Jackson (ed.), *Health and the Modern Home* (Routledge, New York, 2007), 128–52.

[86] Still, *Common Disorders*, 550.

[87] Cautley, *Diseases of Infants*, 756.

[88] Cautley, *Diseases of Infants*, 8.

The Signs of Nervous Pain

Mathew Thomson has suggested that, in the adult context, the success of diagnoses in terms of 'nerves' lay in the fact that it covertly made the development of psychotherapeutic medicine acceptable and provided an escape from the dead end of asylum-based psychiatry.[89] Seen from some distance, hysteria and neurasthenia have so many common features that it is impossible not to include some remarks on their relationship and the transition from one to the other. However, a closer look at the data suggests a messier landscape. In fact, cultural historian Elaine Showalter has asserted that most neurasthenic patients in the United States were women and that in Britain the diagnosis was associated mainly with young women.[90] Beyond gender distribution, the extent of this diagnosis before the discovery of psychoanalysis and modern psychology could be said to have preserved intact the principles of the clinical tradition a little longer. Historian Mathew Thomson and Javier Moscoso have described how terms such as 'neurasthenia' and 'hysteria' were often used – to different degrees in different countries – as a kind of catch-all or loose umbrella terms for a range of 'nervous' disorders. Thomson suggests that the term 'neurasthenia' (more popular in the United States than in the United Kingdom) was seen as an attractive diagnosis because it 'offered a somatic location – the nerves – for a vast range of conditions which had no other obvious organic origin'.[91]

To a certain extent, a similar process happened in the context of the emerging specialism of paediatrics, as paediatricians such as Still and Garrod published textbooks about children's nervous disorders, including neurasthenia, hysteria, neuralgia, nervous tic and hyperesthesia. Very often, the distinction between hysteria and neurasthenia is merely nominal, as they came to be used almost interchangeably. On certain occasions, pain without illness diversified into a wide spectrum: neuralgia, nervous tics and rheumatism, both acute and chronic. One work of special significance is Garrod's *Diseases of Children*, published in 1913. Garrod, who pioneered the field of inborn errors of metabolism, argued that 'all neurotic children are liable to aches and pains'.[92] For this English physician, rheumatism was 'generally held to be the chief cause of neuroses in mid-childhood', but the prominence of the neuroses did not always coincide with the severity of rheumatism.[93] While 'localised pain' was probably at the bottom of all hysterical paralyses and contractures in childhood, the pain was often the result of rheumatism, a slight

[89] Thomson, 'Neurasthenia in Britain', 79. [90] Showalter, *The Female Malady*, 137.
[91] Moscoso, *Pain*, 172–81; Thomson, 'Neurasthenia in Britain', 79.
[92] Garrod et al., *Diseases of Children*, 679. [93] Garrod et al., *Diseases of Children*, 679.

strain or 'incipient tuberculous disease'.[94] Garrod mentioned other factors involved in the production of functional neuroses: a sudden emotional shock, fear, dread, worry, anxiety, over-pressure, a life of unhealthy excitement or an environment that was uncongenial for one reason or another. Again, Garrod's study links the concepts of physical and emotional pain and the interplay of bodies and minds, which calls into question the 'bodies to minds' narrative put forward by recent studies of the history of childhood.

James Taylor also documented the relationship between neurasthenia and rheumatism in his book *Paralysis and Other Diseases of the Nervous System in Childhood and Early Life*, published in 1905, specifying the site of pain 'in the joints and down the limbs'.[95] Sir Dyce Duckworth, physician to the Prince of Wales, also held that rheumatism played an important role in causing nervousness and a very important part in the causation of children's nervousness and especially in the proliferation of 'various neuralgic affections' in children. In the most serious cases, the illness could degenerate to the point of producing a total paralysis of the child's nervous system. Robert Hutchison called this type of paralysis 'true hysterical paralysis' and illustrated the diagnosis with the case of one of his patients who presented with a complete 'loss of power in the whole arm'.[96] The twelve-year-old boy had attended the practice with a previous diagnosis of infantile paralysis. On examination, wrote Hutchison, the patient was found to be a healthy child whose health had previously been good, and no cause had been found for 'the onset of the paralysis'. 'The right arm was quite motionless' and showed considerable atrophy, 'especially in the small muscles of the hand. It was blue and cold, as in a case of infantile paralysis', but it was completely insensitive to touch, pain and temperature. Hysteria was therefore diagnosed, and 'a strong faradic current applied with vigorous suggestion'.[97] This provoked an emotional outburst, but the child regained power in the arm immediately and returned home the next day 'perfectly well' except for atrophy in the arm resulting from its lack of use.[98] In this case, it was 'the existence of the anaesthesia and its characteristic distribution' that enabled Hutchison to make his diagnosis. Unlike doctors who referred to heredity or the failures of modern society, Hutchison preferred to see conditions such as hysteria and neurasthenia as physical illnesses that could be treated successfully within the framework of medicine.

As well as pains of a rheumatic type, the doctor had to consider the presence of a disproportional pain in attending to the diagnostic signs of childhood nervousness. Thus, Garrod considered that the neurotic temperament was characterised by hyperesthesia – excessive physical sensitivity – and 'unduly active response to all forms of stimuli', both physical and

[94] Garrod et al., *Diseases of Children*, 728. [95] Taylor, *Paralysis and Other Diseases*, 227.
[96] Hutchison, *Lectures*, 228. [97] Hutchison, *Lectures*, 229. [98] Hutchison, *Lectures*, 229.

mental.[99] An excessive sensitivity of the skin linked to exaggerated reflexes and tendon jerks, tremors, tics, spasms and convulsions pointed to a diagnosis of physical hyperesthesia. 'Emotional hyperesthesia', on the other hand, was characterised by exaggerated sensitiveness and reaction to environmental stimuli.[100] Garrod, who described emotions according to the Darwinian paradigm, argued that the neurotic and emotional child presented an excessive sensitivity that made any experience, whether physical or emotional, painfully unbearable. For William Osler, hyperesthesia was usually associated with other manifestations of hysteria and neurasthenia, and patients with this condition usually complained of 'excruciating pain' in the stomach. The behaviour of the patient with hyperaesthesia could be characterised by a chronic and intractable stomach pain, a pain that, in severe cases, ended up with the patient 'reduced to an extreme degree by starvation'.[101]

For Osler, the most extraordinary manifestations of children's nervousness – whether they involved hysteria, neurasthenia or other manifestations of nervous instability – always resulted in 'grave sensory disturbances in the region of the stomach, in addition to the general nervous symptoms'.[102] Once again, physical suffering is presented as a clear diagnostic sign. Thus, Osler mentions 'Achylia Gastrica Nervosa', a condition often associated with hysteria and neurasthenia and characterised by a lack of the normal amount of acid in the stomach. And he added to this 'gastralgia' or 'severe pains in the epigastrium', which occurred 'as a manifestation of a functional neurosis, independent of organic disease, and usually associated with other nervous symptoms'.[103] For Luther Emmett Holt, the manifestations of gastralgia or 'sudden, severe attacks of abdominal pain' were more marked in older children than in infants. In many cases, the pain was so severe 'as to lead one to think that the stomach is the seat of disease' when in reality it was a nervous problem.[104] Whereas in mild cases the pain was intermittent without the presence of other symptoms, in severe cases, 'the pain may be so great as to cause pallor, faintness, cold perspiration, and very marked prostration'.[105] This American doctor recommended a treatment that involved putting the patient to bed, applying a 'counter-irritation' over the stomach, by means of a turpentine stupe or mustard paste. Patients should be given hot water containing brandy or gin, together with five drops of spirits of chloroform, and all food should be withheld.

Following Holt, Sir James Frederic Goodhart considered that the 'griping abdominal pain of a paroxysmal kind' and the pain in the side experienced by

[99] Garrod et al., *Diseases of Children*, 666. [100] Garrod et al., *Diseases of Children*, 667.
[101] William Osler, *The Principles and Practice of Medicine* (D. Appleton and Company, New York, 1920), 603.
[102] Osler, *The Principles and Practiçe*, 603. [103] Osler, *The Principles and Practice*, 603.
[104] Holt, *Diseases of Infancy*, 290. [105] Holt, *Diseases of Infancy*, 290.

many children he saw in his practice were not caused by temporary conditions, such as problems with their diet.[106] On the contrary, 'these varied pains and aches' were often 'an evidence of nervous instability, and they are found in nervous children or nervous families'.[107] According to Goodhart, 'the insignificance of the exciting causes, the suddenness of the attack, the suddenness of its subsidence, the nature of the attack in many cases, even the presence of an excess of mucus' were all compatible with enfeebled nerve control.

In *The Diseases of Infants and Children*, Cautley added to the physical pains that were characteristic of neurasthenia and hysteria, the psychological pains that were produced in cases of psychasthenia, 'a variety of neurasthenia in which the mental symptoms predominate'.[108] Cautley described psychasthenia as a mental illness that presented a high degree of irritability, caused by an imbalance of the imagination that led to anxious feelings, such as fear, in the child. While in neurasthenia the chief symptoms were somatic and physical and always of a harmful nature – headache, vomiting, palpitations and arrhythmia – children with psychasthenia showed a large degree of moral suffering. 'The child develops morbid scruples, increasing mental uncertainty and hesitation, lack of initiative power or acting promptly, auto-analysis, and excessive emotional reactions',[109] wrote Cautley. The next stage, he argued, was that the child either started to carry out 'imperious strange acts' – such as frequent handwashing, 'aimless rummaging' and 'verification of unimportant matters' – or remained 'in a state of rumination or reverie'.[110] Finally, the child developed 'fixed ideas, persistent obsessions, and phobias'. For Cautley, the child's uncontrollable actions depended on these uncontrollable ideas and 'the will is enfeebled and irresolute, the child being incapable of fixing either attention or energy'.[111] Such children were eccentric in manner and clumsy in action, and the 'joyousness of youth is replaced by melancholy or hypochondriasis'.[112]

Pain from the Unconscious Mind

Historians of medicine generally agree that a shift in medical paradigms at the beginning of the twentieth century led to the decline of neurasthenia and of beliefs that the physical condition of the nervous system was the location of a wide range of illnesses. As a result of this shift, the origin of certain physical symptoms was displaced from mental to somatic spheres.[113] Neurologists

[106] James Frederic Goodhart, *The Diseases of Children* (J & A Churchill, London, 1899).
[107] Goodhart, *Diseases of Children*, 112. [108] Cautley, *Diseases of Infants*, 776.
[109] Cautley, *Diseases of Infants*, 777. [110] Cautley, *Diseases of Infants*, 777.
[111] Cautley, *Diseases of Infants*, 777. [112] Cautley, *Diseases of Infants*, 777.
[113] Moscoso, *Pain*, 172–81; Thomson, 'Neurasthenia in Britain', 82.

continued to try to demonstrate that these illnesses had a specific organic origin and were treatable with traditional medicine, while other doctors recognised the influence of the unconscious mind on bodily functions, the susceptibility of the mind to suggestion and the psychotherapeutic role played by the doctor. Bodily symptoms were translated into mental problems that resulted from the struggle of an individual to adapt to a changing environment. As Mathew Thomson has shown, the implications for the diagnosis and treatment of neurasthenia and other nervous disorders were potentially very radical.

With this shift, there was an increasing recognition of the psychotherapeutic role of the doctor. According to the historians of childhood who have described the translation process from bodies to minds, for child welfare work, a 'space' for psychodynamic ideas was created in British medical science in the interwar period. This 'New Psychology', which involved new definitions of parental adequacy and led to new forms of family intervention, focused on feelings and emotions rather than behaviourist concerns with health and habits.[114]

From the 1920s, British experts became more interested in children's emotional problems as manifested in such behaviours as eating disorders, bed-wetting, anger, fear and anxiety. At the same time, there was a change in their interpretation. For instance, fear was now seen as a natural feeling rather than as an expression of a child's lack of self-control. Similarly, treatment shifted from a disciplinary approach of correction towards understanding the motives behind the feeling.[115] Analogously, lying or self-willed children were now seen as potential victims of emotional neglect rather than simply labelled as naughty.[116] However, not all interpretations of this shift see it in positive terms and some note that these changes took place alongside the 'psychologisation' of medical discourse.[117] David Armstrong, adopting Foucauldian terminology, sees an extension of the clinical gaze into the intimacy of the mind.[118]

After the Freudian concept of 'neurosis' burst onto the scene after the First World War, it coexisted with the more traditional notion of 'nervousness'.[119] Freud traced a clear connection between the failure of

[114] Angela David, 'British child psychology and the evacuation of children during World War Two', Centre for Medical History Seminar Series, 2 February 2012, University of Exeter (2012), 1.

[115] For a cultural history of fear see Joanna Bourke, *Fear: A Cultural History* (Virago, London, 2006).

[116] See Bakker, 'A harmless disease', 383–401.

[117] Urwin and Sharland, 'From bodies to minds', 44; Shapira, *The War Inside*, Introduction; Harry Hendrick, *Child Welfare: Historical Dimensions, Contemporary Debate* (Policy, Bristol, 2003).

[118] David Armstrong, *Political Anatomy of the Body: Medical Knowledge in Britain in the Twentieth Century* (Cambridge University Press, Cambridge, 1983), 7–9, 21, 26.

[119] See T. A. Ross, *An Enquiry into Prognosis in the Neuroses* (Cambridge University Press, Cambridge, 1936).

neurology's corporeal approach to provide an explanation for the proliferation of symptoms that were being observed by contemporary doctors. He argued that it was impossible to deny that there were many people with an abundance of symptoms that could not be explained by any morphological injury or complaint. Freud held that all patients manifesting an excess of ailments were suffering from the same illness, and he claimed that they could not be treated as people with located somatic illnesses. Contrary to the anatomo-clinical principle, he saw no reason to claim a connection between the symptoms and nervous or functional illnesses; instead, he shifted the causal logic to infer that all observable and conscious pathological symptoms stemmed from the disrupted and unconscious flow of the patient's psychic existence.[120] Together with physical discomfort, Freud postulated the existence of psychological pain from the unconscious mind, which enabled neurotic symptoms and behaviour to be considered.

Two of the main personalities who determined the fate of children-focused psychoanalysis in British society and democracy during the Second World War (see Chapter 5) were present at Freud's address at the fifth meeting of the International Psycho-Analytical Congress, held in Budapest in 1918 in the context of the First World War, which allowed Freud to tie shell-shock symptoms to unconscious conflicts.[121] Significantly, both of these people were women. Melanie Klein (1882–1960), after finding herself 'enraptured' by Freud's essay on dreams when she read it in 1914, started an analysis with Sandor Ferenczi in her early thirties that brought her into direct contact with shell-shocked soldiers. She happened to be based in Budapest when Freud made his remarks in 1918. She came to London in 1926 and then became a pioneer in British psychoanalysis, alongside Anna Freud (1895–1982), Sigmund Freud's sixth and last child, who had been an analysand of her own father, and with whom Klein started an analysis in 1918.[122] Two years later, Anna Freud started an informal group on child analysis and later took up the analysis of children of close friends that provided material for *Introduction to the Technique of Child Analysis*, published in 1928, ten years before her exile to London.[123]

As Klein recalled later, Sigmund Freud's address made a deep and lasting impression and, as a result, 'the wish to devote myself to psychoanalysis was strengthened', while Anna Freud believed that by introducing psychoanalysis into the field of child studies, she was serving her father's goal of broadening

120 Sigmund Freud, 'On the psychical mechanism of hysterical phenomena' (1893), in *Freud, The Standard Edition of the Complete Psychological Works*, vol. II (Hogarth Press, London, 1955), 27–39.

121 Elisabeth Young-Bruehl, *Anna Freud: A Biography* (London, Macmillan, 1988), 81.

122 On the role of Anna Freud and Melanie Klein in the development of child analysis see G. Donaldson, 'Between practice and theory: Melanie Klein, Anna Freud and the development of child analysis', *Journal of the History of the Behavioural Sciences*, 32 (April 1996), 160–76.

123 Young-Bruehl, *Anna Freud*, 166.

the reach of psychoanalysis.[124] Soon, the victims of war neurosis disappeared from public view, but there was now a new object of psychoanalytic investigation: the anxious child. Nelleke Bakker has argued that, as a diagnosis for children, 'nervousness' became unpopular, while Freud's concept of neurosis grew rapidly.[125] However, before the 1920s, psychoanalysis had paid little attention to children, and Freud himself had never conducted analysis on a child. His famous study of little Hans, a five-year-old boy with a phobia of horses, was based on consultations with the child's father – Freud did not treat Hans himself.[126] Nonetheless, child analysts used this 1909 essay as a benchmark.[127]

This section of the chapter accepts the terminological shift from 'nervous conditions' to 'neurosis', and it develops it in relation to the history of childhood and the history of pain. It explores the sources to test Thomson's hypothesis that views of neurasthenia varied considerably between elite clinicians and general practitioners.[128] However, instead of comparing different levels of expertise within the same discipline, this section explores different disciplines to show that during the interwar period, there was considerable debate about the location and causation of nervous illnesses and the interplay between bodies and minds.

The rise of the New Psychology did not immediately lead to the abandonment of long-established concerns about habit, will and character. In fact, the embrace of psychological medicine in Britain between the wars was rather tentative, as can be seen from the fact that, as late as 1922, paediatrician Henry Dwight Chapin published the book *Heredity and Child Culture*, which still covered topics including 'organic inheritance', 'social inheritance' and 'nerve culture'. While some clinicians and paediatricians advocated for the incorporation of psychology into medical practice, viewing it as essential for a more comprehensive approach to healthcare,[129] there was much resistance to the new psychological accounts from British doctors (particularly certain neurologists), who continued to emphasise physiological explanations, along with the primacy of innate factors.[130] Nonetheless, the idea that *both* mental *and*

[124] Phyllis Grosskurth, *Melanie Klein and Her Work* (Alfred A. Knopf, New York, 1986), 71; Russell Viner, 'Melanie Klein and Anna Freud: the discourse of the early dispute', *Journal of the History of the Behavioural Sciences*, 32 (January 1996), 6.

[125] Bakker, 'A harmless disease', 320.

[126] P. Gay, *Freud: A Life for Our Time* (Papermac, London, 1995), 255–61.

[127] Viner, 'Melanie Klein and Anna Freud', 6. [128] Thomson, 'Neurasthenia in Britain', 78.

[129] C. Lawrence, 'Still incommunicable: clinical holists and medical knowledge in interwar Britain', in C. Lawrence and G. Weisz (eds.), *Greater than Their Parts: Holism in Biomedicine, 1920–1950* (Oxford University Press, Oxford, 1998), 94–111.

[130] Trevor Turner, 'James Crichton-Browne and the anti-psychoanalysts', in Hugh Freeman and German Berrios (eds.), *150 Years of British Psychiatry, Volume II: The Aftermath* (Athlone, London, 1996), 144–55.

somatic factors were important was implicitly, if not explicitly, accepted. As we have seen in the previous section, paediatricians were already aware of the importance of emotions and environment in the aetiology of nervous illnesses long before the interwar period, anticipated by Charles West's work in the last decades of the nineteenth century, in which he discussed the importance of taking children's emotions into account to diagnose illnesses.

The Nervous Child

Historians have noted that the diagnosis of neurasthenia began to disappear from European and American treatises of psychiatry and neurology around 1920. Despite this, both neurasthenia and hysteria seem to have been given a second lease of life in literature about children's medical conditions and education, although the word 'neurasthenia' was soon replaced by popular equivalents such as 'nervousness', which was also used as a loose umbrella term for a wide range of conditions. But, as shown by the title of the section of Still's book, these conditions would soon move from their roots in the nervous system to pathological signs of a new diagnosis: nervous children.[131] 'Nervousness' not only survived into post-war paediatric discourse, but also gained in popularity.[132] There seem to be two main reasons for this. First, the term proved a more useful label for deviant behaviour in childhood than alternatives. For paediatricians and parents alike, nervousness may have been an attractive label for a problematic child, as it spared children with mental illness the stigma of insanity.[133] The second reason is related to the increasing popularity of 'mental hygiene' in schools. In the economically depressed years of the 1920s, juvenile delinquency became a major concern in Britain. Educationally backward children were seen as both a drain on resources – either by hindering other pupils or by taking up teachers' time and energy – and as those most likely to become disruptive and delinquent. According to

[131] On the nervous child see Roper, 'From the shell-shocked soldier', 39–69; Oppenheim, *Shattered Nerves*, 233–64.

[132] On nervousness, see Laura Salisbury and Andrew Shail (eds.), *Neurology & Modernity: A Cultural History of Nervous Systems, 1800–1950* (Palgrave Macmillan, Basingstoke, 2010); Edward Shorter, *How Everyone Became Depressed: The Rise and Fall of the Nervous Breakdown* (Oxford University Press, Oxford, 2013); Bonea, *Anxious Times*.

[133] Trevor Turner has shown how the word 'nervous' increasingly replaced 'insane' in an attempt to reduce the stigma, particularly among private patients, of being labelled mentally ill. See Turner, 'The early 1900s', 20. Edward Shorter has also emphasised the fact that nervous illness, unlike psychiatric illness, was considered non-inheritable, thus providing an opportunity to avoid the implications of hereditary illness and degeneracy. See Edward Shorter, *A History of Psychiatry: From the Era of the Asylum to the Age of Prozac* (Wiley, New York, 1997), 113. Several contributors to the book edited by Gijswijt-Hofstra and Porter, *Cultures of Neurasthenia from Beard to the First World War*, have advanced similar arguments.

Julienne Ford, Denis Mongon and Maurice Whelan, the medicalisation of deviant behaviour enabled the education service to defend its interests against pupils who interfered with both its 'open' and its 'hidden' curricula.[134] Nervousness was recognised as a major risk from the 'mental overburdening' of school children.[135]

From the 1920s, paediatricians began to recognise the impact of children's unconscious problems and the impact of the environment upon children's physical and mental health. These doctors were interested in children's psychological responses both to the normal pressures of growing up and to the abnormal strains of serious illness, and they paid particular attention to nervous children. The most authoritative textbook on nervous children, *The Nervous Child at School* by the paediatrician Hector Cameron (1878–1958), discussed nervousness in the context of the classroom.[136] Published in 1919, it was based on Cameron's experiences in the children's department at Guy's Hospital. As Leonard Guthrie had done previously, he explored the borderline between emotional and physical health, arguing that both normal and abnormal children needed to be studied to gain a full understanding of children's nervousness, as it was not possible to separate physical and psychological disabilities, and he further developed the topics of nervous pain and emotional suffering. In the opening section of the book, titled 'Doctors, mothers and children', Cameron urged his colleges to take into account a child's character when making a diagnosis, arguing that many child patients did not recover because the 'hygiene of the mind' was often overlooked.[137] For Cameron, it was essential to take into account this other aspect because of 'the certainty that physical disturbances of one sort or another will follow upon nervous unrest'.[138] Cameron noted how in most cases, the patients who arrived at hospital wards ended up going home with an incorrect diagnosis, as doctors focused only on physiological signs, forgetting the importance of the child's environment and the mental and emotional state of the patient in the development of the illness. To validate the importance of paediatrics in the study of the child, he commented that only the good physician, open to understanding the child as a whole, could appreciate and estimate the 'influences which proceed from parents and nurses of different characters and temperaments, and the reaction which is produced by them in the child'.[139]

Cameron placed pain as a privileged object in research and in medical practice with nervous children. Thus, he describes the case of 'a child of two

[134] Julienne Ford, Denis Mongon and Maurice Whelan, *Special Education and Social Control: Invisible Disasters* (Routledge and Kegan Paul, London, 1982), 34.
[135] Bakker, 'A harmless disease', 317; Shuttleworth, *Mind of the Child*, 138.
[136] Hector Cameron, *The Nervous Child* (Oxford University Press, London, 1919), 25.
[137] Cameron, *The Nervous Child*, 2. [138] Cameron, *The Nervous Child*, 2.
[139] Cameron, *The Nervous Child*, 5.

or three years of age who was brought to him with the complaint that defaecation was painful' and whose constipation had resisted several remedies.[140] Whenever the child was placed upon the potty, he started to cry, and it was impossible to console him. 'It is not sufficient for the doctor in such a case to make an examination which convinces him that there is no fissure at the anus and no fistula or thrombosed pile', argued Cameron, who concluded that all the symptoms presented by the child had a psychological origin.[141] Cameron held that many diseases involved 'a combination of organic disturbance' and 'emotional trouble'. For example, an eighteen-year-old girl had on-and-off pains in the left arm dating from a fracture of the olecranon 'when she was two years old'. Although she presented an organic injury – stiff joints and deformity in the arm – the pain always increased whenever 'she was tired or unhappy'.[142] In cases such as these, Cameron held that the treatment should seek to control both factors: the organic issue should be removed, psychological faults corrected. He believed that all kinds of emotional states including grief, anger, anxiety and excitement inhibited normal physiological processes or interfered with their action, so that these outbursts were usually followed by symptoms of a harmful character. The child patients who came to the paediatrician's practice complaining of a nervous condition presented palpitation, migraine, neuralgia, precordial pain, tachycardia of a functional nature, abdominal pains and diarrhoea, and hypersensitivity of taste, hearing, sight, smell and touch.

While Cameron's text shows the influence of the emerging literature that recognised the power of the subconscious mind and the emotions over the body, it nonetheless finds itself halfway between the assertion of the somatic reality of nervous suffering and the psychoanalytical and New Psychology literature, which accepted the mental origins of somatic conditions. In fact, Cameron continued to locate symptoms in an unstable nervous system, demonstrating the influence of authors such as Maudsley.[143] In 1923 – in a discussion on the subject of nervous children that he chaired at the British Medical Association's annual conference – despite taking into account the impact of 'intense emotions' in the development of nervous symptoms, Cameron continued to emphasise that the problem resided in the fact that a child's 'nervous system is unstable' and that 'this is made very manifest in sickness, and certain symptoms thus aroused may long act as a reminder'.[144]

In 1920, many physicians were still more attracted to the older model of the somatic reality of patients' suffering: besides the fact that it was readily

140 Cameron, *The Nervous Child*, 2.
141 Cameron, *The Nervous Child*, 3.
142 Cameron, *The Nervous Child*, 3.
143 See Chapter 3.
144 British Medical Association, *British Medical Journal* (24 November 1923) in Roper, 'From the shell-shocked soldier', 60.

understood, it had the advantage of absolving them to an important extent of individual responsibility.[145] This model led to a treatment regime based on somatic therapies, with less overt psychotherapeutic dimensions, which satisfied many of the physical and emotional needs of their child patients.[146] Thus, Dr J. Stewart Mackintosh sent a letter to the *British Medical Journal* in 1923 in which he criticised Hector Charles Cameron's *The Nervous Child*. For this doctor, the most frequent cause in the aetiology of childhood nervous disorders was 'disturbance in the character and distribution of the intestinal flora', with the most common manifestations involving 'chronic gastrointestinal catarrh with recurrent febrile exacerbations'.[147] While Cameron argued that nervous instability was almost always the cause of psychological pain – which is to say, that the emotions had an impact on the body – this commentator held that 'this type of nervous instability is a graft on the 'catarrhal diathesis'.[148] The letter ended by emphasising this point and criticising Cameron, saying that while he 'duly notes this association [...] the special opportunities of a family actor have enabled me to observe that the order of precedence is invariable – the catarrh comes first'.[149] In Mackintosh's view, by the time the state of 'malnutrition', 'toxic absorption', 'disturbed digestive functions', 'endocrine perversion' and 'muscular hypotenuse' was established, the child was already deeply immersed in an environment of perpetual concern, which created the nervous problems, adding psychic maladjustment 'to the other troubles'.[150] He added that even when the cause of psychological unease was physiological, an understanding of child psychology and psychotherapy was needed, 'for the sense of inferiority is all too readily acquitted, as are also the various fixations and complexes that impede or pervert psychic development'.[151] In other words, while Cameron believed that the emotions influenced the development of a nervous character and that this type of character had a greater tendency towards somatic illness, Mackintosh held that the order of causation was precisely the opposite: that physiological weakness created the nervous problems in the child. This difference of opinion is an example of the gulf between expert opinion and general practitioners, many of whom remained ignorant of psychological theories, as Mathew Thomson has shown.[152]

In 1927, Cameron published an article that discussed the connection between ketonzemia (cyclical vomiting) and certain nervous disturbances. The symptoms the mothers of these children reported were most usually

[145] Thomson, 'Neurasthenia in Britain', 84.
[146] This also happens in the adult context, see Shorter, *How Everyone Became Depressed*.
[147] J. Stewart Mackintosh, 'The nervous child', *British Medical Journal* (15 December 1923), 1183–84.
[148] Mackintosh, 'The nervous child', 1183.
[149] Mackintosh, 'The nervous child', 1183.
[150] Mackintosh, 'The nervous child', 1183.
[151] Mackintosh, 'The nervous child', 1184.
[152] Thomson, 'Neurasthenia in Britain', 82.

significant: rapid loss of weight, pallor with puffiness and lividity under the eyes, prostration, muscular laxity, constant yawning or sighing, constipation, bad breath, excessive perspiration and breathlessness on exertion, giddiness or faintness on getting up in the morning, a persistently irregular temperature and, above all, 'joints and muscular pains'.[153] Cameron described such pains as always intermittent and usually of short duration, 'lasting perhaps but half-an-hour at most, and [. . .] often relieved by warmth, by lying down, or by any measure which improves the skin circulation'.[154] Following the model of causality he had defended in relation to nervous children, Cameron argued that often these pains had an emotional origin, as they were as 'apt to be induced by fright as by a visit to the doctor', or by psychological exhaustion. However, he also acknowledged excitement, overexertion and starvation as possible causative factors. While this doctor commented that children who presented a nervous metabolism had a greater predisposition to develop this kind of ailment, he referred to the teachings of Sir James Mackenzie, saying that what 'seems to me most true and most fundamental is the recognition of the importance for each one of us, in our little way, and in the measure of our opportunities, to busy ourselves in studying the trifling beginnings of ill-health'.[155]

For the professor of psychiatry and neurology Beverley Tucker, this type of child did not need to visit the psychologist or psychoanalyst, but rather a 'competent neurologist'.[156] In line with thinking developed at the end of the nineteenth century, which held that physical disorders generated mental problems, this medic considered that congenital syphilis was one of the most likely causes of nervousness in children. In the same way, continued illnesses or pain produced nervousness in their aftermath, while some shorter illnesses – such as scarlet fever, measles, whooping cough, malaria and other acute infectious diseases – left the child's nerves temporarily or permanently impaired. In addition, Tucker claimed that injury – whether at birth or later – to the brain, spine or nerves could make a child nervous or leave him or her with 'an organic nervous disease', while constitutional conditions – such as 'debility, improper food assimilation, rickets, rheumatism, and kidney disease' – also played a role in nervous children.[157] It is interesting to note how the same symptoms led to very different diagnoses: there was much variation in the perspective of neurology, paediatrics and a new type of literature influenced by the emerging discipline of psychoanalysis.

153 Hector Cameron, 'Ketonæmia, cyclical vomiting and some nervous disturbances in children', *Archives of Disease in Childhood* 01/1927; 2(7) (1927), 55–61.

154 Cameron, 'Ketonæmia', 56. 155 Cameron, 'Ketonæmia', 58.

156 Beverley R. Tucker, *Nervous Children: Prevention and Management* (R. G. Badger, Boston, MA, 1916), 15.

157 Tucker, *Nervous Children*, 15.

In Vienna and Berlin, psychoanalysis was pioneering the study of children. In 1913, Hermine Hug-Hellmuth had published her first book on the topic and Karl Abraham started to analyse his daughter Hilda.[158] The 1920s saw rapid developments to the extent that, by 1925, Freud was able to remark that 'children have become the main subject of psychoanalytic research and have thus replaced in importance the neurotics on whom its studies began'.[159] In Britain, David Eder (1865–1936), one of the cofounders of the British Psychoanalytical Association, started to apply psychoanalytic theories to children. Eder's article 'The unconscious mind in the child', written jointly with his wife Edith and published in *Child Study* in 1918, shocked the readership to such an extent that it was withdrawn.[160] Conscious of the terrible physical conditions and poverty in which many children lived, Eder argued that the state could provide services that would benefit children's mental and spiritual self-development, with the latter seen as the higher aim of socialism. Although he syringed ears, performed tonsillectomies and weighed babies, Eder also made notes on 'the nervous traumas hidden in the starved little bodies of [his] child patients'. This new emphasis on the self and the emotions offered an alternative perspective on the advance of child welfare during this period.

The rapid growth of psychoanalysis inspired child guidance clinics, which started to become established across the Western world from the 1920s to treat children's mental health.[161] The transformation in the understanding and regulation of childhood physiological and emotional states can be seen in the context of the growth of child-centred intervention, with the development of ideas coming from both psychoanalysis and the various approaches of New Psychology, often in contradictory terms: the latter differed sharply in emphasis from the former, particularly over the centrality and necessity of Freud's psychoanalytic concepts. Freud's ideas were not completely accepted

[158] Claudine Geissmann and Pierre Geissmann, *A History of Child Psychoanalysis* (Routledge, London, 1998), 34–36.

[159] Quoted in Young-Bruehl, *Anna Freud*, 101.

[160] Mathew Thomson, 'The solution to his own enigma': connecting the life of Montague David Eder (1865–1936), socialist, psychoanalyst, zionist and modern saint', *Medical History*, 55 (2011), 71.

[161] On Child Guidance see: Horn Margo, *Before It's Too Late: The Child Guidance Movement in the United States, 1922–1945* (Temple University Press, Philadelphia, PA, 1989), 39; John Stewart, 'The scientific claims of British Child Guidance, 1918–1945', *British Journal for the History of Science*, 42 (2009), 407–32; John Stewart, *Child Guidance in Britain, 1918–1955: The Dangerous Age of Childhood* (Pickering & Chatto, London, 2013); Deborah Thom, 'Wishes, anxiety, play, and gestures: child guidance in Inter-War England', in Cooter (ed.), *In the Name of the Child*, 200–19; For previous studies focusing on the development of child guidance clinics in Britain, see: George Behlmer, *Friends of the Family: The English Home and Its Guardians, 1850–1940* (Stanford University Press, Stanford, CA, 1998); Olive Sampson, *Child Guidance: Its History, Provenance and Future* (British Psychological Society, London, 1980).

in Britain, and child guidance clinics usually referred to nervous rather than neurotic children. Unlike the Freudian concept of neurosis, neurasthenia or nervousness was a supposedly somatic condition, which meant that parents were freed from feeling guilt in relation to their children's distress, a form of 'cognitive off-loading' to medical technologies and the complexity of their offspring's physicality.[162]

In 1926, *The Lancet* published Millais Culpin's essay 'The nervous child', which explored both physical and emotional factors, arguing that nerves were things that could be seen and handled and that diseases that affected these nerves could be called 'nervous diseases', but that the term 'nervous', when applied to children, meant something quite different.[163] Until recently the lack of medical and psychological knowledge about human 'thoughts or feelings or emotional reactions' meant that, when these processes were disturbed, experts put these disturbances in the category of bodily events. This was despite the fact that these nervous signs had nothing to do with nerve tissue, but concerned unconscious cognitive activities and psychological traumas.[164] Culpin's perspective on nervousness suggests how broad the influence of psychoanalysis and the idea of the unconscious was: nervousness was an 'uncalled-for emotion' beyond the child's control and awareness.[165] 'Nervousness can produce physical symptoms', Culpin argued, claiming that the sequence had been seen the wrong way round, with nervousness regarded as being caused by the physical complaint when it was the emotional pain that caused the physical trouble.[166] Thus for Culpin, the theory of the unconscious was essential to understanding children's neuroses, although he continued to use the term 'nervous' rather than adopt 'neurotic'. Thus, symptoms such as vomiting, headaches and back pain arose from a 'difficulty of adjustment' and 'may be used as a means of escaping that difficulty and thereby become perpetuated'.[167] Even a mental symptom such as night terrors served a purpose, that of 'enforcing the presence of a loved person'.[168] Therefore, children's neuroses and the bodily signs that accompanied them were symptomatic of psychological trauma.

Pain and Mental Illness in Neurosis

After the First World War, pain and psychological illnesses began to be related to studies of childhood in different ways. First, physical suffering was present as a clear diagnostic sign and psychogenic pain – physical pain caused by

[162] Bakker, 'A harmless disease', 323.
[163] Millais Culpin, 'The nervous child', *The Lancet*, 208 (1926), 785–88.
[164] Culpin, 'The nervous child', 785.
[165] Culpin, 'The nervous child', 785.
[166] Culpin, 'The nervous child', 785.
[167] Culpin, 'The nervous child', 785.
[168] Culpin, 'The nervous child', 785.

mental, emotional or behaviour factors or increased or prolonged by them – played a central role in debates about neurosis in children.

Already by the end of 1923, Margaret Lowenfeld had obtained a Medical Research Council scholarship and the Muirhead Fellowship, which enabled her to work under Professor Leonard Findlay at the Royal Hospital for Sick Children, Glasgow, on a study of the relationship between acute rheumatism in children and home conditions.[169] This study was one of the first epidemiological investigations to concentrate on illness in children and to attempt to relate it to lifestyle and material circumstances. Ultimately the study gave rise to the monograph *Social Conditions and Acute Rheumatism*, published in 1927.[170] The survey confirmed a general relationship between rheumatism and the kinds of poor living standards produced by poverty, and it confirmed that there was no simple hereditary mechanism involved. But Lowenfeld did not go as far as to assert that emotional life had an impact on the development of rheumatic pains. Some years later, she developed the concept of the relationship between physical and mental pain in the article 'A new approach to the problem of psychoneurosis in childhood', which was published in 1931.[171] This article, which presented cases of psychoneurosis at the Children's Clinic for the Treatment and Study of Nervous and Delicate Children, argued that 'neurosis represents the reaction of the whole child to his whole circumstances'.[172] Thus, when treating these children, various factors needed to be taken into account, including bodily constitution, physical heredity, mental capacity, emotions and desires. For Lowenfeld, the physical constitution of childhood was quite fluid, which meant that disappointment 'can be the cause of a severe rise of temperature, and the onset of organic disease can be shown, not in pain, but in depression and tears. [. . .] It is often difficult in the case of a child to separate a physical form from an emotional cause'.[173] Unlike an adult, a child does not have a self-awareness that is separated from his or her body, so that pain is felt by the body as a whole. Furthermore, 'mental and physical pain' also tend not to be separated, as 'the child can give no accurate description of either'.[174]

169 On Margaret Lowenfeld, see Cathy Urwin and John Hood-Williams (eds.), *Child Psychotherapy, War, and the Normal Child: Selected Papers of Margaret Lowenfeld* (Free Association Books, London, 1988). PP/LOW/I/22: Box 24, Cathy Urwin, Short article on life of Margaret Lowenfeld, 1999, Archives and Manuscripts, Wellcome Institute.

170 Medical Research Council, *Child Life Investigations: Social Conditions and Acute Rheumatism*, Special Report Series, Archives and Manuscripts, Wellcome Institute No. 114 PPLOW/A/A/2.

171 Margaret Lowenfeld, 'A new Approach to the Problem of Psychoneurosis in Childhood, British Journal of Medical Psychology', 11 (1931) 194–227.

172 Urwin and Hood-Williams, *Child Psychotherapy*, 194.

173 Urwin and Hood-Williams, *Child Psychotherapy*, 195.

174 Urwin and Hood-Williams, *Child Psychotherapy*, 195.

In 1931, the English paediatrician and psychoanalyst Donald Winnicott (1896–1971) tackled the relationship between psychological suffering and rheumatic pain in his first book, *Clinical Notes on the Disorders of Childhood*.[175] In this first attempt to take account of emotional factors in the study of childhood disorders, Winnicott argued that in the case of children with rheumatism, it was possible to look at the problem from 'the point of view of other than rheumatic diseases'.[176] Thus, 'the aches and pains' felt by these children were not rheumatic, argued Winnicott, who held that the 'common pains of childhood' – whether they were felt in the thighs, in the calves, groins, loins, across the chest, in the epigastrium, in the back or in the head – 'may be taken as part of the picture resulting from common difficulties in emotional development'.[177] Such pains were closely connected to other anxiety symptoms, such as lying awake at night, night terrors, excessive sweating, phobias and fidgetiness.[178] He provides the example of eight-year-old Frank C., who was sent to a hospital rheumatism clinic 'as a case of possible rheumatic heart diseases'.[179] The child, a twin in a healthy family of five children, came to Winnicott's practice with a history of recurring illness with pains. Winnicott concluded that, considering that the child did not present swollen joints – an organic injury or condition – the diagnosis was incorrect and that these symptoms and attacks were 'anxiety phenomena'.[180]

Similarly, C. L. C. Burns, director of the Birmingham Child Guidance Clinic, argued in his article 'Neurosis in schoolchildren', published in *The Growing Child and Its Problems* (1937), that one of the most common symptoms of the 'nervously ill' child 'is of course pain'.[181] According to this psychologist, the distinction between the pain of rheumatism and 'neurotic pain' was of considerable importance in the school environment. Thus, those pains 'which come and go, which are felt vaguely in the muscles rather than the joints', and which were not accompanied by other clinical signs of rheumatism, were more likely to be of a psychogenic type and would warn the specialist that he was dealing with a hypersensitive child.[182]

Winnicott developed Lowenfeld's theory further in a paper published in the 1939 *Survey of Child Psychiatry*, edited by Dr Ronald Gordon and published by the Child Guidance Council, and in the very first book that used the words

175 On Winnicott, see Jan Abram (ed.), *Donald Winnicott Today* (Routledge, London, 2013).
176 Donald W. Winnicott, *Clinical Notes on Disorders of Childhood* (William Heinemann (Medical), London, 1931), 66.
177 Winnicott, *Clinical Notes*, 66.
178 Winnicott, *Clinical Notes*, 66.
179 Winnicott, *Clinical Notes*, 67.
180 Winnicott, *Clinical Notes*, 67.
181 C. L. C Burns, 'Neurosis in schoolchildren', in Emmanuel Miller (ed.), The Growing Child and Its Problems (Routledge, Trench, London, Trubner & Co, London, 1937), 175.
182 Burns, 'Neurosis in Schoolchildren', in Miller, The Growing Child, 185.

'child psychiatry' in its title.[183] In this survey, several prominent British writers discuss the emerging clinical discipline under the special headings of physical illness, mental illness, sociologic aspects and special syndromes.[184] This latter category mainly comprised sleep disorders, tics, enuresis, stammering and sexual difficulties.[185] The dialectic between the physiological and the psychological weaves its way throughout the book, from the influence of physical factors and diseases on a child's mental apparatus to the role of the environment in the appearance of mental conditions with physical consequences. In the first section of the book, Winnicott's paper on 'The psychology of juvenile rheumatism' put forward a psychoanalysis of pain, suggesting that the potential depressive child had often been mistaken for a rheumatic and that doctors needed to acknowledge in their practices that many of the physical pains of childhood were not rooted in the body, but in the mind and the emotions.[186]

In 'The physiological approach to psychiatric problems', R. D. Gordon discussed whether it was possible to correlate anatomy, physiology and physical pathology with children's psychiatric problems. To illustrate this question, he quoted 'certain cases of conduct disorder which were presumably of organic origin, followed closely organic illnesses, but which could be paralleled quite easily in any clinic dealing with psychogenic cases'.[187] William Moodie, in his book *The Doctor and the Difficult Child* (1940), also drew a distinction between neuroses that were learnt, and which could be addressed through advice and teaching, and those that resulted from infection or physiological disorder.[188] In 'Hysteria in children', John Bowlby (1907–90) identified pain as one of the most frequent symptoms of hysteria, commenting that 'as in

[183] Richard Bowlby, *Fifty Years of Attachment Theory* (Karnac on behalf of the Winnicott Clinic of Psychotherapy, London, 2004), 5.

[184] R. G. Gordon, on behalf of the Child Guidance Council (ed.), *A Survey of Child Psychiatry: Contributed by Contemporary British Authorities* (Oxford University Press, Humphrey Milford, London, 1939).

[185] The issue of enuresis (bed-wetting) was much associated with evacuees at the time and features repeatedly in recent literature about the health of evacuees. See: Virginia Berridge, 'Health and medicine', in F. M. L. Thompson (ed.), *The Cambridge Social History of Britain 1750–1950, III: Social Agencies and Institutions* (Cambridge University Press, Cambridge, 1990), 239, cited in John Welshman, 'Evacuation, hygiene, and social policy: our towns report of 1943', *The Historical Journal*, 42 (1999), 785; Anne Digby, *British Welfare Policy: Workhouse to Workforce* (Faber & Faber, London, 1989), 55, cited in Welshman, 'Evacuation, hygiene, and social policy', 785; Jennifer Crane, 'Rethinking how evacuees influenced post-war British thinking on health', *Retrospectives*, 2 (2013), 22–41.

[186] Donald Winnicott, 'The psychology of Juvenile Rheumatism', in Gordon, *A Survey of Child Psychiatry*, 28.

[187] R. G. Gordon, 'The physiological approach to psychiatric problems', in Gordon, *A Survey of Child Psychiatry*, 2.

[188] William Moodie, *The Doctor and the Difficult Child* (Commonwealth Fund, New York, 1947), 7–8.

adults the hysterical pain of childhood can almost be of any variety'.[189] Even when some of these symptoms were acquired by the process of identification, something that made them more transitory, in children who suffer from more serious neuroses, pains may become a serious problem and, if not treated properly, 'may interfere with the child's social and school life'.[190] Thus he mentions the case of a thirteen-year-old boy who had 'four attacks of exceedingly severe pain, which caused him to scream'. Sometimes the pain was in the abdomen and other times there were 'terrible pain across his eyes', which made him unable to see.[191] Apart from these attacks of pain, the child was chronically neurotic. During this boy's treatment, the aetiology of his hysteria was unravelled. Bowlby did not see the problem in the child's nervous system but in the quality of his emotional life. On one occasion, the boy had accidentally smashed an electric light bulb. After his father's death, Robert assumed that it resulted from the explosion of the broken bulb, a sense of guilt that Bowlby used to explain his symptoms: the emotional trauma had created the physical pain. Bowlby stressed the need to look for physical causes when diagnosing hysteria, as well as considering the child's personality and the emotional atmosphere in the home.[192]

The Survey of Child Psychiatry thus presents the problems of the children it describes as having been caused by a complex interaction between social, mental and physical conditions. In addition, if each case resulted from a unique combination of these conditions, it would appear that medicine was the only field able to come up with a diagnosis and treatment. However, practitioners also recognised their limitations with regards to difficult cases: in some situations, psychological suffering had no apparent explanation. Thus, in 'Psychoses in children', R. D. Gillespie refers to children who wish to avoid everybody, who experience short depressive phrases at least three times a year, who refuse to eat and to leave the house and who at times 'would laugh or cry without apparent reason'.[193]

Gillespie's account shows how experts started to recognise the difficulty of correcting behavioural problems through education and the cultivation of healthy habits of self-control, and it speaks to the gradual change from religious or moral interpretations to a psycho-medical perspective that saw these behaviours as manifestations of deviations from healthy emotional development. 'Difficult' children were no longer seen as being guilty of the illness that afflicted them, and the importance of the external conditions was recognised. Causation, which until recently had been located in the nervous

[189] John Bowlby, 'Hysteria in children', in Gordon, *A Survey of Child Psychiatry*, 81.
[190] Bowlby, 'Hysteria in children', in Gordon, *A Survey of Child Psychiatry*, 81.
[191] Bowlby, 'Hysteria in children', in Gordon, *A Survey of Child Psychiatry*, 81.
[192] Bowlby, 'Hysteria in children' in Gordon, *A Survey of Child Psychiatry*, 81.
[193] R. D. Gillespie, 'Psychoses in children', in Gordon, *A Survey of Child Psychiatry*, 66–79.

system, was now externalised. Psychoanalysis, in particular, considered the interaction between parents and children during early childhood as the most important cause of neurosis. Thus, Winnicott presented 'nervousness' as the expression of a neurotic child or one who had an Oedipal conflict.[194] In 'Personality deviations in children', Clifford Allen of the Institute of Medical Psychology argued that the path to the development of an adequate personality in a child was a 'slow, painful and dangerous one'.[195] For this medical psychologist, certain conditions needed to be fulfilled for a child to develop a suitable personality. Among these was the need for parents with appropriate personalities, so that when the child modelled itself on them it would have a 'store of reliable responses obtained from them'.[196] Given its 'malleable' condition, the mind of the child was regarded as being particularly vulnerable to infection by 'nervous aches and pain' or neurotic ones.

Second, if the main symptom of children with personality disorders was that of pain without any physical injury, one of the causes of such disorders could be that the child lived in an atmosphere 'which has been emotionally painful to it'.[197] In not having encountered the conditions for emotional development, the intellect of these children 'has never been able to show itself as it really is', producing the personality disorder of the 'sad type', often regarded as a mentally defective child and 'treated accordingly all its life'.[198]

Following Freud, the idea that the repression of traumatic experiences is at the base of neurotic behaviour ran through a good part of the period's literature about childhood neurosis. Thus, Hugh Crichton-Miller highlighted the importance of exposing fears and addressing the dangers of emotional repression:[199] 'When we repress, a rather complicated process occurs' in which certain ideas become 'for some reason painful to the conscious mind' of the child and cannot be thought of without being accompanied by 'some painful emotion'. The repression of these thoughts and emotions leads to a neurotic process, claimed Crichton-Miller, for whom the repression of painful emotions was the main cause of a neurotic child. In his *The New Psychology and the Teacher* (1923), he described neurosis as 'the choice of physical suffering instead of mental suffering', showing once again the dynamic complications between emotional and physiological pain, and the relationship between body, mind and emotions in the causation of neurosis.[200] Crichton-Miller believed that

194 Papers by Donald Winnicott, 1979, Archives and Manuscripts, Wellcome Institute GC148/21/21.
195 Clifford Allen, 'Personality Deviations in Children', in Miller, The Growing Child, 115.
196 Allen, 'Personality Deviations in Children', 115.
197 Allen, 'Personality Deviations in Children', 124.
198 Allen, 'Personality Deviations in Children', 124.
199 Hugh Crichton-Miller, *The New Psychology and the Parent* (Jarrolds, London, 1922), 137.
200 Hugh Crichton-Miller, *The New Psychology and the Teacher* (Jarrolds, London, 1923), 38.

psychodynamic methodologies could prevent these first minor nervous disorders from developing into serious long-term mental and social problems.

While emphasising the role of the domestic environment in the aetiology of neurosis, Crichton-Miller also recognised that there was often more than 'bad parenting' behind antisocial and undesirable behaviour in the young. He highlighted modernity, arguing in a 1926 paper that many cases of neurosis could have resulted from social changes as Britain moved from strictly defined Victorian behavioural rules and expectations to more liberal values, which created the potential for intergenerational conflict.[201] Following this line of thinking, Paterson Brown, the medical director of the North-Western London Child Guidance Clinic, considered that the development of manias and nervous habits could be caused by a process through which the child 'may compensate for some painful condition in the environment, or in the child'. Some lines later, Brown noted how the 'most important' and difficult-to-understand mechanism a child has for relieving anxiety is 'seeking pain or self-punishment'.[202]

The relationship between pleasure and pain takes us to the third way in which psychological illnesses were related to pain. In a paradoxical move that would have been impossible in the clinical tradition, the combination of trauma and recollection appeared connected to a form of pleasure that a modern reader might label as 'masochistic' or 'self-pity'. In *The Problem of the Nervous Child* (1919), the psychoanalyst Elida Evans developed this subject in the chapter 'Pleasure in pain', in which she argued that 'the habit of experiencing painful emotions is acquired through the pleasure which is associated with pain itself'.[203] For this American psychoanalyst, 'any discharge of accumulated vitality is accompanied with a distinct sense of pleasure'.[204] But should the pleasure of discharge be 'associated with an adventitious pain administered by parents', a link between pleasure and pain would be established.[205] Evans deployed this argument to criticise the use of corporal punishment, because if a child learnt to associate unpleasantness with duty, 'he is not only given a mental twist which makes him see everything wrongly, but one which prevents him from acting wholesomely in every most intimate relation of a later love life'.[206] She comments that 'it cannot be too strongly emphasized that the pleasurable emotions are the creative ones, which build up, or furnish the most favourable conditions for building up, the tissues of the body and thus making for both mental and physical health', while 'the

201 Hugh Crichton-Miller, 'Psychology and social hygiene', *Journal of Social Hygiene*, 12 (1926), 14–24.

202 W. Paterson Brown, 'The family neurosis', in Gordon, *A Survey of Child Psychiatry*, 121.

203 Elida Evans, *The Problem of the Nervous Child* (Kegan Paul, Trench Trubner, London, 1919), 30.

204 Evans, *The Problem*, 30.

205 Evans, *The Problem*, 30.

206 Evans, *The Problem*, 45.

unpleasurable emotions are destructive and make for both physical and mental illness'.[207] Hence, consequences for both physical and mental health in children were established for the negative emotions generated by physical pain inflicted by parental authority.

The theme of negative emotions and their repercussions would be developed in the United Kingdom by Melanie Klein who, initially inspired by Freud, developed her own theory of object relations and created a new school of psychoanalysis.[208] In Kleinian theory, the maternal figure represents a world that is satisfying and frustrating to the infant at the same time.[209] The frustration – when hungry, for instance – arouses 'sadistic feelings' and impulses directed to 'his external object', the mother.[210] Klein believed that children should be allowed to express their aggression and violent fantasies and that, to enable this, it was important for the analyst to tackle the subject of early hatred of the mother.[211] She also suggested that guilt and anxiety, which often manifested in aggressive behaviour, might sometimes be an unrecognized problem in children who seemed to be well behaved and docile.[212]

Winnicott, too, acknowledged the importance of Freud's instinct theory and agreed with Klein that psychoanalysis needed to go further in examining the pre-verbal, pre-Oedipal phase of development. But he also rejected some of Klein's ideas (on the death instinct, for instance) and developed his own model in which the psychic pain of psychopathology is caused by the failure of the earliest environment, and the vagaries of emotional growth are overcome through the internalisation of a 'good enough' psychic environment. Winnicott's celebrated article 'Hate in the countertransference' (1949) portrays hate as a developmental achievement rather than (as Klein would have it) an affect emanating from the death instinct.[213] Winnicott emphasises the responsibility of the mother's ordinary devotion towards her infant that will facilitate good enough development.

One of Klein's beliefs was that infants are beset by the fear of being destroyed or losing loved ones and that this preoccupation with destruction

[207] Evans, *The Problem*, 30.

[208] On Melanie Klein, see Shapira, *The War Inside*; Julia Kristeva (trans. Ross Guberman), *Melanie Klein* (Columbia University Press, New York, 2002); Meira Likierman, *Melanie Klein: Her Work in Context* (Continuum, London, 2001).

[209] Melanie Klein, 'Weaning', in John Rickman, *On the Bringing Up of Children* (Paul, Trench, Trubner, London, 1936), 33.

[210] Melanie Klein, 'Early stages of the Oedipus conflict and of super-ego formation', in John Rickman (ed.), *The Psychoanalysis of Children* (The Hogarth Press, London, 1975), 148.

[211] Melanie Klein, 'Symposium on child-analysis', *International Journal of Psychoanalysis*, 8 (1927), 339–70.

[212] Klein, 'Symposium on child-analysis', 370.

[213] D. W. Winnicott, 'Hate in the counter-transference', *The Journal of Psychotherapy Practice and Research*, 3 (1994), 348–56.

and death is expressed in children's play, where anguish is expressed towards the external object. In 'The nursery as a community' – published in the book *On the Bringing Up of Children*, edited by John Rickman and Susan Isaacs (1885–1948) – Isaacs also discussed this theme, arguing that neurotic aggression was produced in the child who had felt detached from his mother who 'thus [became] to him[self] almost entirely an object of disappointment and pain'.[214] Isaacs important work is discussed in the next chapter.

The child then resorts to an excessive hate and defiance against the 'internal pain or remorse and guilt', projecting this aggression towards the being he loves, his mother.[215] A year earlier, in the lecture 'Rebellious and defiant children', Isaacs had shown how children who displayed a tendency to enjoy inflicting pain on others had 'a special sensitivity to those issues of love and hate, hidden behind their outer shell of apparent hardness and lack of remorse'.[216] Thus, 'the pain and frustration' for the child of hating the person he loves is almost unbearable and is lessened or removed by the aggressive expression of inflicting pain upon others. Like Winnicott and Melanie Klein, Issacs outlined a psychoanalytic theory in which the interplay between body, mind and emotions can be extremely complex, collapsing the distinction between physical and emotional pain.

Conclusion

Historians of childhood have recently paid attention to the question of the relationship between body and mind from the perspective of diachronic change. In their influential text, 'From bodies to minds in childcare literature', Cathy Urwin and Elaine Sharland made a stark division between mind and body, the physical and the psychological, by arguing that in the United Kingdom between the wars there was a shift 'from bodies to minds' in perceptions of children and childhood.[217] By extending this line of argument to the history of pain, this chapter has questioned the extent to which one can apply a clear distinction between the suffering of the body and that of the mind. It has also explored the intertwining of somatic and psychic pain, the boundaries between which are anything but distinct.

This chapter presumes that this transition from bodies to minds was not a sudden paradigm shift, but rather a slow and sometimes tentative process of change. It has argued that the history of nervous pain (painful symptoms without a lesion located in the body's nervous system) and the history of

[214] Susan Isaacs, 'The nursery as a community', in John Rickman, *On the Bringing Up of Children* (Paul, Trench, Trubner, London, 1936), 187.
[215] Isaacs, 'The nursery', 187. [216] Isaacs, 'The nursery', 187.
[217] Urwin and Sharland, 'From bodies to minds', 174–99.

psychogenic or unconscious pain (where the same symptoms were understood on the basis of a psychological localisation in the mind) took place in parallel, across separate but coexisting disciplines. In line with the preceding chapters, this one has shown that pain is a concept with multiple meanings that is interpreted by different communities through social practices and rituals that can coexist at the same historical moment. Thus, very different diagnoses can be made based on the same symptoms depending on whether they are observed from the perspective of neurology, paediatrics, child psychology or psychiatry. Leading neurologists such as Thomas D. Savill, who subscribed to the general principles of the anatomo-clinical tradition, generally dismissed the idea that pain could exist without a material lesion and postulated a 'seat of disease' in the nervous system for many kinds of pain without apparent lesions. However, paediatricians such as Hector Cameron and psychoanalysts such as Donald Winnicott came to believe that a psychological illness could cause physical pain unrelated to physical injury – so-called psychogenic pain. Those psychologists and psychoanalysts who, starting from the First World War, studied the subject of psychogenic pain did not work on the basis of a mind–body dualism and did not trace a clear dividing line between body and mind. Like neurologists, they also found extensive evidence that physical pain could not only accompany or exacerbate psychological illness, but also, in some cases, cause it.

The identification of 'uncaused symptoms' and their assignment to a scientific nomenclature created a conflict between the predominant anatomo-clinical tradition and the emerging theories of psychoanalysis, which both sought to understand illness and childhood. While the former still applied the principle that there were correspondences of a morphological nature between symptoms and organic lesions – even to the extent of making ad hoc adjustments to explain an invisible lesion and thereby keep the principle intact – the latter had no hesitation in dropping that principle and shifting causation to the dangers of development amid environmental pressures. However, for psychogenic pains to appear in the study of childhood nervous conditions, it was first necessary that interpreters defined the illnesses as functional accidents that led to forms of somatisation or behavioural patterns of a psychological origin. Thus, while running in parallel, the physiological discourses on 'nervousness' may have been a major condition for the possibility of conceiving psychoanalytical discourses on 'neurosis'.

Concerning childhood, it was necessary that the symptoms of the young patient were studied within a medical and psychological framework specific to infancy, rather than on the basis of theories about adult constitutions. While neurologists studied the figure of the child in relation to the adult, paediatricians sought to expand their focus to include psychogenic as well as somatic pain, thereby creating new diagnostic models that went beyond those of the neurologists. Meanwhile, psychoanalysts, like paediatricians, studied childhood neuroses from within their own theoretical and diagnostic framework. We should not forget the importance of the figure of the child in the field of psychoanalysis and the Freudian idea that adult neuroses originated in childhood traumas. Thus, following the nineteenth-century Wordsworthian idea that 'the child is father of the man', a double process came about in which childhood psychoanalysis was promoted as a way to understand adult neuroses, just as adult patients were encouraged to regress to their childhood to solve their problems.

5 The Pain of Separation

In March 1941, Patrick, 'a boy of three years and two months, of pleasing appearance, well built and rather big for his age', was sent to the Hampstead War Nurseries – set up by the exiled Viennese psychoanalyst Anna Freud in 1941 to provide foster care for child victims of the war – after a previous attempt at evacuation to the country had proven unsuccessful.[1] The little boy had started to wet the bed and, as a result, the billet to which he had been sent during the Blitz 'would not keep him' and he had to return home only a couple of days later. Unfortunately, the reunion with his mother did not last very long. Soon after his return, Patrick came down with measles, forcing a second separation from his mother. After he recovered, the mother took the child to Anna Freud at the Hampstead War Nurseries. Leaving him there, she told him to behave like 'a good boy' and said she would come and visit him, but only if he promised not to cry. As in many other similar clinical cases, 'the state of affairs that developed after she left "was a most unhappy one"'.[2] Young Patrick struggled to keep his word. He did not cry but kept nodding his head and repeating a litany, saying that his mother 'would come for him, she would put on his overcoat and would take him home with her again'. After a couple of days, the nodding became more compulsive and Patrick started to add to the list of clothes his mother would bring: 'She will put on my overcoat and my leggings, she will zip up the zipper, she will put on my pixie hat.'[3] A worker at the clinic urged the boy to change his attitude, so – trying to comply with his mother's demand that he behave like a good boy – Patrick stopped repeating the formula aloud. But the small movements of his lips demonstrated that the compulsion had not ceased. Soon the spoken words were replaced by 'gestures that showed the position of his pixie hat, the putting on of an imaginary coat, the zipping of the zipper etc.'. Finally, Patrick entered a state of nervous compulsion, with a weak and rapid pulse,

[1] Freud and Burlingham, *War and Children*, 26.
[2] Freud and Burlingham, *War and Children*, 26.
[3] Freud and Burlingham, *War and Children*, 26.

with no interest in the outside world and 'with an absolutely tragic expression on his face'.[4]

In this way, Anna Freud and Dorothy Burlingham described, in their 1943 book *War and Children*, the shock they felt on seeing an apparently healthy and 'normal' boy develop a 'compulsive tic' in front of their very eyes. For the exiled Viennese psychologist, who was among the first to document how children suffered when separated from their parents during the war, Patrick's trauma was directly related to 'the pain of separation'. Like most of the literature coming from the sphere of psychoanalysis, *War and Children* was based on the assumption that, if essential needs – such as 'the need for personal attachment, for emotional stability, and for permanency of educational influence' – were not met, then it was probable that there would be lasting psychological malformations.[5] While the general consensus was that the conditions the war imposed upon the lives of children would cause lasting bodily malformation in later years, according to Freud and Burlingham, 'it is not generally recognised that the same is true for the mental development of the child'.[6] Based on this argument, and combining clinical cases with theoretical suppositions, Freud and Burlingham offered a study that went beyond the material and physical effect of the war on children to consider the impact of loss, separation and familial break-up on the emotional and psychological development of young children.

This chapter deals with the emotional pain inflicted on children in the UK during the Second World War through the forced evacuation of the underage urban population to rural areas. The topic of evacuation represents a continuation of Chapter 4, because it was psychoanalysis – thanks to the work of some remarkable pioneering women who had been directly influenced by Freud's practice – that proved to be the medical discipline most able to address the complexity of the problem in its different layers, including social policy, national health and civic education. If psychoanalysis decoded the figuration of the evacuee, the Second World War proved to be the moment when the new discipline consolidated itself. Several historical studies have investigated the evacuation schemes and the experiences of children who were relocated. Prominent among these are Richard M. Titmus, John Macnicol, John Welshman and Jennifer Crane.[7] But while the topic has been widely

4 Freud and Burlingham, *War and Children*, 26.

5 Freud and Burlingham, *War and Children*, 6.

6 Freud and Burlingham, *War and Children*, 6.

7 See Richard M. Titmuss, *Problems of Social Policy* (His Majesty's Stationary Office, London, 1950); John Macnicol, 'The effect of the evacuation of school children on official attitudes to state intervention', in H. L. Smith (ed.), *War and Social Change: British Society in the Second World War* (Manchester University Press, Manchester, 1986); Robert Holman, *The Evacuation: A Very British Revolution* (Lion, Oxford, 1995); and John Welshman, 'Evacuation and social

explored – because of the importance of the Second World War, the visible results in social policy and the catastrophic consequences of evacuation – so far, no scholar has investigated the issue within the framework of the history of pain, focusing on the suffering of the evacuated children and how their suffering was framed by the various scientific and medical communities involved.

This chapter is organised around two themes. It first explores how the sight of children's suffering – the aesthetics of pain – was used in different ways by the authorities. The second section contrasts such official discourse on children's suffering with the different ways that the child's body was rendered in two main domains: traditional medical discourse and psychoanalytic theory and practice.[8] The first section of the chapter first surveys the socialised making and remaking of the child image during this agonising wartime period, focusing on the forced evacuations, which were conceived of as a preventive action against the bombings.[9] As Mathew Thomson has argued, the literature of 'total war' provides two powerful and contrasting images that have frequently been deployed to illustrate what became the dominant narrative of Britain's war. On the one hand, there is the evacuee, distraught and abused, torn from home and family. On the other, there is the child of the Blitz, playing in the ruins of the city, a symbol of hope and defiance amid destruction.[10]

policy during the Second World War: myth and reality', *Twentieth Century British History*, 9 (1998), 28–53.

8 Work that used psychoanalysis to connect psychology and ethics before and during the war included: Edward Glover, *War, Sadism and Pacifism* (George Allen & Unwin, London, 1947); William Brown, *War and Peace: Essay in Psychological Analysis* (A. & C. Black, London, 1939); Roger Money-Kyrle, 'Towards a common aim: psychoanalytic contribution to ethics', *British Journal of Medical Psychology*, 20 (1944), 105–17; Roger Money-Kyrle, *Psychoanalysis and Politics: A Contribution to the Psychology of Politics and Morals* (Duckworth, London, 1951). See also Evan Durbin, *The Politics of Democratic Socialism* (Routledge, London, 1940); John Carl Fluger, *Man, Morals and Society: A PsychoAnalytical Study* (International Universities Press, New York, 1945); Donald W. Winnicott, 'Some thoughts on the meaning of the word democracy', *Human Relations*, 3 (1950), 175–86; Wilfred R. Bion, 'Psychiatry at a time of crisis', *British Journal of Medical Psychology*, 21 (1948), 81–89; H. V. Dicks, 'In search of our proper ethics', *British Journal of Medical Psychology*, 21 (1948), 1–14; Ernest Jones, 'The psychology of quislingism', *The International Journal of Psychoanalysis*, 22 (1941), 1–12; Ernest Jones, 'How can civilization be saved?', *The International Journal of Psychoanalysis*, 24 (1942), 1–7.

9 Notable academic publications on evacuation include: Martin Parsons, *I'll Take That One: Dispelling the Myths of Civilian Evacuation, 1939–1945* (Beckett Karlson, Peterborough, 1998); Holman, *The Evacuation*; Macnicol, 'The effect of the evacuation of school children'; John Stewart and John Welshman, 'Culture, behaviour and poverty: the evacuation of children in Scotland, 1939–1945', *Journal of Scottish Historical Studies*, 26 (2006), 100–20; Welshman, 'Evacuation, hygiene, and social policy', 781–807; Welshman, 'Evacuation and social policy', 28–53.

10 Thomson, *Lost Freedom*, 1–21.

This section provides an analysis of the child in Second World War Britain: 'the bombed child', who suffered the physical and mental trauma of the air raids, and 'the uprooted child', who was evacuated from the bombed cities to rural 'safety' but who suffered the pain of separation. These categories overlap: the threat of the bombs was a pervasive danger that inflicted significant psychological damage on children, especially when separated from parents and relatives left behind in the cities that were being bombed. The figure of the uprooted child is explored not only in the medical literature but also in political discourse and propaganda. In contrast with the debates between different medical professions covered in earlier chapters of this book, the discussion on the uprooted child actively engaged public opinion and was closely monitored by – and sometimes entering into conflict with – politicians and policymakers. While psychoanalysts saw an image of fragile children suffering from emotional disturbance because of both the bombs and the policy of evacuation, certain social groups in the rural areas that received the evacuees saw only unruly urban children who spread diseases through their dirty habits, and other circles of opinion saw the same children as victims of poverty and social injustice.[11]

This chapter then examines the resulting texts and how they relate empirically to the compiled data, and it considers the scientific discourses that framed the understanding of emotional damage from these two different, yet interwoven, causes: bombing and separation. Through literary readings and explorations of the scientific and medical discourses of the era, this chapter reconstructs the controversy over the consolidation of the child with emotional pain as an object of study in psychology, psychoanalysis and medicine. This process involved evaluation, normalisation, symptomology, inclusion in a taxonomic system and the attribution of diagnostic value. It started with evaluating signs, which were then converted into symptoms on the basis of which the new medical category of separation anxiety was created, leading in turn to diagnoses of children as suffering from this new illness and to the creation of a new diagnostic category: the child with separation anxiety.

However, there was disagreement about this new diagnostic category, extending the debate over somatic and psychogenic conditions that was analysed in the previous chapters. Doctors debated whether the physical shock of the bombs provoked psychological disturbances or whether it was the other way around – that the fear and anxiety provoked by the bombing caused organic illnesses. Meanwhile, psychologists and psychoanalysts argued that,

[11] Sarah Hayes has argued that by 1927 a medical model had developed in Britain relating to maladjusted children which consisted of two polarised categories of children: psychological 'rabbits' and delinquent 'rebels.' See 'Rabbits and rebels', in Mark Jackson (ed.), *Health and the Modern Home*, 128–52.

while the evacuated children may have been saved from physical harm, they had also been subjected to considerable emotional harm as a result of separation from their homes and families, and in particular from their mothers. Psychoanalysts used their reflections on the nature and consequences of the pain of separation as part of a project to legitimise psychoanalysis as a discipline that could preserve healthy citizens and their contributions to the democratic regime. A comparison of the discourse of doctors, psychoanalysts and psychologists shows the depth of disagreements about the extent to which children were affected when separated from their mothers, the relationship between the age of a child and the development of a neurotic behaviour, and symptomology. This diversity of opinion is reflected even more in the analysis of the problems related to the classification, causality and interpretation of signs through which separation anxiety was woven. Similar symptoms provoked different diagnoses, depending on whether they were observed from the position of paediatrics, from the view of exiled continental analysts, such as Melanie Klein and Anna Freud, or by native analysts such as John Bowlby and Donald Winnicott.

Thus, Patrick's case was read and understood in different ways by different interest groups and scientific bodies. By considering the child's appearance and how these same symptoms were seen across a range of other cultural sites – such as psychoanalysis and medicine – this chapter argues that the expression of children's emotional suffering, represented chiefly by signs such as enuresis and behavioural problems, was subject to different interpretations depending on the different professional bodies invested with the performative authority required to shape its meaning.[12] Thus, there were those such as the Tavistock Institute psychotherapists Theodora Alcock and W. E. Mons who saw these symptoms as indications of 'war strain' or 'air raid shock', a form of stress reaction that today would probably be diagnosed as post-traumatic stress disorder. At the same time, psychoanalysts interpreted the very same symptoms as indicating separation anxiety.

This chapter argues that the new psychological category of the child with separation anxiety was yet another form of disciplinary objectification. While there was rarely any suitable treatment available, this category allowed the children to be catalogued and both their public behaviour and private experience to be studied. The following pages define the historical and sociological context of the discussions about separation anxiety in relation to two axiological institutions: the family and democracy. While the emerging role of psychoanalysis served the conservative function of preserving the centrality of

[12] The issue of enuresis (bed-wetting) was much associated with evacuees at the time and features repeatedly in recent literature about the health of evacuees. See Welshman, 'Evacuation, hygiene, and social policy'; Crane, 'Rethinking how evacuees', 22–41.

these two central constructs for social coexistence, it also changed quite radically the notion of a normally functioning individual and the nature of social bonds, serving as an ancillary discipline to the emergence of social democracy. The chapter reconstructs the controversy over the impact of the Second World War on children's mental and physical health, exploring how children's signs of emotional pain – bed-wetting, anxiety and bad habits – were conceived, conceptualised, contested and diagnosed.

At the same time, a dialogue is established between the sources used by social historians interested in the 'slum mentality' of the evacuee and those used by cultural historians and historians of psychiatry interested in the genealogy of separation anxiety, thereby highlighting the coexistence of two different figurations of childhood during the Second World War, both based on the figure of the evacuee. On the one hand, there was the dirty, ill-trained child whose symptoms were framed within the myth of the 'slum mentality'; on the other hand, there was the 'uprooted' child, whose symptoms reflected a deep emotional pain. Yet the construction of both figurations was based on the same bodily signs. The different accounts of the symptoms and their inclusion in competing taxonomic systems produced a conflict between rival cultural and social visions of childhood.

In addition to scientific and psychoanalytic sources previously analysed in published works that reviewed the crystallisation of theories of attachment as a result of the Second World War and the evacuation policy – based on key texts such as the *Cambridge Evacuation Survey* and Anna Freud's writing – this chapter draws on psychological, medical and other relevant publications on children's evacuation, beginning with Katherine M. Wolf's *Evacuation of Children in Wartime – A Survey of the Literature, with Bibliography*.[13] The aim has been to access perceptions from beyond the higher reaches of psychoanalysis (the likes of Anna Freud and John Bowlby) to include other perceptions of children's pain from lay figures as well as specialists.

The story of separation anxiety has been written in the context of the 'subjectification' (to use Foucault's term) that took place in psychoanalytic practice around the time of the war. In fact, a key aspect of Foucault's concept of subjectification was precisely the representation of childhood, motherhood, fatherhood, parental conduct and family life through expert discourses that 'infuse[d] and shape[d] the personal investments of individuals'.[14] This took place not only through government institutions but also through the media of books about childcare, radio broadcasts and women's magazines, as well as through mothercraft training.

[13] Katharine M. Wolf, 'Evacuation of children in wartime – a survey of the literature, with bibliography', *Psychoanalytic Study of the Child*, 1 (1945), 389.

[14] Nikolas Rose, *Governing the Soul: The Shaping of the Private Self* (Routledge, London, 1998).

Some social and cultural historians have investigated the profound interest provoked by the mother–child bond during the Second World War and the post-war period.[15] Some of these studies referred to the sociopolitical interests that underlay the confinement of women to domesticity and maternity, the personal interests that guided professionals and the cryptic nature of the language of psychology, with its jargon expressions such as 'maternal deprivation', the 'bond' between mother and child and 'maternal instinct'.[16] Feminist historians have wrestled with the legacy of some psychoanalytic theories that were developed during this period, which seemed to load the collective responsibility for the emotional sanity of the society onto the mother–child dyad.[17] As Juliet Mitchell noted, given the effect of locating the remedy for social ills in a heterosexual, two-parent family, with a traditional division of labour according to sex and with a separation between the private, feminine world of care and the public, masculine sphere of business, 'the developments of child psychoanalysis contributed very neatly to the political demands of the epoch'.[18]

Historians have also portrayed the evacuation policy as a defining point in modern British social history. According to James Hinton, placing urban working-class (and often impoverished) children in the countryside 'involved the negotiation of profound cultural differences, not only between town and country but also between class and class'.[19] Discussing the attitudes of the Women's Voluntary Service, an important voluntary organisation, he further argues that the 'rifts and chasms of Britain's social fabric revealed by the early experiences of evacuation had long-term consequences for both working-class and middle-class perceptions of social inequality'.[20] Sonya Rose similarly claims that the evacuation process 'produced a discourse concerning "the social question" that underscored the dire consequences of urban poverty and brought national attention to its victims'. It also highlighted, in her view,

15 Rose, *Governing the Soul*; Hendrick, 'Children's emotional well-being', 213–42; Shapira, *The War Inside*, 1–23; Urwin and Sharland, 'From bodies to minds'; Davis, 'British child psychology and the evacuation'; Marga Vicedo, *The Nature and Nurture of Love: From Imprinting to Attachment in Cold War America* (University of Chicago Press, Chicago, 2013); Frank C. P. van der Horst, *John Bowlby – From Psychoanalysis to Ethology: Unraveling the Roots of Attachment Theory* (Wiley-Blackwell, Chichester, 2011).

16 Angela Davis, *Modern Motherhood: Women and Family in England, 1945–2000* (Manchester University Press, Manchester, 2014), chapter 5.

17 Denise Riley notes that feminist interpretations of 'Bowlbyism' have taken it as no coincidence that after the war childcare facilities for the children of working mothers were withdrawn at the same time as Bowlby's ideas were widely promulgated. Denise Riley, *War in the Nursery: Theories of the Child and Mother* (Virago, London, 1983).

18 Juliet Mitchell, *Psychoanalysis and Feminism* (Basic Books, New York, 1974), 229.

19 James Hinton, *Social Leadership, and the Second World War: Continuities of Class* (Oxford University Press, Oxford, 2002), 147–48.

20 Hinton, *Social Leadership*, 147–48.

the 'focal point between what were imagined to be two opposing ways of life – urban and rural'.[21] The historian of childhood Harry Hendrick remarks that evacuation was 'one of those rare moments when prejudice, mainly shaped and articulated by sections of the rural and small-town middle class, unveils itself unashamedly'.[22]

Some recent studies have examined the centrality of theories of attachment to the constitution of the democratic project during the Second World War. Hendrick has argued that 'the specific issue of hospital visiting became one of the areas where 'separation anxiety', as a psychoanalytic condition in young children, was held to constitute a direct threat to national fitness' and to the idea of the democratic subject.[23] He is not the only one to have drawn such a conclusion. Michal Shapira has recently investigated, in *The War Inside*, how the major social function for psychoanalysis at this time was to educate British citizens in the effort of recognising and managing the 'war inside', which was seen as a fundamental element of human nature that also mirrored the external engagement of democracy against the barbaric forces of totalitarianism.[24] Shapira argues that the mental health and psychology of young children gained extraordinary importance during the Second World War, as 'psychoanalytic experts made the understanding of children and the mother–child relationship key to the successful creation of social democracy'.[25] Both Hendrick and Shapira are right to note that expert discussion turned its focus to the mental health and psychology of children, yet it is important to emphasise that the figure of the child in pain during the Second World War was not an exclusively or predominantly a scientific figuration. Instead, the sciences – whether medical science or the newer psychological and social sciences – drew on wider cultural domains to which they also contributed and which they sometimes contradicted. Attention to the actual symptoms of separation anxiety in relation to the different renderings of the child body in psychoanalytic practices, British medicine and social discourse and welfare during the Second World War is a novel contribution that this book makes to the academic debate.

Pain as Propaganda

The cover of the US magazine *LIFE* published on 23 September 1940 did not take long to establish itself as one of the great icons of the battle against the

[21] Sonya O. Rose, *Which People's War? National Identity and Citizenship in Wartime Britain 1939–1945* (Oxford University Press, Oxford, 2003), 56, 208.
[22] Hendrick, *Child Welfare: Historical*, 124.
[23] Hendrick, 'Children's emotional well-being', 213–42.
[24] Shapira, *The War Inside*, 1–23.
[25] Shapira, The War Inside, 1.

Third Reich.[26] In the picture, a little girl clutches a worn-out stuffed toy while staring straight at the camera in an innocent, slightly sad, almost heart-melting way. The text that accompanies the photograph adds to the narrative and renders the story possible: 'The wide-eyed young lady on the cover' is Eileen Dunne, a young victim of the Blitz who is recovering from her injuries in a bed in a hospital in the north of England. 'A German bomber whose crew had never met her dropped a bomb on a North England village' and 'a splinter from it hit Eileen'.[27] A 'plucky chorus of wounded children' had just finished singing "Roon, Rabbit, Roon' [a northern-dialect version of 'Run, Rabbit, Run'], when the British photographer Cecil Beaton released the shutter of his camera, immortalising the image of Eileen and of many other British children who lived through the Blitz (Figure 5.1).[28] At the time the photograph of Eileen was published, Winston Churchill's Ministry of Information, a fully propagandistic instrument of the government, was behind Beaton's commission to furnish a positive photographic representation of the struggle on British soil. At that moment, the country was losing the propaganda war against a very well-organised German machine and needed artists who could transmit the pain of military violence and the struggle of the British people through the media of mechanical reproduction.[29] His photographs, which tried to reflect the devastation of the Blitz and the capacity for resistance of ordinary British people, were published in pamphlets and magazines that were distributed both nationally and internationally, as objects of information and consumption.

During these years of strife, Kenneth Clark, the director of the National Gallery, established a consultative committee of artists which, for the purposes of propaganda, built up the myth of the Blitz. Created with the blessing of the Ministry of Information, the War Artists' Advisory Committee (WAAC) sent artists – from painters and printmakers to photographers – to the cities in flames. The ministry believed that the work of the artists would leave a valuable testimony of the difficult times, and that they would in turn give moral support to the British public. The artists and photographers of the WAAC had to portray all that was useful and interesting for the purposes of propaganda in the United Kingdom and in neutral countries, for the history of art, and for military history. To achieve this, Clark relied on certain guidelines that determined what should be photographed and the way it should be done to fulfil each of the Ministry of Information's objectives. Ideas for

[26] Hilary Roberts, *Cecil Beaton: Theatre of War* (Jonathan Cape, London, 2012), 25.

[27] *LIFE Magazine*, 23 September 1940, 21. [28] *LIFE Magazine*, 23 September 1940, 21.

[29] On war artists and the Second World War See Brian Frederick Foss, *War Paint: Art, War, State and Identity in Britain, 1939–1945* (Yale Books, New Haven, CT, 2007); Brian Frederick Foss, 'British artists and the Second World War. With particular reference to the War Artists', Advisory Committee of the Ministry of Information' (Unpublished PhD thesis, University College London, 1991).

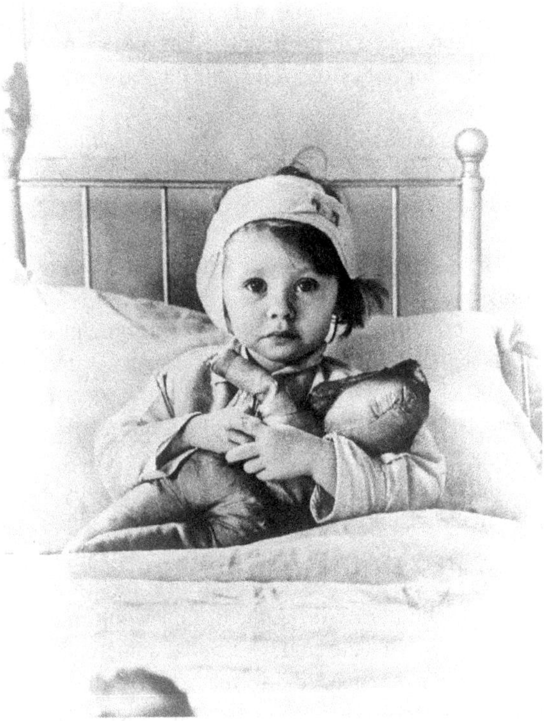

Figure 5.1 Cecil Beaton, *Copy negative made from vintage print. Eileen Dunne, aged three, sits in bed with her doll at the Great Ormond Street Hospital for Sick Children, after being injured during an air raid on London in September 1940* (1940), MH 26395, Ministry of Information Second World War Official Collection, Imperial War Museum.

commissioning pictures of bombed buildings were promoted – especially during 1940 – as well as photographs of children and civilians suffering and enduring the consequences of the Blitz. According to a letter published in the British magazine the *Connoisseur* (1940), such images were both a 'permanent record for posterity' and propaganda aimed at the American public, 'whose sympathy with Britain's cause is growing daily, [and who] would have the opportunity of seeing exactly what the enemy has done to our symbols of mutual culture'.[30] One of these missions led to Cecil Beaton's visit to the north of England and to his picture of Eileen Dunne. Published more than a year before the United States entered the war, this moving photograph was one of

[30] A. E. Cooper and Adrian Bury, 'Glorious London', *Connoisseur*, 106 (1940), 265.

the most potent examples of visual propaganda produced during those years. The image was widely reproduced in pro-war media in the United States and became an icon of the call for help from the UK to its brothers and sisters on the other side of the Atlantic.

Two days before the publication of *LIFE*'s issue, the *Illustrated London News* published a slightly different version of the Beaton photograph on its inside front cover. In the *LIFE* photograph, Eileen held the toy forcefully pinned to her body, carrying the pain with stoicism and showing a much more traumatic experience of the Blitz, indicating that there was no justification for her pain and suffering.

The second image, in contrast, did not present a girl tormented by physical suffering but more as an icon in line with the normative representation of Romantic childhood. The photograph published in the *Illustrated London News* transmitted a much more combative message, reinforced by the caption: 'Bombers' prey. Goering's attacks on London achieve little but the maiming and slaughtering of children.'[31] In this way, while the photograph published with the title 'Air raid victim' made visible the pain of the child, seeking to make the American population aware of the effects of the Blitz and its impact on the civilian population, the image directed at the British public had a slightly different message: despite children's suffering, Britain would never surrender. This message fitted perfectly with the policy adopted sometime earlier by the Ministry of Information, which engaged in creating and maintaining myths through which the British would continue to be committed to the war effort. In his diaries of the war years, *The Years Between*, Beaton explained his motivation in taking his photographs: 'Besides the vandalistic damage we must show the tenacity and courage of the people and we do not have to look far.'[32] With the advent of aerial warfare, civilians – typically defined by contemporaries as women and children – became the primary war targets. *The Times* reported on 28 April 1941 that Winston Churchill had spoken about this home-front battlefield in and around London in his latest broadcast. He reportedly said:

> The sublime but also terrible experiences and emotions of the battlefield, which for centuries have been reserved for the soldiers and sailors, are now shared for good or ill by the entire population. All are proud to be under the fire of the enemy. Old men, little children, the crippled, the veterans of foreign wars, aged women, the ordinary hard-pressed citizen [. . .] the sturdy workman with his hammer in the shipyard or who loads the ships, and the skilful craftsman, the members of every kind of A.R.P. service, are proud to feel that they stand in the line together with our fighting men.[33]

[31] *The Illustrated London News*, 21 September 1940, 3.

[32] Cecil Beaton, *The Years Between: Diaries, 1939–44* (Holt, Rinehart & Winston, New York, 1965), 40.

[33] Winston S. Churchill, *The Unrelenting Struggle* (Cassell and Company, London, 1942), 92.

The role of the 'ordinary citizen' in the war was fundamental to the view of the British government. As Katherine E. Fisher has argued, as the hinge at the centre of Churchill's long list of citizen soldiers, which ranges from children to air-raid wardens, is the ordinary citizen whose key role in the war effort is thereby emphasised.[34] As in the publication of the photograph of Eileen Dunne, Churchill's rhetorical placing of non-combatants on the front line along with traditional combatants highlighted civilian spaces as scenes of combat. The photograph of Eileen Dunne is one of many notable depictions of civilian suffering during the Second World War. However, in both its versions – even with the second's direct reference to 'mutilated and slaughtered children' – the photograph hardly registers pain. The artificiality of the images is even more evident if they are compared with photographs of injured children in the hospital taken by the British press. The idea that children were under attack fuelled resentment that had to be carefully managed to make sure that it was aimed against the barbaric enemy rather than against a state that could no longer protect its own civilian population. The photograph of Eileen Dunne was commissioned as part of the Ministry of Information's propaganda activities. Its main objective was to present the British cause in a way that both provided information about the war effort and boosted public morale. The primary focus of wartime literature following the onset of the Blitz was to uphold public morale by employing positive, yet truthful, propaganda to portray Britain in the best possible light as it endured and persevered against the German onslaught, and children played a central role in this dramatisation.[35] Given that the child's face functions here as a symbol of collective resistance, her pain must be represented according to a series of norms and moral conventions.

The contradictions inherent in the presentation of a real image that also functioned as a kind of icon to strengthen public morale forced Beaton and other photographers to adapt the conventions of studio-portrait photography to create what could be considered as a false world of injured children.[36] In the photograph, the injuries provoked by the war are represented through the bandage that the girl wears around her head, one of the most common conventions for the iconography of the wounded since the First World

[34] For a discussion of the centrality of civilians – in particular, women and children – in the physical spaces and landscapes of wartime Britain, see Katherine E. Fisher, *Writing (in) the Spaces of the Blitz: Spatial Myths and Memory in Wartime British Literature* (University of Michigan Press, Ann Arbor, 2014), 40; Susan R. Grayzel, *At Home and under Fire: Air Raids and Culture in Britain from the Great War to the Blitz* (Cambridge University Press, Cambridge, 2014).

[35] Grayzel, *At Home and under Fire*, 259.

[36] For a discussion on the relationship between portrait photography, medicine and war, see Sheehan, *Doctored*, chapters 1 and 2.

War.[37] The spectacle of children's suffering could not reflect the actual severity of the lived experience. Actual injuries, broken bones, bleeding and similar displays of bodily damage were never displayed at the time, in accordance with socially accepted sensitivity. Far from reflecting reality, this form of representation constructed an iconic model with highly pedagogic and propagandistic content. This guided manner of representation of the damage to children would remain engraved in the collective imagination. Eileen Dunne was not the only child captured by Beaton's lens. Her portrait formed part of a series of photographs taken in the children's ward in a hospital in the north of England.

Beaton made another series, featuring children in the Great Ormond Street Hospital in London, which – as this book has already shown – had a long-standing tradition in the social utilisation of child photography (Figure 5.2). Only one of the four children portrayed in these two series displayed signs of the wounds of war. However, it is not surprising that it was one of these images that should end up as representing the struggle of Britain against Germany. The power of this iconography – and, in particular, of the photograph eventually chosen, that of Eileen – resides in its capacity to combine notions of innocence and suffering. The photograph contains a group of signs proper to the middle class, which helped to awaken the sympathy of those to whom it was addressed. At the same time, through the wound of the war, little Eileen embodied not only the experience of civilian victims of the Blitz but also that of all those who were fighting in the war. Eileen's pain became an icon of Britain's fight against the destruction of National Socialism. Over time, it has become one of the most recognised symbols of British civil resilience in wartime.[38]

As with the photograph of Eileen Dunne, media coverage emphasised the victimisation of children to highlight both the cruelty of the war and the vulnerability of civilians under the new warfare.[39] At the heart of these photographs is the confidence that this material would convince decent people that the war had to stop, because the end to the conflict would return the most innocent – the children – to their true nature, that of childhood. News accounts showed the effects of the air raids on British children and supported the representation of children's behaviour mainly as a form of stoicism. On 10 September 1940, *The Times* told how London was carrying on its daily life despite 'destruction wrought by the blind and wanton night attacks of

[37] For a discussion of the iconography of war during the First World War, see Suzannah Biernoff, 'The face of war', in Andrei Pop and Mechtild Widrich (eds.), *Ugliness: The Non-Beautiful in Art and Theory* (I. B. Tauris, London, 2014), 34–48; Suzannah Biernoff, 'The rhetoric of disfigurement in First World War Britain', *Social History of Medicine*, 24 (2001), 666–85; Beatriz Pichel, *Picturing the Western Front: Photography, Practices and Experiences in First World War France* (Manchester University Press, Manchester, 2021).

[38] Roberts, *Cecil Beaton: Theatre of War*, 25.

[39] Grayzel, *At Home and under Fire*, 258–59.

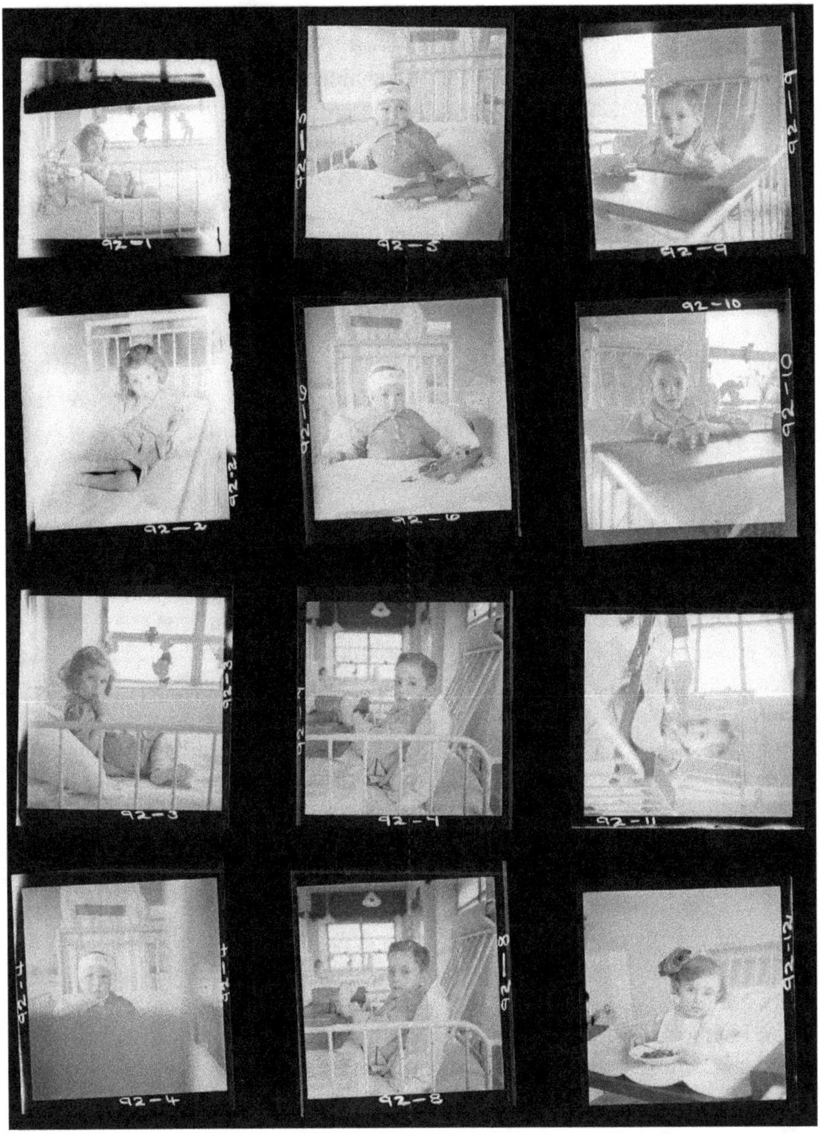

Figure 5.2 Cecil Beaton, *Children in hospital series* (c. 1940), GOS_01 jpg Cecil Beaton 2, Great Ormond Street Archives.

German bombers,' pointing out that the bombs had fallen on 'humble suburban homes' and 'a maternity hospital'.[40] Reports of attacks on Merseyside focused on the heartrending story of a four-month-old child who survived in a drawer for 25 hours amid the wreckage of a home where the rest of the family had been killed by falling debris.[41] In the film *Christmas Under Fire* (1941), 'brave little Englanders' were portrayed as defying the Blitz and the privations of war to celebrate Christmas. Press coverage of 'Gas Mask Sunday' was nearly unanimous in emphasising the calm that prevailed as families lined up to be given gas masks.[42]

These accounts, like the photograph of little Eileen, portrayed children as living examples of endurance and recovery. Her portrait also showed how pain should be endured. In a normative way, these photographs expressed how children and civilians were expected to behave when in pain, and how they ought to cope with the material consequences of war. That, at least, was the public message. However, some disagreed with the morale-boosting image presented by the government and advocates of the so-called People's War, which sought to encourage volunteer efforts. While these accounts suggested that children coped surprisingly well with the war and air raids – emphasising the stoicism and good morale exhibited by these children – war generated many alternative responses in the minds and bodies of children.

Beaton's image of Eileen Dunne and the childhood she represented was read in different ways by different interest groups and scientific bodies. While the government projected a symbol of British resistance and civilian courage, psychoanalysts saw a much less positive image of fragile children suffering from emotional disturbance caused by both the bombs and the subsequent process of evacuation. The Second World War, the Blitz and the evacuation experience produced extensive literature (psychoanalytic and non-psychoanalytic) about their impact on children. While non-analytic writers tended to adopt a straightforward, descriptive tone, psychoanalysts offered more thorough portrayals of inner life. Their complex theoretical frameworks offered new ways to understand the dynamics of fear, anxiety and aggression in children who had been separated from their families, while also showing how such children could pose a potential threat to the functioning of a democratic society.[43] Writers from various perspectives talked about the problems created by evacuation and by the air raids, yet at the top of the list were always enuresis and anxiety. To put this in its context, the huge

40 'Blind Savagery of Night Attacks', *The Times*, 10 September 1940 in Grayzel, *At Home and under Fire*, 286.

41 Grayzel, *At Home and under Fire*, 258–59.

42 'Sunday Queues for Gas Masks', *Daily Mail*, 26 September 1938, 11.

43 See Rose, *Governing the Soul*, 161.

scale of the evacuation and the conflicts it generated between different social groups need to be understood.

Psychoanalytic Discourse versus Government Propaganda

The outbreak of the Second World War produced an extensive literature on the connection between childhood and democracy, with claims such as: 'While we are making a world safe for democracy, we must preserve in children readiness for democracy – these are the people in whose hands the new world order will be moulded.'[44] Psychoanalytical theories on children's psychological development and the role of the mother within were framed within broader debates about the meaning of democracy and the need to deal with aggression in the age of total war.[45] By arguing that healthy family dynamics during childhood and – more importantly – the formation of a good bond between mother and child were seen to safeguard British society from barbarism and fascism, 'psychoanalysis informed new and changing understanding not only of individuals and their health, but also of broader political questions in the age of mass violence and mass anxiety'.[46] Through the work carried out by the clinics and institutions created to receive these uprooted children, psychoanalysis positioned itself as the science that could resolve the problems of abnormal children and, by raising 'democratic' citizens, thereby reducing their potential risk to the community.

Thus, war proved to be a turning point in the history of psychoanalysis, as planners saw the need to understand the mechanisms of mental health and the dynamics of early childhood relationships to prevent submission to authoritarian leaders.[47] The claims of psychoanalysts that all modern selves have destructive drives that should be studied and controlled became increasingly widespread in the circles of official planners and the public. Michel Shapira has pointed to a process whereby the ideas and practices of child psychoanalysts had a wide impact on public opinion and social policy, by creating a new relationship between the state, the family and the child. In the view of these professionals in children's mental health, the psyche of the child was a site for expert knowledge and for transmitting ideas about the family, citizenship and democracy that would have concrete implications for public debate and social

[44] Clarice Madeleine Dixon, *Keep Them Human* (John Day, New York, 1942), cited in Urwin and Sharland, 'From bodies to minds', 192.

[45] Shapira, *The War Inside*, 1–23; Urwin and Sharland, 'From bodies to minds', 174–99; Davis, *Modern Motherhood*, chapter 5; Davis, 'British child psychology and the evacuation', 3–4.

[46] Shapira, *The War Inside*, 2; Davis, 'British child psychology and the evacuation', 1–2.

[47] Mathew Thomson, 'Before anti-psychiatry: "Mental Health" in wartime Britain', in Marijke Gijswijt-Hofstra and Roy Porter (eds.), *Cultures of Psychiatry and Mental Health Care in Postwar Britain and the Netherlands* (Rodopi, Amsterdam, 1998), 43–59.

policy. Even though analysts collaborated with other experts, bureaucrats and fellow citizens in the war effort and in the later subsequent development of the welfare state – thus having their influence on social policy and public opinion – the narrative that emerges from psychoanalytic practice was highly critical of the policy of evacuation. For these experts, the mass evacuation of children from cities and large towns meant that 'billeted' children did not face physical harm, but they did suffer emotionally as a result of separation from home and family. Consequently, it was not simply the nature of human aggression and human love that was at stake, but the social and political implications of the ways these emotions were handled politically.[48]

However, government policy throughout the war remained impervious to criticism from specialists in psychology of the evacuation policy and the residential children's hostels.[49] In the mass evacuation of mothers and children from the cities, the Ministry of Information never addressed the psychological consequences and avoided representing evacuees' suffering in photographic and propagandistic discourse.[50] Clark and his WAAC colleagues chose not to portray the material and psychological consequences of the evacuation.[51] The ideas and practices of John Bowlby and his colleagues were far too critical of the government to gain visibility outside the professional psychoanalytic and psychiatric communities.

In this way, the series titled 'The civilian evacuation scheme in the Second World War' by a photographer of the Ministry of Information photography division captured the lives of children in reception homes, emphasising the cleanliness and happiness of the children portrayed, while staging a series of everyday activities whose intention was to demonstrate their adjustment to new circumstances.[52] In almost all the photographs in the series, children are surrounded by nature and in most cases there are no adults present. The caption of one photograph – 'Evacuated children from London dance happily on the lawn at the country mansion of a well-known peer. The house was given over entirely to the children' – already contains the narrative that the image seeks to display (Figure 5.3). In this image, the psychological distance that the children maintain towards the reasons that have brought them to the security of the camp is reinforced by the decorative arrangement of their shadows and the game they are playing. By conveying the anxiety and excitement of

48 Urwin and Sharland, 'From bodies to minds', 89. 49 Rose, *Governing the Soul*, 167.

50 The study of the photographs of evacuated children commissioned by the Ministry of Information has still to take place. For a study of paintings and sculptures on the same subject, see Foss, *War Paint*, 66–68 and Foss, 'British artists and the Second World War'.

51 Foss, *War Paint*, 68.

52 See also, Rose M. Kundanis, '"Baby riots" and "Eight-hour orphans": a comparison of the images of child care in British and US popular magazines during World War II', *Women's Studies International Forum*, 19 (1996), 239–42.

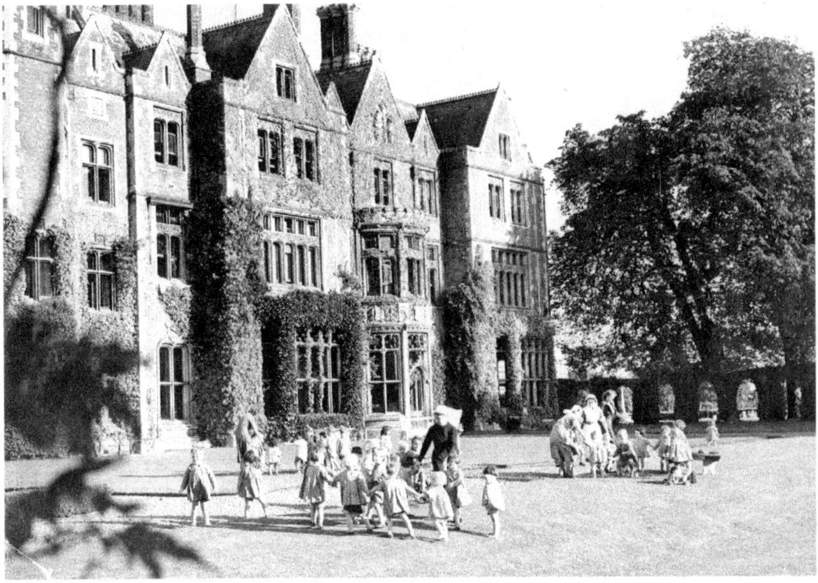

Figure 5.3 Photographer unknown, *Evacuated children from London dance happily on the lawn at the country mansion of a well-known peer. The house was given over entirely to the children* (c. 1940), HU 69020, Ministry of Information Second World War Press Agency Print, Imperial War Museum.

children as they are forced to adjust to a new way of life, the WAAC artists generated a visual rhetoric that was intended to permeate collective imagination. But the issues that were toughest for civilians – the material and psychological consequences of evacuation – were not portrayed.

However, the WAAC images of home-front children involve more than a simple denial of pain and trauma, elements that were too much in evidence to ignore. These images show British children putting themselves above their circumstances – an attitude that connects with the photographs of the bombed children, such as that of Eileen Dunne, and the myth of the Blitz. The happy, well-adjusted children portrayed by the official artists display characteristics such as resilience, courage, unflappability and humour, which were part of this myth. Furthermore, by combining the figure of the uprooted child with the 'we can take it' propaganda, the negative effects of separating children from their mothers were obscured, as the war itself was shown to be a grave threat to the family. In the photographs of air-raid victims, children – who can be seen as representatives of the domestic realm – were portrayed as the main victims of the air attack, and their pain was shown to underline the new vulnerability of the home and how this pain would be endured. In the photographs of evacuated children, there is room for neither physical pain nor psychological trauma, because children – and therefore Britain itself – will 'take it', overcoming the emotional disturbances produced by the war and adapting rapidly to evacuation. A hierarchy of pain was thus created in which some types of pain could be represented, and others were invisible. While the physical pain of the bombs – a pain inflicted by the enemy – is resignified as a warlike discourse and resistance, the pain of evacuation – provoked by the government's own practices – could not be shown.

Evacuation and Its Effects on Children

On 9 September 1939, the *Times Educational Supplement* assessed the first wave of evacuations: 'Nor can one recall a greater piece of non-military planning than the transport and administrative arrangements which made the evacuation possible.'[53] The evacuation of British cities at the start of the Second World War, known as 'Operation Pied Piper', was the biggest forced mass displacement in the UK's history. Already by 26 May 1938 – fifteen months before the war began – Home Secretary Sir Samuel Hoare announced that he had invited Minister for Civil Defence John Anderson to chair an Evacuation Committee,[54] with the aim of drawing up plans to evacuate children in the event of aerial bombing by a 'belligerent' force.[55] Air-raid precautions were needed because there were insufficient means to prevent or deter aerial attacks. Faced with the impossibility of 'envisag[ing] the horrors of intensive air attack', the satisfactory resolution of this plan was repeatedly questioned. In his remarks in the House of Commons, Conservative MP Walter Elliot said: '[W]e cannot [. . .] escape from the fact that in this small and industrialised country, under the possible conditions of air warfare, safety is only relative.'[56] Even so, members of the committee moved towards the implementation of the plan, in the hope that events that had taken place in Spain and in China 'have at least given some indication' as to what was to come and the measures to take. Circulars, albeit very general in nature, started to arrive in local districts. On 25 August 1939, Devon County Council notified the Dawlish Town Clerk by telephone that the evacuation would begin on

[53] *The Times Educational Supplement*, 9 September 1939.

[54] Other committee members were Sir Percy Harris, Liberal MP for South-West Bethnal Green, Mr George Doland, Conservative MP for Balham and Tooting, and Dr Leslie Haden-Guest, Labour MP for North Islington. *Parliamentary Debates (Hansard)*, vol. 336, col. 1380 (26 May 1938), cited in S. J. Hess, 'Civilian evacuation to Devon in the Second World War' (Unpublished PhD thesis, University of Exeter, 2006), 72.

[55] Van der Horst, *John Bowlby – From Psychoanalysis*, 33.

[56] City of Plymouth Evacuation Scheme 1644/375, Walter Elliot speaking in the House of Commons, 18 May 1939, cited in Hess, 'Civilian evacuation to Devon', 72.

1 September.[57] Six days later, on 31 August, Okehampton Town Council received a telegram which read: 'Most immediate Evacuation commences Friday 1 September. Take Action.'[58] On 1 September, Germany invaded Poland, triggering the official evacuations. Two days later, the UK declared war.

In a matter of days, about 827,000 unaccompanied children[59] were evacuated from at-risk areas in England, Scotland and Wales to many British reception areas.[60] The possibility that those involved might change their minds had not been anticipated, which led to confusion in many places. With the numbers much lower than expected, the carefully planned train timetables were no longer relevant and when school parties arrived at major railway stations, they were pushed onto the first available train.[61] As a result, in the subsequent rush to get the trains out as quickly as possible, siblings and parties that were travelling together were split up. Once the authorities saw that the expected air attacks had not materialised and that danger was no longer imminent, many of the evacuated children were able to return to their homes. In many cases, such reunions would not last very long, as a second – smaller – evacuation took place in the spring and autumn of 1940. France had fallen and the first bombs of the Blitz were falling from the English skies. That same year, Cecil Beaton would take the photograph of Eileen Dunne. By June 1941, the devastating aerial attacks had lessened, and some children returned, for a second time, to their homes.

Although bombs did not fall in 1939, the evacuation in September of that year created the greatest expressions of concern, both among experts and in the wider social sphere. Medical journals such as *The Lancet* and the *British Medical Journal* gave details of this operation and how it was affecting children. On 9 September, the *British Medical Journal* spoke of the great efficiency with which 'the evacuation from London of some 650,000 persons' had been achieved.[62] After comparing the journey of 'thousands of Londoners' with that of 'the children of Israel, who made a much more leisurely though less comfortable exodus from Egypt', the article – which was headlined 'A successful exodus' – concluded that 'the whole procedure has taken place smoothly, expeditiously, and without a single casualty'. While the article is positive and has a clearly religious tone, the final paragraph predicts what was to come: 'There remains to be told, when the time comes, the story of how well

57 Dawlish Urban District Council Minutes R2369A/(5/3) C24, 25 August 1939, cited in Hess, 'Civilian evacuation to Devon', 79.
58 Okehampton File 3248A/16/1-2, cited in Hess, 'Civilian evacuation to Devon', 79.
59 Richard Padley and Margaret Cole, *Evacuation Survey: A Report to the Fabian Society* (Routledge, London, 1940), 22.
60 Titmuss, *Problems of Social Policy*, 562.
61 Hess, 'Civilian evacuation to Devon', 79.
62 Editorial 'A successful exodus', *British Medical Journal*, 2 (9 September 1939), 573.

the reception areas have risen to their opportunity.'[63] Despite early expressions of enthusiasm, the process of evacuation faced some resistance, and there were many voices that would not describe it as a 'successful exodus'.

When the bombing did not occur and people had time to reflect on the evacuation, there were criticisms of the 'lack of forethought in high places, and a failure to picture the inevitable results of a rapid, wholesale migration of children'.[64] While the process of evacuation, it was reckoned, had been necessary, those who criticised the way in which it had been carried out indicated that scant consideration had been given to what would happen on the other side. Little time was needed to see that the local authorities, the teaching staff, the voluntary organisations, the host families and the evacuees were struggling to cope with the realities of evacuation in the reception areas.[65] There were problems caused by differences in social provenance, as well as those of local geography or religion. These examples were only part of the mix-ups that led to tensions and disagreements between children and their foster families. Unlike the articles, which assured that 'the evacuated children were happy and were gaining in health' and that 'the hosts, too, were happy',[66] many hosts were resistant to the idea of welcoming a child into their homes, given that they shared prejudices about the conditions in which the children lived and the type of influence – both physical and moral – that they brought from their urban homes.

Especially in the initial wave of evacuation – when medical assessments were not so strict and when the 'phoney war' may have reduced the degree of compassion in some parts of the population – various lurid tales about the physical health and behaviour of the evacuees emerged.[67] Some general practitioners reinforced this myth, warning of such dangers as the spread of parasites and filth, and other undesirable social effects. In a 1939 letter to the *British Medical Journal*, in response to the 'A successful exodus' article, one E. Evans warned of the misfortunes and dangers faced by country people who opened their doors to children from the city. According to this doctor, parasites and the serious consequences that these entailed would spread across the whole countryside: 'When evacuees arrived I was informed many were verminous. One girl volunteer told me she was struck by sores on some children she had to carry and dump on a hostess.' Evans continued, explaining that, as if this were not already serious enough, 'there were women among them who soiled their

[63] 'A successful exodus', 573.

[64] H. C. Dent, *Education in Transition: A Sociological Study of the Impact of War on English Education, 1939–1944* (Routledge & Kegan Paul, London, 1948), 21.

[65] *The Times Educational Supplement*, 9 September 1939.

[66] 'A successful exodus', 573.

[67] See Welshman, 'Evacuation, hygiene, and social policy', 781–807; Crane, 'Rethinking how evacuees'.

beds with urine and faeces'.[68] And he ended by saying that, as a doctor, he was 'deeply humiliated by the lack of foresight and sympathy displayed by the Ministry of Health, which is the responsible authority in the matter under consideration'.[69]

Some lines below, Dr Esther Carling argued that the plan had failed not only because of the irreconcilable differences between city and country, or the difficulties of adapting 'richer to poorer, clean to less clean', but mainly because of the failure to provide a prompt answer to a simple, fundamental question many affected individuals asked themselves: 'what is my duty, where do I belong?'[70] Dr Carling continued by explaining that country people had learned 'by very uncomfortable contact' how the other half of the nation lived, 'and we have seen that the other half appreciates us as little as we appreciate them'. To sum up, the dominant feeling in the destination zones was that 'in many cases the scum of a town has been poured into a clean countryside' with a cruel and extensive indifference towards the consequences of this action and without offering the most basic guarantees for public health.[71] 'There are limits to what people will stand', commented another article, adding that 'in too many cases these limits have already been reached'.[72]

What is interesting about these opinions is that they all have a deliberately ambiguous character. On the one hand, everyone assumed that the government was responsible for the terrible situation in which they were living but, on the other hand, a judgement was made about the suitability or unsuitability of the children, with the mother being the one ultimately responsible. The 1940 'Town children through country eyes report'[73] described the 'real shock' when 'many of the guests arrived in a condition and with modes of life or habits which were startlingly less civilised that those that had [been] accepted for a life-time'.[74] Supporters of eugenics and those with a reformist agenda welcomed evacuation, which led to a perception – as exaggerated as it was persistent – that 'the evacuees [...] provided a close-up view of the conditions which many of the poor accepted as normal: children with head lice, impetigo and scabies, often unwashed and without any knowledge of elementary hygiene'.[75]

68 E. Evans, 'Problems of evacuation', Letter to the editor, *British Medical Journal*, 2 (28 October 1939), 884.

69 Evans, 'Problems of evacuation', 884.

70 E. Carling, 'Evacuation of women and children', *British Medical Journal,* 2 (28 October 1939), 896. This article is in the section called |Letters, Notes, Etc.|

71 Carling, 'Evacuation of women and children', 896.

72 I. C. Keir, 'Evacuation', Letter to the editor, *British Medical Journal*¸2 (7 October 1939), 745–46.

73 National Federation of Women's Institutes, *Town Children through Country Eyes* (Dorking, 1940).

74 *Town Children*, 4.

75 John Stevenson, *British Society 1914–1945* (Penguin, London, 1984), 141.

Before the first wave of evacuation took place, some had already expressed concern about billeting 'dirty children'. The evacuation of large numbers of people raised concerns about the risk of viral epidemics and skin diseases such as scabies and impetigo. Such diseases thrived in war conditions, particularly in crowded underground air-raid shelters where people would not be able to wash properly. On 24 May 1939, Sir Percy Harris, MP for an area of the East End of London, told Parliament that these opinions were based on 'pure ignorance'. London children, even those coming from the poorest districts, were, he said, 'delightful and charming', well brought-up, well taught, 'clean and tidy'.[76]

Despite these opinions, a Ministry of Health circular of September 1939 admitted that there were problems with the state of some of the children who had been evacuated from the most deprived areas: 'In a limited number of districts the influx of persons in a dirty or verminous condition or suffering from skin trouble and similar ailments has presented a somewhat serious and distressing problem.'[77] The *Summary Report by the Ministry of Health* for 1 April 1939 to 31 March 1941 acknowledged that despite the exaggerations, too many children were suffering from conditions such as pediculosis and skin diseases that were directly related to a lack of cleanliness and bad habits. Like the people who made their complaints on the pages of *The Times*, the Ministry of Health recognised that living conditions in big cities were partially the cause of the problem, but once again, the report ultimately blamed mothers for the health of their children. Consequently, the report recommended a series of measures and courses to teach mothers the 'beautiful and important task' of being 'good' mothers, with the aim of solving the problem for good.[78]

Historians of the evacuation have correctly indicated that the process ignited a kind of mass panic.[79] Despite this, more than a few people during the conflict were aware of the exaggerated nature of these stories. Some members of Parliament and various publications about the evacuation admonished the unfortunate exaggerations, and the teachers' guild said that the 'exaggeration of the Press has made teachers physically sick'.[80] One woman told her vicar of the despair in her village of the mothers of these children when reading 'the

[76] *Parliamentary Debates (Hansard),* vol. 347, col. 2330 (24 May 1939), cited in Hess, 'Civilian evacuation to Devon', 72.

[77] *Ministry of Health Circular 1871* (12 September 1939), found in *Okehampton 3248/16/2*, cited in Hess, 'Civilian evacuation to Devon', 72. See also Titmuss, *Problems of Social Policy*, 125, and Parsons, *I'll Take That One*, 195, 197.

[78] *Summary Report by the Ministry of Health, Exeter City Council, Town Clerk's Papers, ARP Evac Group G*, Box 1/8, cited in Hess, 'Civilian evacuation to Devon', 80.

[79] While John Macnicol labels the 'evacuee stereotype' a 'dirty, lice-ridden and foul-mouthed urchin who wet the bed with monotonous regularity', John Welshman refers to the prevalence of this myth in current literature. See Macnicol, 'The effect of the evacuation of school children', 15. See Welshman, 'Evacuation and social policy', 33.

[80] *L.S.A. Bulletin* (March 1940), 3, cited in Rose, *Which People's War?*, 208.

wholesale strictures on their [the children's] condition and conduct'. Although mothers could write to *The Times* 'to defend their children', the vicar empathised with the women whose reputations were being sullied while their children were being mistreated. The article adds that the vicar was informed by the local evacuation officer that only 25 out of 1,000 children had problems, and it ended: 'Pray too for a heart of grace, that you too may look with compassion, and not with criticism, on these children who very possibly are the victims of circumstance.'[81] According to the London County Council Education Department, 'unfortunately it was always the unusual incident of evacuation that attracted the attention of the press and public',[82] while the Ministry of Health said that claims that a significant percentage of the children were unclean and infested with vermin was 'a gross exaggeration, expressed in this general form'.[83]

Bad habits, lice and bed-wetting were bodily signs pointing to a moral problem. It was upon this semiotic duplicity of body and mind that the myth of the evacuated child was constructed. Pediculosis and skin disease were added to the list.[84] In 1940, the Scottish socialist author and journalist Ritchie Calder criticised this kind of collective panic and affirmed that the 'lousiness' and 'dirty habits' of the children had been very much exaggerated.[85] 'Dirty habits' is a description of a deliberately ambiguous character. On one side, medical journals and letters to newspapers and periodicals such as *The Times* and the *British Medical Journal* saw them as a physical problem. On the other side, commentaries coming from the sphere of psychology and social education understood them to be a natural reaction to a psychological shock.[86] What was for the former a clear motive for reprimand and punishment was understood by the latter as a social alarm, which called into question the nation's stability. In both cases, whether through education or nature, the child appeared as inept in the control of his habits or sphincter movements.

'A Cruel Psychological Experiment': Scientific Literature on Evacuation

The bombing of British cities during the Blitz and the policy of evacuating children from these areas to the countryside provoked considerable medical

[81] Letter from the Vicar of Littleham-cum-Exmouth, *Express and Echo* (4 November 1939). Also in *The Western Times* (10 November 1939), cited in Hess, 'Civilian evacuation to Devon', 242.
[82] Richard Samways (ed.), *We Think You Ought to Go* (London Metropolitan Archives, City of London, 1995), 14.
[83] *MH 78/230* 'Notes on unsatisfactory aspects of evacuation compiled from reports of observers in Action Stations in England and Wales', letter sent from MOI to Ministry of Health, dated 16 September 1939 cited in Hess, 'Civilian evacuation to Devon', 281.
[84] Welshman, 'Evacuation and social policy', 39.
[85] Ritchie Calder, 'The school child', in Padley and Cole, *Evacuation Survey*, 148.
[86] Crane, 'Rethinking how evacuees'.

and scientific debate about the effects on both the behaviour of children and their mental health. The bad behaviour of some evacuees and the spectre of juvenile delinquency raised questions about the psychological mechanisms that might be involved and the role of children's experience of both air raids and the separation from their families entailed by evacuation. The emerging discipline of psychoanalysis challenged much conventional thinking, in particular by suggesting that children who were evacuated might suffer greater mental problems than those who were bombed, precisely because of the effect of separation from their mothers.[87] As it provided a wealth of case studies and a grand experimental theatre with many thousands of subjects, the policy of evacuation provided a fundamental opportunity for the emergence of psychoanalysis as a professional discipline in the United Kingdom and for the engagement of psychoanalysts in the design of social policies.

As early as 1939, the *British Medical Journal* had reflected the concerns of some citizens about the emotional well-being of children. In a letter to the editor, a certain Yates observed that if many evacuated children presented the grave problems already mentioned in earlier letters – 'the chief of these being bed-wetting and unmanageableness'[88] – these symptoms did not belong either to the physiological or the moral arena. On the contrary, the discussion needed to be moved towards psychological disorders and nervous conditions. 'So much has been written about the physical advantage to children of being out of big cities', wrote Mary Burbury in the article 'Effects of evacuation and of air raids on city children' (1941), that it seemed worthwhile to try 'in some way to assess and reduce to terms the psychological effects of evacuation on them'.[89] While the main social anxieties provoked by evacuation – and nurtured by sensationalist press coverage – arose from the revelations about urban poverty, psychiatrists and psychologists were more concerned with the effects on children of separation from their parents.[90]

The experience of evacuation generated an extensive literature about the effects of the process on the mental health of children. In her article

87 See Shapira, *The War Inside*, 48–68; Davis, *Modern Motherhood*, chapter 5; Davis, 'British child psychology and the evacuation', 1–10.

88 S. L. Yates, 'Problems of evacuation', Letter to the editor, *British Medical Journal*, 2 (28 October 1939), 883–84.

89 W. M. Burbury, 'Effects of evacuation and of air raids on city children', *British Medical Journal* (8 November 1941), 660.

90 See John Bowlby, 'Psychological aspects of the evacuation', in Padley and Cole, *Evacuation Survey*, 186; John Bowlby, *Maternal Care and Mental Health* (World Health Organization, Geneva, 1952); Dorothy Burlingham and Anna Freud, *Children in Wartime* (Medical War Books, New York, 1940); Donald Winnicott, *The Child and the Outside World* (Tavistock, London, 1957); Donald Winnicott, 'Children's hostels in war and peace', *British Journal of Medical Psychology*, 21 (1948), 175–80. See also, Wolf, 'Evacuation of children in wartime', 389–404.

'Evacuation of children in wartime' (1941), Katharine M. Wolf considered it 'a cruel psychological experiment on a large scale', although in the arena of children's mental health, the war brought more innovation than in other areas. As a result, there were increased expectations of better services for everyone and an understanding that the state would be more involved in their provision.[91] Medical professionals – including psychoanalysts – started calling for more state responsibility for the people's welfare and for improved health services.[92] The changes brought by war had their roots in developments in the 1930s. While general practitioners warned that evacuation would lead to the spread of uncleanliness and vermin, psychologists and psychoanalysts argued that the emotional impact of confronting possible separation from or loss of one or both parents and the break-up of the family unit was of greater concern. Both psychology and psychoanalysis had developed as disciplines since the end of the First World War, and children's mental health and psychology became the domain of experts.[93] As Michel Shapira has observed, although psychoanalysis contributed to this shift 'from bodies to minds', its key role started to emerge just before the Second World War, with its insistence on the centrality of the child psyche and of children's relationships with their parents to the normal development of future adult citizens.[94] Before the war had started, British analysts had already begun to examine how they could contribute as individuals to society and help in dealing with panic and mental breakdown caused by the anticipated air raids on the civilian population.[95] The bombing of British cities and the evacuation of British children provided them with an abundance of work with civilians, helping to shift the nature of their profession in a way that crystallised earlier interwar developments.[96]

However, the main contribution of psychoanalysts during the war – beyond their conceptualisation of anxiety and aggression – was the work they did with

[91] Shapira, *The War Inside*, 56. [92] Shapira, *The War Inside*, 57.

[93] Hendrick, *Child Welfare: Historical*, 149–76.

[94] Shapira, The War Inside. See also: Urwin and Sharland, 'From bodies to minds', 174–99; Nikolas Rose, *The Psychological Complex: Psychology, Politics and Society in England, 1869–1939* (Routledge and Kegan Paul, London, 1985); Rose, *Governing the Soul.*

[95] Pearl King, 'Activities of British psychoanalysts during the Second World War and the influence of their interdisciplinary collaboration on the development of psychoanalysis in Great Britain', *International Journal of Psychoanalysis*, 16 (1989), 15–32.

[96] The perceived psychological effects of the Second World War in general, and on the home front in particular, are understudied when compared to those of the First World War. Furthermore, as Sonya Rose notes, despite the central place that evacuation occupied in the popular memory of the war, it has still not been analysed extensively. See Rose, *Which People's War?*, 124; John Welshman, *Churchill's Children: The Evacuee Experience in Wartime Britain* (Oxford University Press, Oxford, 2010); Titmuss, *Problems of Social Policy*; and Angus Calder, *The People's War: Britain, 1939–1945* (Pantheon Books, New York, 1969), 35–50.

children, the home front's most visible victims.[97] As Michal Shapira has suggested, psychoanalysis presented itself as a new science of 'normal' mental health that sought to maximise the positive potential of individuals while minimising the troubles that debilitated them, and which was able to tackle the problem of the 'abnormal' child who represented a 'potential threat to the whole community'.[98] The war provided an environment in which psychological and psychoanalytic ideas could be developed in new and inventive ways. The new psychological thinking was seen by government officials and others as preferable to what was now an old-fashioned class-based vision of the 'bad habits' of the urban poor. While it is true that the evacuation did at times reinforce this classist idea of juvenile delinquency as being linked to both poor socioeconomic conditions and a lack of parental discipline, and to the idea of the 'problem family', on the other hand, it encouraged debates about children's mental health. In particular, the use of evacuation hostels and nurseries – some run by psychoanalysts (including Anna Freud) – stimulated the setting up of more progressive institutions that would eventually expand to other vulnerable segments of the population, such as the elderly and the mentally ill, thus anticipating later welfare-state innovations in 'community care'.[99]

Psychoanalysts were among the many critics of the policy of evacuation – and they did not lack arguments. On 2 December 1939, *The Lancet* published a letter from John Rickman under the heading 'Evacuation and the child's mind', which said that the continuous separations and break-ups to which children were exposed during the process of evacuation could have serious consequences for their mental health. In the words of this British psychoanalyst, 'at a time when his need for security, and the comforting assurance of familiar faces, is great', the child's separation from his parents 'will tax him severely'.[100] For Rickman, separation had a direct impact on the child's mental health, which would be set off towards the development of a 'disaffective character' and 'unsatisfactory or unhappy social relationships later in life'.[101] For him, as for other psychologists, evacuation had been anything but a great success when considered from the point of view of the mental health of the children involved. In another letter, to *The Lancet*, Rickman wrote: 'Even a situation of emergency should not be allowed to divert our attention for the basic needs of the mental and social development of our future fellow citizens.'[102]

[97] On analysts' work in the British military, see Tom Harrison, *Bion, Rickman, Foulkes and the Northfield Experiments: Advancing on a Different Front* (Jessica Kingsley, London, 2000).

[98] Shapira, *The War Inside*, 17.

[99] Welshman, 'Evacuation and social policy', 3–31.

[100] John Rickman, 'Evacuation and the child's mind', Letter to the editor, *The Lancet*, 234 (2 December 1939), 1192.

[101] Rickman, 'Evacuation and the child's mind', 1192.

[102] Rickman, 'Evacuation and the child's mind', 1192.

Two weeks later, similar reservations were expressed by John Bowlby, Emanuel Miller and Donald Winnicott in a letter to another prestigious journal, the *British Medical Journal.*[103] This trio of psychologists argued that children older than five could cope with both the physical and psychological shock of evacuation, but younger children were marked for life by the shock involved in separation, an experience that was much more than a profound sadness. The inability to find a safe and secure reference provided such a shock to these children that, in many cases, it provoked an emotional 'blackout', fertile ground for the later creation of a serious disorder in personality development and the potential for juvenile delinquency. According to Bowlby, Miller and Winnicott: 'If these opinions are correct it follows that evacuation of small children without their mothers can lead to a very serious and widespread psychological disorder.'[104] The government was putting at risk both the health of British children – who ran the risk of developing a 'severe disturbance of the personality which may persist throughout life' – and the health of the nation, as this situation could 'lead to a big increase in juvenile delinquency in the next decade'.[105]

For Bowlby, the experience of evacuated children served only to confirm what he had already witnessed. Between 1936 and 1939, while working for the Child Guidance Clinic in London, Bowlby had carried out a series of investigations on the family lives of young thieves.[106] All the patients had in common the fact of having been brought up by strangers at different moments within the first five years of life. For Bowlby, the study revealed that it was possible to support a causal link between early separation and juvenile delinquency. The effects of separation created a disaffective character, a personality disorder that was the root of the antisocial behaviour. This antisocial behaviour was a *symptom* of a psychodynamic disorder, which, in turn, was the *consequence* of a disturbance that occurred in the early stages of the relationship between the child and the mother.[107]

In the opinion of another of the letter's signatories, the English paediatrician and psychoanalyst Donald Winnicott: 'Evacuation is a story of tragedies; either the children are emotionally disturbed, perhaps more than they can recover from, or else the children are happy and it is the parents who suffer, the implication being that they are not needed even by their own children.' Thus, the only success that the scheme could claim 'is that it could fail'.[108]

103 John Bowlby, Emmanuel Miller and Donald W. Winnicott, 'Evacuation of small children', Letter to the editor, *British Medical Journal*, 2 (16 December 1939), 1202–3.

104 Bowlby et al., 'Evacuation of small children', 1202–3.

105 Bowlby et al., 'Evacuation of small children', 1203.

106 John Bowlby, 'Forty-four juvenile thieves: their characters and home-life', *The International Journal for Psycho-Analysis*, 25 (1944), 19–53, 125.

107 Bowlby, 'Forty-four juvenile thieves', 19–53, 125.

108 Donald W. Winnicott, *Deprivation and Delinquency* (Tavistock, London, 1984), 22.

When the war came, Winnicott – who worked as a psychiatric advisor on the government's evacuation plan in Oxfordshire and, within that plan, on the Oxfordshire Evacuation Hostel Scheme – 'could not avoid the delinquency issue any longer'. He was deeply affected by the confirmation of the confusion that the generalised disintegration of family life had generated, as well as the effects of separation and loss, destruction and death. Together with his future wife, the social worker Clare Britton, he helped to fund evacuation hostels to care for some three hundred 'difficult children' whose 'anxious' state prevented them from adapting to their foster families.[109] In the framework of these hostels, the gestures and words of these patients were interpreted in two ways – one individual, the other social. On the one hand, there was concern for the child who was afflicted by anxiety and other ailments of a neurotic character. On the other hand, there was a focus on the potential risk of juvenile delinquency and its effect on the future stability of the democratic regime.

These hostels acted as substitutes for the family and helped to relieve children's anxiety and to generate the conditions necessary for implanting the desired state of 'social adjustment'.[110] In the opinion of Winnicott and Britton, the child who does not feel wanted 'becomes a burden on society, hardening into an anti-social character, or developing some other sort of mental illness'.[111] In the widely distributed pamphlet *Children's Communities: Experiments in Democratic Living*, Winnicott and Britton expressed their concern for the children whose lives were spent in institutional spaces. Unlike much other research into children interned in clinics and institutions, this study focused on children who had not suffered any previous pathology. The conditions of anxiety and stress in which the lives of these children had developed had demonstrated the fragile emotional life of infancy, the authors claimed. According to these two experts, the child who was deprived by the circumstances of the war of a normal family life 'tends to lack something not only in personal happiness, but also in the development of character and in the qualities of citizenship'.[112] The discussions generated by the hostels showed a growing concern about the aggressiveness that was being exhibited by the evacuated children. The hostel programme to restore these children's health included introducing them into a familiar

[109] Brett Kahr, *D. W. Winnicott: A Biographical Portrait* (London, Karnac, 1996), 83–85. During the war, the government had to open special hostels for children who were 'unbilletable'. See Hendrick, *Child Welfare: Historical*, 109.

[110] Michal Shapira, 'The psychological study of anxiety in the era of the Second World War', *Twentieth Century British History*, 1 (2012), 31–57.

[111] Donald W. Winnicott and Clare Britton, 'The problem of homeless children', in Joel Kanter, *Face to Face with Children: The Life and Work of Clare Winnicott* (Karnac, London, 2004), 97.

[112] Winnicott and Britton, 'Problem of homeless children', 6.

emotional framework, but for children who presented a strong antisocial character, the treatment 'cannot avoid being dictatorial'. Children 'must gradually be brought up against the consequences of their own destructive actions'.[113] The possibility of cooperation between citizens, and the future of democracy itself, was based on the restoration of these values. Emotions, if not managed correctly, posed a problem for democracy. The social relevance of the hostels lay in their instrumentality towards the resolution of this conflict, guaranteeing a stable and healthy emotional life to these future members of democratic society.

The same line of argument was adopted in the article 'The school and the child guidance clinic', published in the book *Educating for Democracy* (1939). Its author, the British psychologist Raymond B. Cattell, wrote that the war had demonstrated that 'the variety of abnormality requiring specific assistance and treatment is very great'.[114] After listing the types of disorder that were referred to the 'average' child guidance clinic – rebelliousness, disobedience and offences against authority, nervousness and exaggerated or irrational fears, general backwardness in school, chronic stealing, truancy from school and home, excessive lying, emotional instability and inability to get on with other children, difficulties over feeding, problems with specific school subjects, enuresis and bed-wetting, stammering, masturbation, unusual jealousy, and destructiveness – Cattell grouped these disorders into three categories of 'unusual children'.[115] First, he placed 'delinquency and behaviour disorders', followed by 'personality disorders and nervous symptoms in the wider sense', and finally by 'scholastic disabilities and difficulties in learning'. He noted that there were 'surprising differences in their relative incidence in various economic and social groups, schools, or residential areas and in various levels of intelligence within the school'. Thus, while personality problems were more frequent among the 'brighter' children and those from higher social classes, 'delinquency showed the reverse distribution'.[116]

Cattell's words were written as part of the debate about scholastic backwardness and the fierce disputes as to whether the child guidance clinic should concern itself at all with it. In Cattell's opinion, drawing 'a sharp line between

[113] Winnicott and Britton, 'Problem of homeless children', 6. See also, A. T. Alcock, 'War strain in children', *British Medical Journal*, 1 (25 January 1941), 124. Winnicott worked closely with the child guidance officer Theodora Alcock, who claimed that, while the physical conditions of children might improve in the countryside, their mental strain was great and resulted from their separation from their homes and from their mothers.

[114] Raymond B. Cattell, 'The school and the child guidance clinic', in J. I. Cohen (ed.), *Educating for Democracy* (Macmillan and Co., London, 1939), 169–83.

[115] Cattell, 'The school and the child guidance clinic', 174.

[116] Cattell, 'The school and the child guidance clinic', 173.

cases of emotional disability and mental defect' was impossible until an examination had been made. Thus, it would be 'natural' for the clinic to 'examine, diagnose, and classify all types of psychological and educational abnormality'.[117]

For Martha W. MacDonald, psychiatric services adviser to the Children's Bureau at the US Department of Labor in Washington, DC, the fact that the 'nations of the world' were becoming concerned about links between war and juvenile delinquency was 'indicative of the present-day constructive attitude toward delinquency in children'.[118] According to MacDonald, the war had shown that both juvenile delinquency and other psychological disorders were symptoms of 'nutritional deficiency', a deficiency in the child's spiritual nurturing that affected moral development.[119] The delinquent child, the psychiatrist concluded, is a 'sick child' whose behaviour could be seen as an expression of protest against deprivation – in this case the deprivation of love. Love was not merely a romantic ideal – it was the medium in which children developed as normal or pathological.

Psychiatrists and psychoanalysts had to battle against the view that the origins of crime and vice should be traced to parents' failure to instil morality in their children, combined with contagion from the bad habits that infected the corrupt environment of urban life. However, psychologists such as Winnicott, MacDonald and Cattell understood that the processes involved in the emotional development of the child were very fragile and delicate, vulnerable to multiple distortions that could lead to pathologies that ranged from bad behaviour and delinquency to sheer madness. As Michel Shapira has indicated, the debate generated by psychoanalysis about the relevance of the mother–child bond for the adequate development of the child not only produced a general re-evaluation of the experience of separation but also generated influential responses to certain questions relating to the possibility of maintaining harmonious and cooperative human relationships in the twentieth century.[120] British psychoanalysis – which from the beginning was tied to a sense of obligation to ensure 'a specific understanding of social democracy' in periods of both war and peace – developed as it engaged in treating social problems.[121] War and the development of the welfare state posed moral, theoretical and practical questions to the psychoanalysts in a way that restructured their discipline. At the same time, their responses framed the modern democratic individual in the United Kingdom.

[117] Cattell, 'The school and the child guidance clinic', 174.

[118] M. W. MacDonald, 'Impact of war on children and youth intensification of emotional problems', *American Journal of Public Health*, 33 (1943), 336.

[119] MacDonald, 'Impact of war', 336. [120] Shapira, *The War Inside*, 1–23.

[121] Shapira, *The War Inside*, 1–23.

'War Strain' or 'Air-Raid Shock'

However, there were other attempts to provide psychological explanations for the delinquent or pathological behaviour of some evacuated children besides the effort to draw a causal link between misbehaviour and the trauma of parental separation. Another school of thought is represented by Theodora Alcock (1888–1980), a child psychoanalyst who introduced the Rorschach test to the United Kingdom and who worked for the Ministry of Health in the reception area of Huntingdonshire, where she gave guidance to 'difficult' children evacuated from London and the East Coast. Alcock saw the problem not in terms of evacuation and separation from the mother, but rather in terms of the physical shock of the bombs, which produced disturbances to the psyche. In an address at the Tavistock Clinic on 'war strain' in children, she argued that the disturbance of the 'difficult evacuated children' was the result of a physical agency, 'such as bombing', and that children who had been bombed 'seemed to react much more in the way of unruly behaviour'.[122] Alcock argued that 'children whose chief strain was due to separation from home seemed to account for most of the psychosomatic and psychoneurotic cases, while those in whom the principal disturbance was due to a physical agency, such as bombing, seemed to react much more in the way of unruly behaviour'.[123] Agreeing with Alcock, Rosemary Pritchart and Saul Rosenzweig also maintained that separation led to 'psychosomatic or psychoneurotic disorders', while bombing led to 'unmanageable' behaviour and aggressiveness.[124] It is worth noting that these experts did not substitute one univocal causal link with another. They did not shift the cause of the bad behaviour of evacuated children from the trauma of separation to the shock of the air-raid experience. Rather, they distinguished between two separate types of pathology, arguing that the effects of separation turned against the organism of the child, who experienced the type of somatic and neurotic pathologies discussed in Chapter 4, while the impact of bombing caused the type of misbehaviour that was socially labelled as unruly.

However, in practice, the second type of effects was prioritised over the first. One of Alcock's colleagues at the Tavistock Clinic, W. E. Mons, saw the need to remind parents frightened of evacuating their children to the countryside that 'exposure to even a single "harmless" air raid can do great damage to a child's psyche be he ever so "normal" and "fearless" on the surface'. There were reasons to believe, Mons argued, 'that the child who has been exposed to

[122] Alcock, 'War strain', 124. [123] Alcock, 'War strain', 124.
[124] R. Pritchard and S. Rosenzweig, 'The effects of war stress upon childhood and youth', *Journal of Abnormal Psychology*, 37 (1942), 329.

the experience of one or more air raids is in a class by itself'.[125] Contrary to what happened with war neurosis, which particularly affected those with a strong predisposition, 'air-raid shock' was not considered to be a neurosis in the true sense, as it affected children who had not previously revealed the slightest trace of abnormality. In the same way, Mons argued in 'Air raids and the child' (1941), that after the experience of only a single air raid, 'previously good and intelligent children become suddenly obstreperous, destructive, mischievous, lazy, truant from school, and, in short, unmanageable in the billet to which they have been evacuated'. The article maintained that this behaviour reflected a 'deep resentment against the adults who have failed to provide that security and protection which is every child's birth right'.[126] Faced for the first time with the reality of death, children experienced the most profound agony in realising that 'parental authority is no longer a safe shield against this direct threat of extinction'.[127]

For Mons, the stoic surface of these children had its origin in psychological pathologies rather than in strength of character. Considering the impact of raids to be of an essentially unconscious nature, he argued that as the child was unaware of the air-raid trauma, in most cases 'he tends to make light of his experiences, denies having been frightened, and behaves in that casual manner characteristic of an adult'. But 'these children are no longer what they used to be'.[128] Mons, along with Alcock, reported that the Rorschach responses of children who had been bombed revealed more disturbances in 'deeper layers of personality' than the responses of children who had not been bombed.[129] Publications such as *The Lancet* and the *British Medical Journal* echoed psychologists' and educationalists' opinions that many children had suffered in ways that did not appear on the surface and that parents and teachers did not recognise. Unlike earlier research on children interned in clinics and institutions, these studies focused on children who had not suffered any previous pathology and did not come from families where such pathologies had been experienced.

If for Mons the physical shock of the bombs produced psychological disturbances, for Susan Isaacs, fear and anxiety – far more general causes – produced organic illness. Regardless of whether the trauma was physical or psychological, both Mons and Isaacs strengthened the idea that fear experienced by many young children faced with the threat that their homes and their parents might be bombed was unconscious. Susan Isaacs worked at Malting House School and, from 1933, was Head of the Department of Child

[125] W. E. R. Mons, 'Air raids and the child', *British Medical Journal*, 2 (1 November 1941), 625.
[126] Mons, 'Air raids and the child', 625. [127] Mons, 'Air raids and the child', 625.
[128] Mons, 'Air raids and the child', 625.
[129] A. T. Jersild and M. F. Meigs, 'Children and war', *Psychological Bulletin*, 40 (1943), 562.

Development at the Institute of Education in London. While there, she shifted her focus from how to manage children to how to understand their inner mental and emotional processes.[130] Through pamphlets and responses to parents' inquiries in the journal *Home and School*, Isaacs's work was widely disseminated and included in the education of young schoolteachers. Her book for parents, *The Nursery Years* (1929), was reprinted four times before the outbreak of the Second World War, which suggests its popularity.

According to Isaacs, the child's limited understanding encouraged a selective perception of reality. With the end of resolving the internal anxiety provoked by the lack of safety of their parents and homes, these children clung to the idea that war and air raids were only real in those places that had been evacuated. In turn, argued Isaacs, the significance of the exterior reality of the war was connected for each child with how the ambiguity of their own sentiments had been handled. On the one hand, love and dependence on the parents and, on the other hand, impulses of greed, jealousy and destruction. Following this inner logic, many children deduced that the expulsion from the home was a punishment for their feelings of hatred and jealousy. There were also cases where children blamed themselves for the danger their loved ones faced, believing that these feelings were what was really threatening the well-being of their parents.[131]

But for every argument, there was a counterargument. Mons's view of the vulnerability of a child's psyche to the effect of a single air raid was not shared by educational psychologist Philip Ewart Vernon, of the University of Glasgow, who in an article devoted mainly to adult reactions argued that 'the raids had even less effect on children than upon adults'.[132] In contrast to Isaacs, Vernon was surprised that these children had not reacted in a more drastic manner 'to the operation of a "fear instinct" which is stimulated by loud noises'.[133] Although they were sometimes scared by sirens and explosions, nearly all the children he and his colleagues had been able to observe in the clinic went 'to sleep again remarkably easily'.[134] Like Isaacs, Vernon believed that children had limited capacity to understand and reason, but he believed that it was precisely this lack of awareness that kept them safe from the shock of the war. Connecting the possibility of trauma with the state of the child's development, Vernon's article

[130] Urwin and Sharland, 'From bodies to minds', 190.

[131] See Susan Isaacs, 'Children of Great Britain in wartime', *Child Study* (Winter 1941–1942); Susan Isaacs, 'Cambridge evacuation survey', *The Fortnightly* (June 1940), 619; Susan Isaacs (editor, with the cooperation of S. C. Brown and R. H. Thoules), *The Cambridge Evacuation Survey a Wartime Study in Social Welfare and Education* (Methuen & Co., London, 1941).

[132] Philip E. Vernon, 'Psychological effects of air-raids', *Journal of Abnormal and Social Psychology*, 36 (1941), 457–76.

[133] Vernon, 'Psychological effects', 469.

[134] Vernon, 'Psychological effects', 469.

concluded: 'It is hardly possible to say at what age consciousness of the danger to themselves and their relatives arises.'[135]

There were many arguments against the diagnoses of psychologists and psychiatrists, under the pretext that they impinged against the objectivity of the clinical method. Thus, William A. Brend, in a text titled 'Air raid shock', made a direct criticism of Mons's article and the new category of 'air-raid shock' he had created. This came to join a list of traumatic psychopathologies that went from 'railway spine' to 'traumatic neurasthenia', passing through 'nervous shock', 'shell shock' and 'bomb shock'. This specialist in clinical neurology concluded by saying: 'May I protest against this latest addition to a mischievous and medically meaningless series?'[136] Like Brend, for Dr Felix Brown, 'no acute emotional-shock reactions among children have been seen'. Brown, a psychiatrist at Guy's Hospital in London, argued that 'the excellent prognosis of the civilian air-raid psychoneuroses and emotional-shock' resulted from the fact that civilians had 'no motive for continuation of symptoms any longer than he can help'.[137]

However, the arguments about lack of observation did not affect many of the leading practitioners of the time, starting with Anna Freud's awareness of a scientific opportunity based on the large number of infants available to the scientific eye, and continuing with Ilse Hellman's reception of the reporting methods used by Freud and Dorothy Burlingham at the Hampstead Nursery. Hellman believed that this method of pooling observations used at the nurseries subsequently developed into an important research tool in psychoanalytic child observation.[138] However, as Nick Midgley has noted, there was already a long history of direct observation of children within psychoanalysis, going back to the early twentieth century and the encounter in Vienna between psychoanalysis and 'child studies'. Anna Freud's role in this expansion to Britain is not to be overlooked.[139]

Evaluating Symptoms

While many doctors refused to read the air-raid symptoms as authentic expressions of mental illness and saw them, rather, as the opposite – as expressions of a purely physiological character – psychologists conducted a conceptual

135 Vernon, 'Psychological effects', 476.

136 William A. Brend, 'Air-raid shock', *British Medical Journal*, 2 (15 November 1941), 712.

137 Felix Brown, 'Civilian psychiatric air raid casualties', *The Lancet*, 237 (31 May 1941), 691.

138 Ilse Hellman, 'Work in the Hampstead War Nurseries', *International Journal of Psychoanalysis*, 64(4) (1983), 435–36.

139 Nick Midgley has argued that Anna Freud remained a central figure in the post-war years. Nick Midgley, 'Anna Freud: the Hampstead War Nurseries and the role of the direct observation of children for psychoanalysis', *International Journal of Psychoanalysis*, 88 (2007), 939–59.

re-evaluation of psychological damage that resulted in the construction of new symptomologies. Child symptoms were interpreted according to a table of signs, in such a way that an individual element could take on relevance only in the context of a codified system. Psychologist M. I. Dunsdon devoted an article to the evaluation of these symptoms, based on a survey of schoolchildren following heavy bombing raids on the city of Bristol; this psychologist concluding that of the 8,000 children that were in the city at the time of the bombardment, at least 300 showed clear signs of strain.[140] For Dunsdon, the main symptom in the first phase of air-raid shock was a 'pronounced apathy'. This state of indifference gave way, during the following four weeks, to the pattern of symptoms of reactive depression. While children aged between five and seven showed 'overt psychological symptoms', those who were older than eleven tended to show more frequently 'psychosomatic disorder'.[141]

Like Dunsdon, Mary Burbury, medical director of the Manchester City Child Guidance Clinic, tried to establish a correct identification of the expressive signs of the child affected by air raids and the rest of his or her physiological circumstances. With regard to the impact of air raids on city children, this psychologist considered that the qualifier 'immediate' should be emphasised because 'we are not yet in a position to assume that we know what the final effect of living in constant risk of this sort of warfare is going to be on either the adult or the child population'.[142] The group of cases in which symptoms exhibited by children were attributed to raids included sleepwalkers, nervous children, truants, enuretics, stammerers and pilferers.

Following Burbury's criteria, Frank Bodman considered that the problem of the symptoms presented by these children was that they did not disappear when the stressful situation ended, and they could accompany the subject well into adulthood.[143] Bodman carried out a two-month follow-up study with fifty-four children aged between two months and twelve years of age, who had been evacuated from the Bristol Children's Hospital during a severe bombing. The first reaction 'is that to sirens and noise in general', but while 'in the walking child' the reaction is to run to safety, 'the talking child' rejects the formulation of the experience.[144] This, noted Bodman, is followed by attempts at describing or rehearsing the incident, 'the description becoming more elaborate as the child is more mature'.[145] Returning to connect the symptomology with the state of the child's development, Bodman claimed that 'the younger children felt the strain and lack of sleep more readily than the older ones, who have

[140] M. I. Dunsdon, 'A psychologist's contribution to air raid problems', *Mental Health*, 2 (1941), 37–41.

[141] Dunsdon, 'A psychologist's contribution', 40.

[142] Burbury, 'Effects of evacuation', 660.

[143] Frank H. Bodman, 'War conditions and the mental health of the child', *British Medical Journal*, 2 (4 October 1941), 486.

[144] Bodman, 'War conditions', 487.

[145] Bodman, 'War conditions', 488.

developed more control and can repress their feelings to conform with adult standards with greater success'.[146] Visible psychological symptoms were predominantly observed in children aged five to seven, whereas the group aged eleven to fourteen exhibited a higher prevalence of psychosomatic disorders.[147] Interestingly, Bodman noted that older children (seven-and-a-half years of age and above) tended to view the air raids as an adventure, while those aged eleven and above showed a sense of responsibility for others. Overall, there was remarkably little reaction to subsequent raids. Of eight children with severe later experiences, only two had episodes of anxiety, which eventually disappeared. According to Bodman, 'the most striking finding of this survey is the extraordinary toughness of the child, and his flexibility in adapting to potentially threatening situations'.[148]

Even though there was no shortage of opinions suggesting a correlation between age and symptomology, there was no agreement about the correspondences or which ages most favoured adaptation. Thus, Bodman argued that the older the child, the greater their understanding of the situation and adaptability, while Dunsdon concluded that 'latent adaptation was strongest' among children aged two to five.[149] Studying a group of preschool children who had experienced bombings, E. M. John of University College London noted after-effects in many 'youngsters' six months after the events.[150] After the experience of only one air raid, forty-two children developed an 'abnormal' fear of noises. Concern grew in acknowledging that none of them 'had revealed until the moment the slightest trace of abnormality'.[151] Fear of the dark among children increased, and John noted that the after-effects of the raids seemed more closely related to the degree of fear at the time of the raid than to the severity of the raid itself. Furthermore, the extent of a child's fear often appeared to be influenced by that of the mother, as John reported a correlation between mothers' and children's fears at the time of the raid.[152] Similarly, Joseph C. Solomon, in an account detailing the responses of San Francisco children to an air-raid alarm shortly after the Pearl Harbor attack, also noted that the contagious effect of adult anxieties played a prominent role in the reactions of children.[153] Again, the effect of parental anxiety on the reaction of children was related to the latter's developmental stage. Thus, while young children might be quite affected by the 'intense emotional reactions' of their

146 Bodman, 'War conditions', 486.

147 J. L. Despert, 'Effects of war on children's mental health', *Journal of Consulting Psychology*, 8 (1944), 206–18.

148 Bodman, 'War conditions', 486.

149 Dunsdon, 'A psychologist's contribution', 40.

150 E. M. John, 'A study of the effects of evacuation and air raids on children of pre-school age', *British Journal of Educational Psychology*, 11 (1941), 173–82.

151 John, 'A study of the effects', 173.

152 Jersild and Meigs, 'Children and war', 162.

153 Jersild and Meigs, 'Children and war', 162.

elders, children 'near or at the teen age may be challenged by the emotional distress shown by a parent or other adult and seek to give help or reassurance'.[154] In his opinion, children 'have adapted themselves exceedingly well to the unfamiliar sights and sounds of air-raids,' while older children 'often actually regard them as a great thrill'. This favourable resolution only occurred, Solomon concluded, 'in cases where the adults in contact with the children have behaved with self-control'.[155]

In 1943, the British educational psychologist Cyril Burt, in his essay 'War Neuroses in British Children', suggested that – provided a child was not physically injured – the mental shock provoked by being bombed was less damaging that being with a hysterical adult.[156] Burt also found that it was children aged between two and five – rather than infants – who 'seemed to suffer most severely from the air raids'.[157] Most cases were relatively mild – emotional disturbance rather than neurosis – but the more severe cases included anxiety neurosis and hysteria. Although children of elementary-school age were often less affected by 'contagious panic', they ran a greater risk of being affected by their own imaginations.

With the aim of encouraging other observers to differentiate between anxiety stemming from genuine danger and anxiety triggered by the intensity of the child's innate impulses, Anna Freud identified five different types or aspects of air-raid anxiety.[158] Like Burt and Solomon, she recognised the degree to which a child's response to air raids was linked to parental reactions: while children who were in the care of their mothers or a familiar mother substitute during the raids did not show signs of traumatic shock, others who had not passed through that experience but who lived with 'hysterical mothers' developed highly pathological behaviours.[159] Following this logic, the most anxious children were not necessarily those who had experienced being bombed. Anna Freud cites the case of a four-year-old boy who had not experienced the bombings but who seemed to be the most nervous of all the children at the Hampstead War Nurseries. In contrast, a four-year-old girl, who had experienced bombing and the roof of her home being blown off, attempted to comfort him, advising him to pull the bedclothes over his head to block out the noise of the anti-aircraft guns.[160] For Freud, this supported several

[154] J. C. Solomon, 'Reaction of children to blackouts', *American Journal of Orthopsychiatry*, 12 (1942), 62.
[155] Solomon, 'Reaction of children', 62.
[156] Cyril Burt, 'War Neuroses in British children', *The Nervous Child*, 2 (1943), 324–37.
[157] Despert, 'Effects of war on children's mental health', 212.
[158] Nick Midgley, *Reading Anna Freud* (Routledge, London, 2013), 72.
[159] Anna Freud and Dorothy Burlingham, *Infants without Families* (International Universities Press, New York, 1944), 163–72.
[160] Freud and Burlingham, *Infants without Families*, 185.

psychiatrists' claim that many people – both adults and children – have more anxiety in relation to the *idea* of being bombed than to the reality: the unknown danger is greater than the known, the fantasy more powerful than the reality. Ultimately, the most tangible threat was not trauma caused by the experience of destruction, but the impracticability of education to counteract the effect of destruction once inherited anxieties severed the children's sense of safety.

Like Susan Isaacs, Freud and the rest of the staff at the Hampstead War Nurseries believed that these children feared air raids only to the extent that they could understand what was happening. However, many young children could simply ignore the facts whenever they became unpleasant. For children in the first stage of the development of their 'inner conscience', raids were simply new symbols, substitutes for conventional 'old fears'.[161] Children of preschool age, however, understood the fear reactions of their mother and shared them: 'observers seldom appreciate the depth and seriousness of this grief of a small child'.[162]

At the Hampstead Nurseries, Anna Freud and her staff aimed to observe the mechanisms through which children either expressed or defended themselves against what she called 'the pain of separation', and to address the perceived mental harm already inflicted upon the children.[163] While some children found relief in speech – often after considerable periods of silence – play was a more available form of expression and therapy for others. Many severe cases expressed their maladjustment in deviant behaviour or neurotic regressions to more infantile modes.[164] For example, after being separated from her parents, the seventeen-month-old Carol kept on repeating 'mum, mum, mum in a deep voice for almost three days'.[165] In the cases of children aged three or four – in whom it would be normal to have ambivalent feelings about their parents – separation often seemed to confirm the child's negative feelings. After being told that his mother had been admitted to the hospital, Billie, aged three-and-a-half, remembered how he had kicked her and became anxious that it was his fault that she was ill. In Billie's case, as separation was seen by the child as a consequence of his negative thoughts and actions, he needed to perform actions that compensated for what he had 'made' happen. In normal parental settings, a young child's hostile and aggressive thoughts are

161 Freud and Burlingham, *War and Children*, 30.

162 Freud and Burlingham, *Infants without Families*, 183.

163 For the role of observation in the Hampstead War Nurseries. See Midgley, 'Anna Freud: the Hampstead War Nurseries', 939–59. See also, Shapira, *The War Inside*.

164 For a discussion on regression in the context analysed in this book, see S. Bar-Haim, 'Regression and the maternal in the history of psychoanalysis, 1900–1957', *Psychoanalysis and History*, 16(1) (2014), 69–94.

165 Freud and Burlingham, *War and Children*, 184.

counterbalanced by the experience of the parents' 'survival' of such feelings. But a sudden separation from the parents could serve to confirm a child's deepest anxieties. 'The child is frightened by the parents' absence, and suspects that their desertion may be another punishment or even the consequences of his own bad wishes', argues Freud. 'To overcome this guilt he overstresses all the love which he has ever felt for his parents. This turns the natural pain of separation into an intense longing which is hard to bear.'[166]

Like her colleagues, Anna Freud dedicated herself to observing these bodily signs. However, she criticised the fact that the diagnosis of separation anxiety and other children's disturbances induced by war was highly focused on symptoms while ignoring the age or developmental phase of the children. This 'reliance on manifest symptoms, inevitably led into confusion in assessment and subsequently to erroneous therapeutic inferences', she argued, especially when children were involved, because their symptoms were often transitory and could indicate different things depending on the circumstances. Freud believed that a similar symptom in different children could in one case stem from a developmental disturbance while in another denote an internal conflict. In contrast, different symptoms in different children might be caused by similar underlying pathological dynamics.[167] Anna Freud's words cast light on the shadow of making an incorrect diagnosis and the consequent poor treatment or care of the child, something that is more evident when the vagueness of the definition of neurotic disturbances is appreciated. Overall, descriptions of changes in children's behaviour and symptoms were superficial, whether they were merely negative variants of normal behaviour or variations that had to be recognised as the formation of neurosis.[168]

Anna Freud was a leading voice challenging the official thesis on the evacuation and protection of children from the dangers of wars. Her research showed that much more striking than the way they responded to war was the reaction of these young children to a sudden separation from their families. In fact, there was widespread agreement with Freud's view that it was a greater shock to children to be separated from their parents than to experience a bombardment. Thus, Burbury found the formation of neurotic symptoms or an exacerbation of already present symptoms in 52 per cent of evacuated children, while only 20 per cent of bombed children showed such a negative influence on their adaptation to reality.[169] Alcock held that children who showed symptoms induced by the shock of bombing usually lost them quite

[166] Freud and Burlingham, *War and Children*, 189.
[167] N. Midgley, 'Test of time: Anna Freud's *Normality and Pathology in Childhood* (1965)', *Clinical Child Psychology and Psychiatry*, 16 (2011), 475–82.
[168] Wolf, 'Evacuation of children in wartime', 393.
[169] Wolf, 'Evacuation of children in wartime', 394.

quickly; on the other hand, the symptoms associated with separation from home were much more persistent.[170]

The doctor W. J. T. Kimber commented how 'he had been struck by the effect on children of the threat to the parents left behind and the feeling of guilt in having "run away"'.[171] This fear was vague but nonetheless real, he argued, even in small children, and it produced continuous anxiety. R. P. Garrow, another doctor, agreed that the evacuated child was in some respects in a worse situation that the child who stayed in London because of the separation from the home environment.[172] Following the same logic, Susan Isaacs argued that the effect of the loss of the father on the psychological development of children was more severe than the physical privations that resulted from war. 'For vast numbers of children', she claimed, 'the loss of the father is added to all the strain[,] confusion and suffering of war, of ruined homes and divided families.'[173] When addressing mothers who 'succeeded in keeping their evacuee over a period of years', Winnicott said that although 'the bodily care of a child is a big thing', it is only part of something larger. He emphasised that mothers should take care 'of the whole child, the whole child who is a human being with a constant need for love and imaginative understanding'. For Winnicott and for many others, 'the real worry about bombs was not all'.[174] The other 'real worry' was the child's reaction to loss.

Preventing this kind of harm became the object of social policy, and it featured in much literature about parenting in the post-war period. A widely held interpretation of Richard Titmuss's argument in his 1950 book *Problems of Social Policy* is that evacuation led to governmental, professional and public awareness of the problems faced by working-class children in the cities, which led to the creation of the National Health Service, although this claim has been the object of debate among historians.[175]

The Scientific Method during Wartime: A 'Natural Experiment'

Not only did Anna Freud become an authoritative voice on the exposure of the psychological perils of evacuation, but she was also a shrewd proponent of the adoption of the scientific method in the historic opportunity yielded by war. Although primarily responsible for serving the urgent need of the victims of

170 Alcock, 'War strain', 124.

171 'War strain in children: a debate at the Tavistock Clinic', *The Lancet*, 237 (1941), 121–22.

172 'War strain in children', 121.

173 Susan Isaacs, *Childhood and After: Some Essays and Clinical Studies* (Agathon Press, New York, 1970), 186.

174 Donald Winnicott, 'Evacuation of small children', in D. W. Winnicott, R. Shepherd and M. David (eds.), *Deprivation and Delinquency* (Routledge, London, 1941), 42.

175 Titmuss, *Problems of Social Policy*, 507–8.

the Blitz and the evacuation, Anna Freud was convinced that creating a nursery to care for children affected by war was a 'natural experiment' that should be exploited.[176] Among the aims of the War Nurseries was the care of the child of the war, but also research and training.[177] Although Anna Freud described the research at the nurseries as merely a secondary outcome of charitable war work, she acknowledged that the War Nurseries provided an optimal environment for observation.[178] The nurseries allowed staff to study children from birth in various circumstances – whether in contact with their mothers, deprived of maternal care, breastfed or bottle-fed, dealing with separation and reunification. Freud and her team were able to track key developmental processes, such as the stages of emotional development, weaning, toilet training and speech acquisition, as well as the emergence of 'ego functions'.[179]

Anna Freud was not the only one who understood the war and children's bodies as laboratories of observation and experimentation. In *The Cambridge Evacuation Survey*, Susan Isaacs explained the two main aims of the study. First, the authors wanted to alleviate some of the short-term problems of evacuation: 'If it were necessary to sustain this family separation, how could it be done with the least damage and the most benefit to those who were involved.'[180] However, as in the Hampstead War Nurseries, the study's second aim was more long term: to add to existing knowledge about children and about family life to 'improve social service provision after the war'.[181] Although the resulting report, which Isaacs edited, criticised government agencies for being so concerned with the practical details of evacuation that they had not envisaged the psychological impact it would have on the children involved, she also believed that policymakers could learn from the experience of evacuation:

> This sharp lesson in the ineffectiveness and waste of a partial approach to a great human issue, one which from its very nature touches every side of human life, applies by no means only to the temporary crisis of dispersing urban populations during a war. It has an equally direct and urgent bearing upon the whole field of education and of social reconstruction during and after the war.[182]

176 Rose Edgcumbe, *Anna Freud: A View of Development, Disturbance and Therapeutic Techniques* (Routledge, London, 2004), 232.
177 Anna Freud and Dorothy T. Burlingham, *Young Children in War-Time: A Year's Work in a Residential War Nursery* (George Allen & Unwin, London, 1942), 12.
178 Midgley, 'Anna Freud: the Hampstead War Nurseries', 942.
179 Anna Freud, *Observations on child development*, in *The Writings of Anna Freud*, vol. 4, (International Universities Press, New York, 1951), 146.
180 Isaacs, 'Cambridge evacuation survey', 10.
181 Isaacs, 'Cambridge evacuation survey', 47.
182 Isaacs, 'Cambridge evacuation survey', 11.

As well as indicating areas for improvement in government policy, Freud, Isaacs and many of their colleagues thought the experience of evacuation revealed two core areas of interest: the description of normal child development and the boundaries and social recognition of their own discipline. Both residential and day-care nurseries for children became laboratories for child observation. As Nikolas Rose has argued, the everyday lives of 'normal' children could now be viewed through the lens of psychoanalysis.[183] The vagueness of descriptions of children's behavioural changes, and the symptoms through which the figure of the uprooted child was defined, reflects not only a discipline that saw itself as a laboratory but also a new body of knowledge that was seeking legitimisation.

As Michel Shapira has argued, psychoanalysts' wartime experiments in nurseries and clinics shaped a dominant view of emotions and family life. Exploring anxiety during total war was linked to understanding the rise of authoritarian regimes, while healthy childhood family dynamics – especially the bond between mother and child – were viewed as crucial for preserving democracy.[184] Before the start of the war, the British analysts had already started to analyse how they could contribute to the correct management of panic and the mental collapse of the civilian population. But the bombardment of the cities and the experience of evacuation produced a change in the nature of their profession and helped to consolidate a discipline that was still in its infancy. Beyond the general conceptualisation of anxiety and aggression, the key contribution of psychoanalysts during the war was the work they carried out with children, the most visible domestic victims.

Through the work carried out by the clinics and institutions that were designed to receive these uprooted children, psychoanalysis positioned itself as the science that could resolve the problems of abnormal children and thereby reduce their potential risk to the community. By focusing on child psychology, psychoanalysts were able to stress the vulnerability of subjectivity and highlight the link between childhood emotions and anxieties and the unconscious life of adults. The war encouraged not only a new focus on the psychological development of children and the role of the mother in this development,[185] but also a highlighting of the signs and behaviour of these same children. The figuration of the child with air-raid shock or separation anxiety was thus fundamental in the process of legitimising psychoanalysis.[186]

[183] Rose, *Governing the Soul*, 161. [184] Shapira, *The War Inside*, 2–3.
[185] Urwin and Sharland, 'From bodies to minds', 192.
[186] For a discussion on the emergence of child psychoanalysis, see chapter 4.

Conclusion

Catherine Urwin and Elaine Sharland have argued that, in the decade after the Second World War, 'the mother as the primary source of emotional stability was established as a *sine qua non*'.[187] This came with an acceptance of infancy as a period in which specific emotional needs are paramount, and the war served to encourage a new focus on the psychological development of children in their first five years and on the role played by the mother in this development. While ideas about the importance of maternal care for children's physical development go back to the nineteenth century and the negative effects of poor mothering had long been acknowledged, now maternal separation was recognised as a pathogenic factor. This idea had its antecedents in the pre-war years, but this chapter has shown that the war crystallised such thinking by providing an unprecedented opportunity for studying the effects of separation from the mother. These theories had practical implications for childcare policy and had a much wider effect on the creation of different social and cultural ways of understanding childhood.

The figure of the evacuated child became central to multiple debates and disputes between different political, social and cultural perspectives. This chapter has explored three of these conflicted areas. First, the contrast between the bombed child and the evacuated child, between the child who suffered the physical and mental effects of the Blitz and the child who suffered the effects of separation from parents who remained in the cities. The figure of the evacuated child also brought to light the city–countryside dichotomy, in which families in rural areas received children from the East End of London and other poor areas and thereby encountered the social reality of poverty. This provoked disputes about delinquency, poor hygiene, dirty habits and whether these were the result of poor parenting or of social conditioning. Second, the contrast between the forced displacements imposed by the wartime government and the role of care institutions such as the Hampstead War Nurseries. Third, the contrast between traditional medicine, which remained focused on the somatic, and the emerging discipline of psychoanalysis, which prioritised mental and emotional development and which used the experience of the evacuated children to articulate and research its theories about separation anxiety. As I have suggested, the war provided an opportunity for psychoanalysis to establish itself as a means both to heal individuals and to safeguard society by countering juvenile delinquency and encouraging the development of healthy democratic citizens. All this shows that childhood and the figure of the child in pain was a much-contested area and that there were multiple and

187 Urwin and Sharland, 'From bodies to minds', 159.

often contradictory figurations of childhood within British medical discourse in the years around the Second World War.

Outside the realm of medicine, the uprooted child became a figure onto which various social and political meanings were projected, and which was used for propaganda purposes as a call to action. The photographs of the children of the Blitz commissioned by the Ministry of Information help us to explore the ways in which images of youth were consciously composed and manipulated to boost morale, as democratic Britain confronted the 'darkest hour' of the threat to its existence from Nazi Germany. These images also expressed normative judgements about how children should behave when they were in pain. Home-front children were presented as being simultaneously ordinary and heroic in the way they coped with physical and emotional havoc. In psychoanalytical discourses, the child figures as an adult in the making – psychoanalysis reified the child's psyche and parental relationships as something that were at the core of the normal development of the future adult member of society. In social discourses, the child is portrayed as an adult in training, so that through the acquisition of good habits and morals he or she will become a good adult and citizen.

Conclusion

This book has brought to light, for the first time in academic circles, the use and understanding of children's pain in British medical discourse. Manuscript sources, such as hospital records, case notes and medical texts, along with printed sources and non-textual sources such as photography, have been mobilised to investigate a subject that has never before been the exclusive focus of a historical analysis. Previous historiography has advanced the conversation about some of the topics discussed in this book – such as the relationship between evacuated children and psychoanalysis (Michal Shapira, *The War Inside*), children and mental illness in Victorian England (Sally Shuttleworth, *The Mind of the Child*), and infant pain denial (Joanna Bourke, *The Story of Pain*) – but these debates have not been assessed together and considered in relation to the historiography of pain. In exploring medical perceptions of children's pain in late-nineteenth- and early-twentieth-century British medical discourse, I have tried to suggest that it is a much more complex matter than has often been supposed. It is in the endeavour to explain the pain of children that I hope this book becomes more than the sum of its parts. It is not a book that covers first physiology, then paediatrics and then psychiatry, but rather it explores what these diverse areas of medical and scientific theory and practice have in common as justifying and functioning practices in relation to children's pain. Although there was no uniformity of opinion among scientists, medical researchers and the popularisers of science during this period, what does emerge is a clear disciplinary economy of science that informs and delimits both intellectual debate and the possibilities for children's emotional expression and affective practice.

The construction of a history of childhood pain encounters three complex problems. The first problem concerns the conceptualisation of pain: the question of how to define, understand theoretically and pragmatically frame pain is not a simple one. As this book has shown, there have been a multitude of responses – overlapping and contrasting – particularly regarding the credibility of infant pain. The complexity of this first problem is related to the second issue: the lack of scientific unity, which has been analysed throughout the study. The third problem relates to the 'politics of pain' and the transformation of the disciplinary framings of pain into structures of power.

Concerning the first question of the conceptualisation of pain, the problem starts with the disagreement about what pain is. We recall that, in the nineteenth century, Darwin and Preyer described pain as a reflex action and based their conclusions on the observations of infant reactions to pain. As behaviourism became entrenched among later psychologists, researchers concluded that even a clear response of displeasure was irrelevant to the question of whether babies experienced pain, because the response was no more than a reflex action, an automatic response to a stimulus. Well into the twentieth century, we encounter the oft-cited International Association for the Study of Pain (IASP) definition that pain is 'an unpleasant sensory and emotional experience associated with actual or potential tissue damage, or described in terms of such damage' and that 'pain is always subjective. Each individual learns the application of the word through experiences related to injury in early life'.[1] If the virtues of this model – which understands pain as a complex subjective phenomenon that stems from the interaction of the self and culture – have been highlighted because they allowed the visibility and medicalisation of patients with chronic or terminal pain (whose pain had been invisible for such a long time), this new model of pain also codified a prejudice against the non-verbal expression of pain.[2] The IASP definition meant that the experiences of individuals unable to express themselves verbally cannot be classified as painful, because self-expression is considered necessary for the attribution of pain.[3] Recognising this limitation, the IASP amended its definition in 2020, adding an important additional note that specifically addressed the problem of non-verbal expression of pain and childhood pain: 'Verbal description is only one of several behaviors to express pain; inability to communicate does not negate the possibility that a human or a nonhuman animal experiences pain.'[4] Yet, not long before this amendment, debates about the necessity of verbal communication persisted. As late as 1996, Harold Merskey continued to defend the view that 'we can only know if someone has pain if they tell us truthfully that it is present'.[5] The problem of childhood

[1] The first definition is from H. Merskey et al., 'Pain terms', 249–52.

[2] K. J. Anand and K. D. Craig, 'New perspectives on the definition of pain', *Pain*, 67 (1996), 3–6.

[3] See Murad Ahmad Khan, Fauzia Raza and Iqbal Akhtar Khan, 'Pain: history, culture, and philosophy', *Acta Medico-Historica Adriatica*, 13 (2015), 113–30.

[4] Srinivasa N. Raja et al., 'The revised International Association for the Study of Pain definition of pain: concepts, challenges, and compromises', *Pain*, 161 (2020), 1977.

[5] Harold Merskey, 'Response to editorial "New perspectives on the definition of pain"', *Pain*, 66 (1996), 209. Merskey had already, in 1970, suggested that the perception of pain by children was immature and that this capacity was acquired with age.

pain shows the need to question our notions about pain and sensitivity, as well as those relating to the period we call childhood.

Regarding the second problem, the lack of scientific unity, the various texts and practices analysed in this book show that there was a lack of consensus among scientists throughout this whole period.[6] In Chapter 1, we saw how at the same time as the scientific method was turning the child into a scientific and mechanistic object – with the consequent denial of infant pain – paediatricians were looking at sick children as 'children without childhood' and considered that their professional role was therefore not only to re-establish the health of the child, but also to restore the values of innocence and goodness appropriate to a Romantic conception of childhood. Like the experimental physiologists of Chapter 1 and the evolutionary psychologists of Chapter 2, the psychoanalysts of Chapter 5 did not consider the study of childhood only because they were interested in children. They hoped to discover facts that would illuminate their own disciplines. The ascent of the historical sciences and their alliances with diverse theories – such as those of recapitulation, degeneration and psychoanalysis – granted the child an unprecedented position in the field of knowledge: the child ceased being secondary or superfluous and became a source of fundamental knowledge for a good number of disciplines. Nonetheless, it is surprising that just as the child became a matter of considerable interest to these disciplines, its individuality also seemed to disappear – it became an object of science more than a subject with agency – and how along with this, in some cases, the child's pain also disappeared. The detailed scientific notes about the child's first movements and expressions in relation to sensations and pain (Chapter 1) or the studies of the mind of the child (Chapter 3) did not originate in an interest in the child as such, but rather from an interest in the child's function as an index of evolutionary development or in relation to understanding the adult mind.

The main conclusion of this study is that the construction of medical and scientific models of childhood pain reflects and creates a series of paradoxes and tensions in relation to the emergence and consolidation of the scientific disciplines analysed. In the first place, the strategies that emerged to care for and treat children with pain were formulated around and dependent on the interaction of different professionals from varied disciplines – such as psychiatrists, psychologists, physiologists, paediatricians, politicians and photographers. As Chapter 4 emphasised, the research and analysis of children with behavioural and emotional problems produced a coming together of people with different ideas, methodologies, experience and knowledge who tried to work together for the benefit of children. However, despite the emphasis on

[6] See Biagoli and Galison, *The Disunity of Science.*

co-operation, childhood pain was a field of highly controversial professional competition. Diagnosis, the medicalisation of the pain of children and the creation of various figurations of the child served as means for individuals to acquire professional power, status and recognition for their disciplines. This study has highlighted the professional rivalries between different professions, as with those between neurologists and psychologists seeking authority as experts in the care and treatment of nervous children (Chapter 4). The various theories and methodologies, presented as essential for the treatment and control of the different figures of the child in pain, were used to bolster professional and scientific status within the medical and educational systems. The changing responsibilities in the identification, care and treatment of children with pain reflected complex professional relationships among psychiatrists, psychologists, educators, the judiciary, government departments, central and local authorities, and lay charitable organisations.

As a tool of social and professional power, the medical and scientific conceptualisation of pain reflected important areas of conflict between different groups: paediatricians and physiologists, psychiatrists and psychoanalysts, professional and non-professional organisations. In addition, the concern and increasing professional interest in the emotional and physiological well-being of children gave way to an evolution in the understanding of emotional development and behaviour in childhood and infancy. This, in turn, implied a greater control of childhood, creating tension between the individual experience of the child in pain and the medical figuration of childhood. For instance, psychology and child psychiatry (studied in Chapter 5) developed around the unquestioned assumption that the new psychological and educational theories signified progress. A greater understanding was equated with an improvement in social and medical well-being, an assumption illustrated by figures such as the child analyst Anna Freud, who affirmed that the better we understand children, the better we can care for them. The assumption continued to be a characteristic of approaches to child development throughout the twentieth century, reinforced by the constant historical and contemporary references to the 'pioneering' nature of the theoretical achievement, with accounts centred on the role of medical professionals in the development of new theories rather than on the real experiences or perceptions of children with pain. Nonetheless, this study has shown that a greater understanding of the behaviour patterns of both 'normal' and 'pathological' childhood did not necessarily result in an improvement in the circumstances or behaviour of children with problems. Attempts to solve one problem often created problems of a different nature, which were unnoticed or unrecognised by medical professionals. The focus of psychiatry on the study of childhood illnesses examined in Chapter 3, for instance, resulted in the growing pathologisation and marginalisation of children with behavioural disorders. One of the main findings of this book is that the process of evaluating, treating and managing the pain of children was very variable and inconsistent. Children could be classified as having pain by various figures, including parents, medical professionals and medical institutions. Depending on the route by which they were classified, children with pain could be interned in a wide range of institutions, including hospitals, asylums and clinics. The responsibility for their supervision, medical assistance and social well-being could fall upon any one of various types of agents, including psychiatrists, psychologists, psychoanalysts, progressive educators and parents or carers.

Furthermore, the debate about pain in childhood also provides information about the cultural power of certain ideals about childhood. In part, this wide variety in the strategies of child treatment reflects the malleable nature of concepts of both pain and children. Another paradox that has been highlighted by this study is that, despite a process of medicalisation, the categorisation of children with pain depended on factors other than the criteria of medical diagnosis. To a large extent, the various figurations studied in the book – the sick child, the insane child, the nervous child and the uprooted child – reflected social and moral norms, and adults' expectations and aspirations about childhood. The social value of children was evaluated in normative developmental terms that were physiological, behavioural and – in some cases – moral. This book has situated the child in pain in different discourses to show how the concept generated specific forms – the sick child, the insane child, the nervous child – and how these figurations speak to us of the making of scientific worlds and adult cultures.

In turn, this book uncovered variables that reappear in different periods and disciplines. In the various contexts studied, children were not a homogeneous group: within the period of childhood, they were distinguished by size, individual strength and – occasionally – by sex. These results direct attention towards the general importance of age as a category in modern medicine: children are compared with the ages of the whole life cycle, including youth, adulthood and old age. As has been shown, in the context of children's pain, gender distinctions lacked importance during the period covered, largely because in terms of medical perceptions there was little differentiation between the sexes until the onset of puberty. Hannah Newton has argued that historians of medicine have often tended to overlook age as a category, prioritising sex as the organising principle of modern medicine.[7] So there is a need to focus on the importance of age as a category in modern medicine and on the medical perceptions of childhood, adolescence, youth and old age, and the forms in which sex and age intertwine in medical perceptions and treatments.

[7] Newton, *The Sick Child*, 224.

The third problem this book has considered is the *politics of pain*, a concept which has recently led to new theoretical frameworks in which political claims have collided with the history of emotions. If, as Lucy Bending has shown in *The Representation of Bodily Pain in Late Nineteenth-Century English Culture*, the appropriation of physical pain by different interpretations opens the door to potential abuse by the authorities, not only is pain subject to cultural conditioning, but it is also susceptible to be represented or distorted by these power groups.[8] The research on infant pain denial examined in the first two chapters – to highlight one example – can be considered as a paradigm of the forms in which pain can be manipulated and defined by those who wield power. Each time the communicative power of language is weakened or linguistic communication disappears, Elaine Scarry's thesis that the lack of expression of personal pain converts those who suffer it into beings 'more vulnerable to exploitation, oppression, or torture' at the hands of those who hold power takes on a special importance.[9] This book has traced how the question of the pain of others – of children – became a recurrent political battlefield (within both the various medical disciplines and other power groups). The acknowledgement of childhood pain during the studied era extended beyond just a clinical or scientific concern. The understanding of childhood pain necessitated the collaboration and involvement of various sources and communities.

Pain is a political practice, as what pain means depends not only on the children's testimony but also on the criteria that are agreed (by medical professionals, by the culture) regarding our patterns of trust. Agreement is needed not only among doctors but across the board, between different disciplines, professions, medical associations and families in order for pain to be visualised and the complaints of others to be accepted. The political dimension of pain is not simply a social factor that can be added to other dimensions, such as the physiological and the psychological, as pain is embedded in the political concerns and social values of a specific historical context. Chapter 3, for instance, showed how doctors faced various political considerations when evaluating children with mental illnesses, including what level of incapacity should lead to institutionalisation and whether this should take place in asylums or paediatric institutions. As this implies, the problem of pain is tied up with questions of trust, because how it is assessed and treated always depends on who is defining what pain is. This book has indicated that these parameters can differ in distinct medical disciplines at the same time, and how the understanding of childhood pain has emerged through multiple debates. Thus, I hope to have brought the history of childhood in line with

[8] Bending, *Representation of Bodily Pain*, 1–11. [9] Scarry, *Body in Pain*, 27.

the current debate among historians of pain and the generally accepted view that pain is subject to historical changes. This book has sought to explain what these changes involved and how differences were configured. It has been argued that there is no such thing as 'pain' in itself, there are only beings (in this case children) who feel pain, who are joined to a specific society through their own feelings and emotions and whose experience is subject to different regimes of visibility, expression and repression – depending on who delimits these experiences and who imposes discipline. Thus, any historical analysis of pain needs to consider both those afflicted by pain and the observers, which include historians and social scientists whose descriptions of experiences of pain – or the invisibility of pain in their discourses – contribute or hinder the development of new forms of social consciousness. This book has described a meandering history, where pain appears in a succession of debates and where it is not only *whose* pain that is important but also *which* pains are deemed worthy of being expressed (and which are thus accepted socially) and which should be borne in silence.

Finally, as with any other history of human experience, the history of childhood pain demands a historical awareness through which the gap between past and present can be bridged. The history of emotions – despite the inevitable difficulties involved in attempting to approach the experiences of people in the past – needs to investigate the experiences of those whose pain has been ignored because they have been marginalised, repressed or defeated. Twenty-first century historical accounts have often ignored the question of why, until recently, academic histories of pain had not tended to explore the complex and changing social attitudes towards the pain of children. We pay more attention to certain phenomena that affect a small part of the population – conditions such as phantom limbs, for instance – than to something as fundamental and universal as pain in childhood. Just as there is a hierarchy of pain in the medical world, there is also one in history – and there is an urgent need for this to be questioned and resolved.

Bibliography

Archival Sources

Great Ormond Street Hospital Archives

GOS/1/2/12: Hospital's Committee of Management Minute Books (1871–72).
GOS/9/1/2: Hospital's General Admissions Registers (1865–72).
GOS/9/1/3: Hospital's General Admissions Registers (1872–78).
GOS/9/1/4: Hospital's General Admissions Registers (1879–83).
GOS/9/1/12: Hospital's General Admissions Registers (1906).
GOS/9/1/12: Hospital's General Admissions Registers (1908).
GOS/10/1–14: Dr Charles West casenotes (1857–73).
GOS/10/26: Dr W. H. Dickinson's casenotes (1869–82).
GOS/10/229–230: Dr Frederic Still casenotes (1913–16).
Great Ormond Street Hospital B-INT 0478, ward postcards.

The Historic Hospital Admissions Records Project

The Historic Hospital Admissions Records Project (HHARP) database (Great Ormond Street Hospital for Children/University of Kingston).

Wellcome Library London Special Collections

GC148/21/21: Winnicott, Donald, Papers, 1979.
114 PP/LOW/A/A/2: Medical Research Council, *Child Life Investigations: Social Conditions and Acute Rheumatism*, Special Report Series, Archives and Manuscripts, Wellcome Institute No. 114 PP/LOW/A/A/2.
PP/BOW/C.5/4/1: Evacuation 1939–c1942, 'Psychological problems of evacuation', Draft by John Bowlby, 3–4.
PP/LOW/I/22, Box 24: Urwin, Cathy, Short article on life of Margaret Lowenfeld, 1999.

Published Sources

Ablow, Rachel, *Victorian Pain* (Princeton University Press, Princeton, NJ, 2017).
Abram, Jan (ed.), *Donald Winnicott Today* (Routledge, London, 2013).

Abt, Isaac and Fielding Garrison (eds.), *History of Paediatrics* (W. B. Saunders Company, London, 1965).

Adams, Anne Marie, David Theodore and Patricia McKeever, 'Pictures of health: sick kids exposed', in Loren Lerner (ed.), *Depicting Canada's Children* (Wilfrid Laurier, Waterloo, 2009), 259–78.

Adler, Helen, *Hints for the Scientific Observation and Study of Children* (Teacher Company, New York, 1891).

Ahlbeck, Jutta, Paäivi Lappalainen, Kati Launis and Kirsi Tuohela (eds.), *Childhood, Literature and Science: Fragile Subjects* (Routledge, London, 2017).

Ahmed, Sara, 'The contingency of pain', *Parallax*, 8 (2008), 17.

Alcock, A. T., 'War strain in children', *British Medical Journal* (25 January 1941), 124.

Alexander, Kristine, Stephanie Olsen and Karen Vallgårda, *Voices and Sources: Lessons from the History of Childhood, Digital Handbook of the History of Experience* (Research Council of Finland´s Centre of Excellence in the History of Experiences (HEX), 2023).

Anand, K. J., 'Effects of perinatal pain and stress', *Progress in Brain Research*, 122 (2000), 117–29.

Anand, K. J. and K. D. Craig, 'New perspectives on the definition of pain', *Pain*, 67 (1996), 3–6.

Anderson, Olive, *Suicide in Victorian and Edwardian England* (Clarendon Press, Oxford, 1987).

Andrews, Jonathan, 'Case notes, case histories, and the patient's experience of insanity at Gartnavel Royal Asylum, Glasgow, in the nineteenth century', *Social History of Medicine*, 11 (1998), 255–81.

Andrews, K., D. Desai, H. K. Dhillon, D. T. Wilcox and M. Fitzgerald, 'Abdominal sensitivity in the first year of life: comparison of infants with and without prenatally diagnosed unilateral hydronephrosis', *Pain*, 100 (2002), 35–46.

Andrews, K. and M. Fitzgerald, 'Cutaneous flexion reflex in human neonates: a quantitative study of threshold and stimulus-response characteristics after single and repeated stimuli', *Developmental Medicine and Child Neurology*, 41 (1999), 696–703.

'The cutaneous withdrawal reflex in human neonates: sensitization, receptive fields, and the effects of contralateral stimulation', *Pain*, 56 (1994), 95–101.

Anon, 'Backgrounds: Mr. Faulkner's method of making them', *British Journal of Photography* (22 August 1873), 395.

'The child's home background', *The Lancet*, 1 (6 April 1940), 651.

Children's Communities: Experiments in Democratic Living (NEF Monograph, London, 1944).

'Evacuation: a brighter picture', *British Medical Journal*, 2 (10 July 1943), 46.

'Homicidal insanity', *Journal of Psychological Medicine and Mental Pathology*, 1 (1848), 330.

'How I photograph my little ones', *British Journal of Photography* (28 March 1872), 146–47.

'How Mr Faulkner photographs children', *British Journal of Photography* (11 October 1872), 480–81.

The Illustrated London News (21 September 1940), 3.

'On the injurious effects of the inhalation of ether', *Provincial Medical and Surgical Journal*, 11 (1847), 330–31.
LIFE Magazine (23 September 1940), 21.
'Lunatics at home', *British Medical Journal*, 1 (28 May 1870), 552.
'Malingery', *The Lancet*, 165 (1905), 45–46.
'Mr Crichton on lithotomy', *Edinburgh Medical and Surgical Journal*, 9 (1828), 232.
'A successful exodus', *British Medical Journal*, 2 (9 September 1939), 573.
The Times Educational Supplement, 9 September 1939.
'The town child: a critical survey', *British Medical Journal*, 1 (8 May 1943), 571.
'Treatment for bed-wetting', *The Lancet*, 2 (7 October 1939), 794–95,
'War strain in children: a debate at the Tavistock Clinic', *The Lancet*, 237 (1941), 121.
'Westminster Medical Society, Saturday, November 23, 1833. Mr. Pettigew in the Chair', *The Lancet*, 21 (1833), 362–74.
Ariès, Philippe, *Centuries of Childhood: A Social History of Family Life* (Alfred A. Knopf, New York, 1962).
Armstrong, David, *Political Anatomy of the Body: Medical Knowledge in Britain in the Twentieth Century* (Cambridge University Press, Cambridge, 1983).
Armstrong, George, *An Essay on the Diseases Most Fatal to Infants* (T. Cadell, London, 1767).
Armstrong, Thomas, *The Myth of the ADD Child* (Plume Penguin, New York, 1995).
Ashby, Henry, *The Diseases of Children: Medical and Surgical* (Longman Green, New York, 1900).
Ashcroft, Bill, *On Post-Colonial Futures: Transformations of Colonial Culture* (Continuum, London, 2001).
Asher, C., 'Personal environment and enuresis', *British Medical Journal*, 2 (10 August 1940), 206.
Baden Pritchard, H., 'Mr Robert Faulkner in Baker Street', in *The Photographic Studios of Europe* (Piper & Carter, London, 1882), 68–82.
Bakker, Nelleke, 'A harmless disease: children and neurasthenia in the Netherlands', in M. Gijswijt-Hofstra and R. Porter (eds.), *Cultures of Neurasthenia from Beard to the First World War* (Rodopi, Amsterdam, 2001), 309–27.
Ballet, Gilbert (trans. P. Campbell Smith), *Neurasthenia* (Henry Kimpton, London; Alexander Stenhouse, Glasgow, 1908).
Banks, A. L. and L. G. Norman, 'Sick-bays for child evacuees', *The Lancet* (20 September 1941), 357.
Bar-Haim, S., 'Regression and the maternal in the history of psychoanalysis, 1900–1957', *Psychoanalysis and History*, 16 (2014), 69–94.
Barke, M., R. Fribush and P. Stearns (eds.), 'Nervous breakdown in 20th-century American life', *Social History*, 33 (2000), 565–84.
Barkley, R. A., *ADHD and the Nature of Self-Control* (Guilford Press, New York, 2005).
Attention Deficit Hyperactivity Disorder: A Handbook for Diagnosis and Treatment, 3rd ed. (Guilford Press, New York, 2006).
Defiant Children: A Clinician's Manual for Assessment and Parent Training (Guilford Press, New York, 1997).

Barkley, R. A. and K. R. Murphy, *Attention Deficit Hyperactivity Disorder: A Clinical Workbook* (Guilford Press, New York, 2006).

Barkley, R. A., G. Edwards and A. R. Robin, *Defiant Teens: A Clinician's Manual for Assessment and Family Intervention* (Guilford Press, New York, 1999).

Bartlett, P. and D. Wright (eds.), *Outside the Walls of the Asylum: The History of Care in the Community, 1750–2000* (Athlone, London, 1999).

Bashford, Alison and Phillipa Levine (eds.), *The Oxford Handbook of the History of Eugenics* (Oxford University Press, Oxford, 2010).

Batten, Frederick F., Archibald E. Garrod and Hugh Thursfield (eds.), *Diseases of Children: By Various Authors* (Edward Arnold, London, 1913).

Beach, Fletcher, 'Clinical lecture on mental disorders in children', *Treatment: A Journal of Practical Medicine and Surgery*, 2 (1898), 589.

Beaton, Cecil, *The Years Between: Diaries, 1939–44* (Holt, Rinehart & Winston, New York, 1965).

Beekman, Daniel, *The Mechanical Baby: A Popular History of the Theory and Practice of Child Raising* (Dobson, London, 1977).

Behlmer, George K., *Friends of the Family: The English Home and Its Guardians, 1850–1940* (Stanford University Press, Stanford, CA, 1998).

Beier, Lucinda McCray, *For Their Own Good: The Transformation of English Working-Class Health Culture, 1880–1970* (Ohio State University Press, Columbus, 2008).

Bending, Lucy, 'Pain and religion in the Victorian era', in Javier Moscoso (ed.), *Pain: Passion, Compassion, Sensibility* (Wellcome Trust, London, 2004), 1–5.

The Representation of Bodily Pain in Late Nineteenth-Century English Culture (Clarendon Press, Oxford, 2000).

Bennett, Ivy, *Delinquent and Neurotic Children: A Comparative Study* (Tavistock Publications, London, 1960).

Bergenn, Victor W., 'Myrtle B. McGraw: a growth scientist', *Developmental Psychology*, 28 (1992), 384.

Berridge, Virginia, 'Health and medicine', in F. M. L. Thompson (ed.), *The Cambridge Social History of Britain, 1750–1950, III: Social Agencies and Institutions* (Cambridge University Press, Cambridge, 1990), 171–242.

Berrios, German, 'Classic Text No. 37: J.C. Prichard and the concept of moral insanity', *History of Psychiatry*, 10 (1999), 111–26.

The History of Mental Symptoms: Descriptive Psychopathology since the Nineteenth Century (Cambridge University Press, Cambridge, 1995).

'Mood disorders: clinical section', in German E. Berrios and Roy Porter (eds.), *A History of Clinical Psychiatry: The Origin and History of Psychiatric Disorders* (Athlone Press, London, 1995).

Berrios, German E. and Roy Porter (eds.), *A History of Clinical Psychiatry: The Origin and History of Psychiatric Disorders* (Athlone Press, London, 1995).

Berry, Boyd M., 'The first English paediatricians and Tudor attitudes towards childhood', *Journal of the History of Ideas*, 35 (1974), 561–77.

Betts, Eleanor, 'From Juvenile Delinquent to boy murderer: understanding children who killed, 1816–1908' (Unpublished PhD thesis, Queen Mary University, 2016).

Beyer, Judith E. and Mary Lou Byer, 'Knowledge of paediatric pain: the state of the art', *Children's Health Care*, 13 (2010), 150–59.

Biagoli, Mario and Galison, Peter, *The Disunity of Science: Boundaries, Contexts, and Power* (Stanford University Press, Stanford, CA, 1996).

Biernoff, Suzannah, 'The face of war', in Andrei Pop and Mechtild Widrich (eds.), *Ugliness: The Non-Beautiful in Art and Theory* (I. B. Tauris, London, 2014), 34–48.

'The rhetoric of disfigurement in First World War Britain', *Social History of Medicine*, 24 (2001), 666–85.

Bigelow, Henry, *Ether and Chloroform: A Compendium of their History, Surgical Use, Dangers and Discovery* (David Clapp, Boston, 1848).

'Insensibility during surgical operations produced by inhalation', *Boston Medical and Surgical Journal*, 35 (1846), 309.

Billard, Charles-Michel, *A Treatise on the Diseases of Infants, Founded on Recent Clinical Observations and Investigations in Pathological Anatomy, Made at the Hospice des Enfants Trouvés: With a Dissertation on the Viability of the Child*, 2nd ed. (J. & H. G. Langley, New York, 1840).

Bilon, Hippolite, *Dissertation sur la Doleur* (Feugueray, Paris, 1803).

Blandford, George Fielding, *Insanity and Its Treatment: Lectures on the Treatment, Medical and Legal, of Insane Patients* (Oliver and Boyd, Edinburgh, 1871).

Blanton, Margaret Gray, 'The behavior of the human infant in the first 30 days of life', *Psychological Review*, 24 (1917), 456–83.

Bingham, Adrian et al., 'Historical child sexual abuse in England and Wales: the role of historians', *History of Education*, 45 (2016), 411–29.

Bion, Wilfred R., 'Psychiatry at a time of crisis', *British Journal of Medical Psychology*, 21 (1948), 81–89.

Biro, David, *The Language of Pain: Finding Words, Compassion, and Relief* (Norton, New York, 2010).

'Psychological pain: metaphor or reality?', in Rob Boddice (ed.), *Pain and Emotion in Modern History* (Palgrave, London, 2014), 53–65.

Bland, Lucy and Lesley A. Hall, 'Eugenics in Britain: The view from the metropole', in Alison Bashford and Phillipa Levine (eds.), *The Oxford Handbook of the History of Eugenics* (Oxford University Press, Oxford, 2010), 213–27.

Bleichmar, Daniela, *Visible Empire: Botanical Expeditions and Visual Culture in the Hispanic Enlightenment* (University of Chicago Press, Chicago, 2012).

Boddice, Rob, *A History of Attitudes and Behaviours toward Animals in Eighteenth and Nineteenth-Century Britain: Anthropocentrism and the Emergence of Animals* (Mellen, Lewiston, NY, 2009).

Humane Professions: The Defense of Experimental Medicine, 1876–1914 (Cambridge University Press, Cambridge, 2021).

'Hysteria or Tetanus? Ambivalent embodiments and the authenticity of pain', in Dolores Martin Moruno and Beatriz Pichel (eds.), *Emotional Bodies: Studies on the Historical Performativity of Emotion* (University of Illinois Press, Urbana-Champaign, 2019), 19–35.

Knowing Pain: A History of Sensation, Emotion, and Experience (Polity Press, Cambridge, 2023).

Pain: A Very Short Introduction (Oxford University Press, Oxford, 2016).

(ed.), *Pain and Emotions in Modern History* (Palgrave Macmillan, Basingstoke, 2014).

'Species of compassion: aesthetics, anaesthetics and pain in the physiological laboratory', *19: Interdisciplinary Studies in the Long Nineteenth Century*, 15 (2012), 1–22.

'Vivisecting major: a Victorian gentleman scientist defends animal experimentation, 1876–1885', *Isis*, 102(2) (2011), 215–37.

Bodman, A. G., 'Enuresis', *British Medical Journal*, 1 (20 January 1940), 109.

Bodman, Frank H., 'War conditions and the mental health of the child', *British Medical Journal*, 2 (4 October 1941), 486–88.

Boehm, Katharina, *Charles Dickens and the Sciences of Childhood: Popular Medicine, Child Health, and Victorian Culture* (Palgrave Macmillan, London, 2013).

Bohannon, E. W., 'A study of peculiar and exceptional children', *The Pedagogical Seminary: An International Record of Educational Literature, Institutions and Progress*, 4 (1896), 3–53.

Bolwig, Tom G. and Max Fink Bolwig, 'Electrotherapy for melancholia: the pioneering contributions of Benjamin Franklin and Giovanni Aldini', *Journal of ECT*, 25 (2009), 15–18.

Bonea, Amelia et al., *Anxious Times: Medicine and Modernity in Nineteenth-Century Britain* (University of Pittsburgh Press, Pittsburgh, PA, 2019).

Bonet, Theophile, *A Guide to the Practical Physician* (Flesher, London, 1684).

Bonica, J. John, 'History of pain concepts and therapies', in John J. Bonica and Lea Fabiger (eds.), *The Management of Pain* (Lippincott Williams and Wilkings, Philadelphia, PA, 1991), 2–17.

Bonica, J. John and Lea Fabiger (eds.), *The Management of Pain* (Lippincott Williams and Wilkings, Philadelphia, PA, 1991).

Borsay, A. and P. Dale (eds.), *Disabled Children: Contested Caring, 1850–1979* (Pickering and Chatto, London, 2012).

Borsay, A. and P. Shapely (eds.), *Medicine, Charity and Mutual Aid: The Consumption of Health and Welfare in Britain, c.1550–1950* (Ashgate, Aldershot, 2007).

Bound Alberti, Fay (ed.), *Medicine, Emotion and Disease, 1700–1950* (Palgrave, Basingstoke, 2006).

This Mortal Coil: The Human Body in History and Culture (Oxford University Press, Oxford, 2016).

Bourke, Joanna, 'The art of medicine: languages of pain', *The Lancet*, 379 (2012), 2420–21.

Fear: A Cultural History (Virago, London, 2006).

'The history of medicine as the history of pain', *History Today*, 61 (2011), 56–57.

Pain and the Politics of Sympathy: Historical Reflections, 1760s to 1960s (Utrecht University, Utrecht, 2011).

'Pain, sympathy and the medical encounter between the mid eighteenth and the mid twentieth centuries', *Historical Research*, 8(229) (2012), 430–52.

'The Prothero Lecture: "What is pain? A history"', *Transactions of the Royal Historical Society*, 23 (December 2013), 155–73.

'The sensible and insensible body: a visual essay', *19: Interdisciplinary Studies in the Long Nineteenth Century*, 15 (2012), 2–13.

The Story of Pain: From Prayers to Painkillers (Oxford University Press, Oxford, 2014).

Bourke, Joanna and Whitney Wood, 'Conceptualizing gender and pain in modern history', *Gender & History*, 32 (2020), 8–12.

Bowlby, John, 'Forty-four juvenile thieves: their characters and home-life', *The International Journal for Psycho-Analysis*, 25 (1944), 19–53, 107–28.

'Hysteria in children', in R. G. Gordon, On behalf of the Child Guidance Council (ed.), *A Survey of Child Psychiatry: Contributed by Contemporary British Authorities* (Oxford University Press and Humphrey Milford, London, 1939), 80–94.

Maternal Care and Mental Health (World Health Organization, Geneva, 1952).

Personality and Mental Illness: An Essay in Psychiatric Diagnosis, The International Library of Psychology (Kegan Paul, Trench, Trubner and Co., London, 1940).

'Psychological aspects of the evacuation', in Richard Padley and Margaret Cole (eds.), *Evacuation Survey: A Report to the Fabian Society* (G. Routledge & Sons, London, 1940), 186–96.

Bowlby, J., E. Miller and D. W. Winnicott, 'Evacuation of small children', Letter to the editor, *British Medical Journal*, 2 (16 December 1939), 1202–3.

Bowlby, Richard, *Fifty Years of Attachment Theory* (Karnac on behalf of the Winnicott Clinic of Psychotherapy, London, 2004).

Bowler, Peter, *The Mendelian Revolution: The Emergence of Hereditarian Concepts in Modern Science and Society* (Athlone, London, 1989).

Bowley, A. H., 'Child Guidance surveys in wartime', *Mental Health* (July 1940), 176.

Boyd McBride, Kari (ed.), *Domestic Arrangements in Early Modern England* (Duquesne University Press, Pittsburgh, PA, 2002).

Breggin, P., *Talking Back to Ritalin* (Common Courage Press, Monroe, ME, 1998).

Brend, William A., 'Air-raid shock', *British Medical Journal*, 2 (15 November 1941), 712.

Brière de Boismont, Alexandre, 'On the insanity of early life', *Journal of Psychiatric Medicine*, 10 (1857), 622–38.

Bringmann, Wolfgang G., Norma J. Bringmann and William D. G. Balance, 'Experimental approaches to developmental psychology before William Preyer', in G. Eckardt (ed.), *Contributions to a History of Developmental Psychology: International William T. Preyer Symposium* (Mouton, Berlin, 1985), 159.

Brothwell, D. and Sandison, A. T. (eds.), *Diseases of Antiquity: A Survey of the Diseases, Injuries and Surgery of Early Populations* (Charles T. Thomas, Springfield, IL, 1967).

Brown, Felix, 'Civilian psychiatric air raid casualties', *The Lancet*, 237 (31 May 1941), 691.

Brown, Gillian, 'The metamorphic book, children's print culture in the eighteenth century', *Eighteenth-Century Studies*, 39 (2006), 351–62.

Brown, William, *War and Peace: Essay in Psychological Analysis* (A. & C. Black, London, 1939).

Brown, W. Paterson, 'The family neurosis', in R. G. Gordon, On behalf of the Child Guidance Council (ed.), *A Survey of Child Psychiatry: Contributed by Contemporary British authorities* (Oxford University Press and Humphrey Milford, London, 1939), 115–27.

Bruce, J., 'The footprints of Scottish paediatric surgery', *Journal of the Royal College of Surgeons of Edinburgh*, 21 (1976), 136.

Brunner, J., *Freud and the Politics of Psychoanalysis* (Oxford University Press, Oxford, 1995).

Bryder, Linda, '"Wonderworlds of Buttercup, Clover and Daisies": tuberculosis and the open-air school movement in Britain, 1907–39', in Roger Cooter (ed.), *In the Name of the Child: Health and Welfare, 1880–1940* (Routledge, London, 1992), 72–95.

Buckman, Sydney, 'Babies and monkeys', *The Nineteenth Century*, 36 (1984), 727–43.

Bucknill, Sir John Charles and Daniel Hack Tuke, *A Manual of Psychological Medicine: Containing the History, Nosology, Description, Statistics, Diagnosis, Pathology and Treatment of Insanity* (Blanchard and Lea, Philadelphia, PA, 1858).

Budin, Pierre, *The Nursling: The Feeding and Hygiene of Premature & Full-Term Infants* (Caxton Publishing Company, London, 1907).

Burke, Edmund, *A Philosophical Enquiry into the Origins of Our Ideas of the Sublime and Beautiful* (Penguin, London, 1989).

Burke, R. E., 'Sir Charles Sherrington's *The Integrative Action of the Nervous System*: a Centenary Appreciation', *Brain*, 130 (2007), 887–94.

Burke, Peter (ed.), *A New Kind of History from the Writings of Lucien Febvre* (Routledge & Kegan Paul, London, 1973).

La Revolución Historiográfica Francesa: La Escuela de los Annales, 1929–1989 (Gedisa, Barcelona, 1993).

Burlingham, Dorothy and Freud, Anna, *Children in Wartime* (Medical War Books, New York, 1940).

Burman, Jeremy Trevelyan, 'History from within? Contextualizing the new neurohistory and seeking its methods', *History of Psychology*, 15 (2012), 84–99.

Burbury, W. Mary, 'Effects of evacuation and of air raids on city children', *British Medical Journal* (8 November 1941), 660–62.

Burt, Cyril, 'The billeting of evacuated children', *The British Journal of Educational Psychology*, 11 (1941), 85–98.

'The incidence of neurotic symptoms among evacuated school children', *British Journal of Educational Psychology*, 10 (1940), 8–15.

'Under fives in total war', printed for circulation to members of the British Psychological Society (20 December 1941).

'War neuroses in British children', *The Nervous Child*, 2 (1943), 324–37.

'War neuroses in soldiers, civilians, and children' (duplicated summary for private circulation), Psychology Laboratory, University College London (November 1939).

Calder, Angus, *The People's War: Britain, 1939–1945* (Pantheon Books, New York, 1969).

Calder, Ritchie, 'The school child', in Richard Padley and Margaret Cole (eds.), *Evacuation Survey: A Report to the Fabian Society* (G. Routledge & Sons, London, 1940) 147–53.

Cameron, Hector, 'Ketonæmia, cyclical vomiting and some nervous disturbances in children', *Archives of Disease in Childhood*, 2 (1927), 55–61.

The Nervous Child (Oxford University Press, London, 1919).

Canguilhem, Georges, 'The concept of reflex', in François Delaporte (ed.), *A Vital Rationalist: Selected Writings from Georges Canguilhem* (Zone Books, New York, 1994), 179–202.

Cannella, Gaile Sloan, *Childhood and Postcolonization: Power, Education, and Contemporary Practice* (Routledge, New York, 2004).
Carling, E., 'Evacuation of women and children', *British Medical Journal*, 2 (28 October 1939), 896.
Carmichael, James, *Disease in Children: A Manual for Students and Practitioners* (Edinburgh, Young J. Pentland, 1892).
Carpenter, Laura M., 'If you prick us: masculinity and circumcision pain in the United States and Canada, 1960–2000', *Gender & History*, 32 (2020), 54–69.
Castañeda, Claudia, *Figurations: Child, Bodies, Worlds* (Duke University Press, Durham, NC, 2002).
Caton, Donald, *What a Blessing She Had Chloroform: The Medical and Social Response to the Pain of Childbirth from 1800 to the Present* (Yale University Press, New Haven, CT, 1999).
Cattell, Raymond B., 'The school and the child guidance clinic', in J. I. Cohen (ed.), *Educating for Democracy* (Macmillan and Co., London, 1939), 169–82.
Caulfield, Ernest, 'Pediatric aspects of the Salem witchcraft tragedy', *American Journal of Diseases of Children*, 65 (1943), 788–802.
Cautley, Edmund, *The Diseases of Infants and Children* (Paul B. Hoeber, New York, 1912).
Chamberlain, Alexander Francis, *The Child: A Study in the Evolution of Man* (Walter Scott Ltd., London, 1900).
Chamberlain, David B., 'Babies don't feel pain: a century of denial in medicine', *The Journal of Prenatal and Perinatal Psychology and Health*, 14 (1999), 145–68.
Chaney, Sarah, 'Anaesthetic bodies and the absence of feeling: pain and self-mutilation in later nineteenth-century psychiatry', *19: Interdisciplinary Studies in the Long Nineteenth Century*, 15 (2012), 1–19.
Psyche on the Skin: A History of Self-Harm (Reaktion Books, London, 2017).
'Self-mutilation and psychiatry: impulse, identity and the unconscious in British explanations of self-inflicted injury, c. 1864–1914' (PhD thesis, University College London, 2013).
Chapin, Henry, *Diseases of Infants and Children* (W. Wood and Co., New York, 1911).
Chapple, J. A. V. and Anita Wilson, *Private Voices: The Diaries of Elizabeth Gaskell and Sophia Holland* (Keele University Press, Keele, 1996).
Chartier, Roger, *El Mundo como Representación: Estudios sobre Historia Cultural* (Gedisa, Barcelona, 1992).
Churchill, Winston S., *The Unrelenting Struggle* (Cassell and Company, London, 1942).
Clark, Ann, 'Compliance with infant smallpox vaccination legislation in nineteenth-century rural England: Hollingbourne, 1876–88', *Social History of Medicine*, 17 (2004), 175–98.
Clark, Michael J., 'The data of alienism': evolutionary neurology, physiological psychology, and the reconstruction of British psychiatric theory, c.1850–c.1900' (Unpublished PhD thesis, University of Oxford, 1982).
Clarke, Edwin and L. S. Jacyna, *Nineteenth-Century Origins of Neuroscientific Concepts* (University of California Press, Berkeley, 1987).
Clarke, J. Michell, 'A case of obscure fever with pronounced nervous symptoms, apparently due to infection by a leptothrix bacillus', *British Medical Journal*, 1 (13 January 1912), 67.

'Clinical observations on hysteria', *The Lancet*, 141 (20 May 1893), 1185–89.
Hysteria and Neurasthenia (J. Lane, The Bodley Head, London, 1905).
Clouston, Thomas S., *Clinical Lectures on Mental Diseases* (J. & A. Churchill, London, 1883).
Coakley, Sarah and Kay Kaufman Shelemay (eds.), *Pain and Its Transformations: The Interface of Biology and Culture* (Harvard University Press, Cambridge, MA, 2007).
Cobb, Ivo Geikie, *A Manual of Neurasthenia (Nervous Exhaustion)* (Baillière, Tindall and Cox, London, 1920).
Cohen, Esther, 'The animated pain of the body', *American Historical Review*, 105 (2000), 36–68.
'Towards a history of European physical sensibility: pain in the later middle ages', *Science in Context*, 8 (1995), 47–74.
The Modulated Scream: Pain in Late Medieval Culture (University of Chicago Press, Chicago, 2010).
Cohen, J. I., *Educating for Democracy* (Macmillan and Co., London, 1939).
Colón, A. R. and P. A. Colón, *Nurturing Children: A History of Pediatrics* (Greenwood Press, Westport, CT, 1999).
Cone, Thomas E., *History of American Pediatrics* (Little Brown & Co, Boston, 1979).
Conolly, John, 'Recollections of the varieties of insanity', *Medical Times and Gazette*, 1 (1862), 235.
Cooper, A. E. and Adrian Bury, 'Glorious London' (letter to the editor), *Connoisseur*, 106 (1940), 265.
Cooper, Kate and Gregory, Jeremy (eds.), *Repentance, Retribution, and Reconciliation* (The Boydell and Brewer, Rochester, NY, 2004).
Cooter, Roger, 'In the name of the child beyond', in M. Gijswijt-Hofstra and H. Marland (eds.), *Cultures of Child Health in Britain and the Netherlands in the Twentieth Century* (Rodopi, London, 2003), 287–96.
(ed.), *In the Name of the Child: Health and Welfare, 1880–1940* (Routledge, London, 1992).
Cooter, Roger and John Pickstone (eds.), *Medicine in the Twentieth Century* (Harwood, Amsterdam, 2000).
Cope, Doris, 'Neonatal pain: the evolution of an idea', *The American Association of Anesthesiologists Newsletter* (September 1998), 1–2.
Crane, Jennifer, '"The bones tell a story the child is too young or too frightened to tell": The Battered Child Syndrome in Post-war Britain and America', *Social History of Medicine*, 28 (2015), 767–88.
'Rethinking how evacuees influenced post-war British thinking on health', *Retrospectives*, 2 (2013), 22–41.
Cravens, Hamilton, *Before Head Start: The Iowa Station and America's Children* (University of North Carolina Press, Chapel Hill, 1993).
Crichton-Browne, James, 'On dreamy mental states', *Stray Leaves from a Physician's Portfolio* (Hodder and Stoughton, London, 1927), 7–9.
'Psychical diseases of early life', *Journal of Mental Science*, 6 (1860), 284–320.
Crichton-Miller, Hugh, 'Psychology and social hygiene', *Journal of Social Hygiene*, 12 (1925), 14–24.
The New Psychology and the Parent (Jarrolds, London, 1922).

The New Psychology and the Teacher (Jarrolds, London, 1923).

Culley, Sheena, 'Killing pain: aspirin, emotion and subjectivity', in Rob Boddice (ed.), *Pain and Emotion in Modern History* (Palgrave Macmillan, London, 2014), 130–47.

Culpin, Millais, 'The nervous child', *The Lancet*, 208 (1926), 785–88.

Cunningham, Andrew and Perry Williams (eds.), *The Laboratory Revolution in Medicine* (Cambridge University Press, Cambridge, 1992).

Cunningham, Carol, 'Christ's Hospital, infant and child mortality in the 16th century', *Local Population Studies*, 18 (1977), 37–40.

Cunningham, Hugh, *Children and Childhood in Western Society since 1500* (Longman, London, 1995).

'Histories of childhood', *American Historical Review*, 103 (1998), 1195.

The Invention of Childhood (BBC Books, London, 2006).

Dale, Pamela and Joseph Melling, *Mental Illness and Learning Disability since 1850: Finding a Place for Mental Disorder in the United Kingdom* (Routledge, London, 2006).

Danziger, Kurt, 'Mid-nineteenth-century British psycho-physiology: a neglected chapter in the history of psychology', in William R. Woodward and Mitchell G. Ash (eds.), *The Problematic Science: Psychology in Nineteenth-Century Thought* (Praeger, New York, 1982), 119–46.

Darwin, Charles, 'A biographical sketch of an infant', *Mind*, 2 (1877), 285–94.

The Expression of Emotions in Man and Animals (John Murray, London, 1872).

The Expression of Emotions in Man and Animals, annotated by Paul Ekman (Oxford University Press, Oxford, 2002).

Daston, Lorraine, 'The theory of will versus the science of mind', in M. Ash and W. Woodward (eds.), *The Problematic Science: Psychology in Nineteenth-Century Thought* (Praeger, New York, 1982), 88–115.

(ed.), *Biographies of Scientific Objects* (University of Chicago Press, Chicago, 2000).

Daston, Lorraine and Peter Galison, *Objectivity* (Zone Books, Cambridge, MA, 2007).

Daston, Lorraine and Elizabeth Lunbeck (eds.), *Histories of Scientific Observation* (Chicago University Press, Chicago, 2011).

Daunton, M. J., 'Health and housing in Victorian London', *Medical History*, Suppl. 11 (1991), 126–44.

Davidson, M. A. and J. M. Slade, 'Results of a survey of senior school evacuees', *British Journal of Educational Psychology*, 10 (1940), 179.

Davin, Anna, *Growing Up Poor: Home, School and Street in London, 1870–1914* (Rivers Oram Press, London, 1996).

'Imperialism and motherhood', *History Workshop Journal*, 5 (1978), 9–65.

'What is a child?' in Anthony Fletcher and Stephen Hussey (eds.), *Childhood in Question: Children, Parents and the State* (Manchester University Press, Manchester, 1999), 14–36.

Davis, Angela, 'British child psychology and the evacuation of children during World War Two', *Centre for Medical History Seminar Series*, 2 February 2012, University of Exeter (2012).

Modern Motherhood: Women and Family in England, 1945–2000 (Manchester University Press, Manchester, 2012).

Deacon Girdlestone, Edward, *Vivisection: In Its Scientific, Religious, and Moral Aspects* (Simpkin, Marshall and Co., London, 1884).
De Mause, Lloyd (ed.), *The History of Childhood: The Untold Story of Child Abuse* (Psychohistory Press, New York, 1974).
De Zulueta, Felicity, *From Pain to Violence: The Traumatic Roots of Destructiveness* (Jason Aronson, Inc., Northvale, NJ, 1994).
Debus, Allen G. (ed.), *Medicine in Seventeenth Century England* (University of California Press, London, 1974).
Demos, John, *A Little Commonwealth: Family Life in a Plymouth Colony* (Oxford University Press, Oxford, 1970).
Dent, H. C., *Education in Transition: A Sociological Study of the Impact of War on English Education, 1939–1944* (Routledge & Kegan Paul, London, 1948).
Despert, J. L., 'Effects of war on children's mental health', *Journal of Consulting Psychology*, 8 (1944), 206–18.
Dickens, Charles, 'Some account of chloroform', *Household Words* (10 May 1851), 151.
Dicks, H. V., 'In search of our proper ethics', *British Journal of Medical Psychology*, 21 (1948), 1–14.
Digby, Anne, *British Welfare Policy: Workhouse to Workforce* (Faber & Faber, London, 1989).
Dikötter, Frank, 'Race culture: recent perspectives on the history of eugenics', *American Historical Review*, 103 (1998), 467–78.
Dilthey, Wilhelm, *The Formation of the Historical World in the Human Sciences*, in William Dilthey (ed.), *Selected Works*, vol. III (Princeton University Press, Princeton, NJ, 2002).
Dixon, Clarice Madeleine, *Keep Them Human* (John Day, New York, 1942).
Dixon Savill, Thomas, *Clinical Lectures on Neurasthenia* (Henry J. Glaisher, London, 1899, 1902, 1908).
Doleys, Daniel M., *Pain: Dynamics and Complexities* (Oxford University Press, Oxford, 2014).
Donaldson, G., 'Between practice and theory: Melanie Klein, Anna Freud and the development of child analysis', *Journal of the History of the Behavioural Sciences*, 32 (April 1996), 160–76.
Dormandy, Thomas, *The Worst of Evils: The Fight against Pain* (Yale University Press, New Haven, CT, 2006).
Down, Langdon John, *On Some of the Mental Affections of Childhood and Youth: Being the Lettsomian Lectures Delivered before the Medical Society of London in 1887, Together with Other Papers* (J & A Churchill, London, 1887).
Drummond, William, *The Child: His Nature and Nurture* (Dent, London, 1902).
An Introduction to Child Study (Edward Arnold, London, 1907).
Duffy, Jacalyn, *The History of Medicine: A Scandalously Short Introduction* (University of Toronto Press, Toronto, 2000).
Dunn, Peter M., 'Felix Wurtz of Basel (1518–75) and club feet', *Archives of Disease in Childhood*, 67 (1992), 1242–43.
'Sir Frederic Still (1868–1941): the father of British paediatrics', *Archives of Disease in Childhood: Fetal and Neonatal Edition*, 91 (July 2006), 308–10.
Dunsdon, M. I., 'A psychologist's contribution to air raid problems', *Mental Health*, 2 (1941), 37–41.

Dupree, Marguerite, 'Family care and hospital care: the "sick poor" in nineteenth-century Glasgow', *Social History of Medicine*, 6 (1993), 195–211.

Durbach, Nadia, '"They might as well brand us": working-class resistance to compulsory vaccination in Victorian England', *Social History of Medicine*, 13 (2000), 45–63.

Durbin, Evan, *The Politics of Democratic Socialism* (Routledge, London, 1940).

Dwork, Deborah, *War Is Good for Babies and Other Young Children: A History of the Infant and Child Welfare Movement in England, 1898–1988* (Tavistock, London, 1987).

Eckardt, G., W. G. Bringmann and L. Sprung (eds.), *Contributions to a History of Developmental Psychology: International William T. Preyer Symposium* (Mouton, Berlin, 1985).

Eder, M. D,, 'The conflicts of the unconscious in the child', *Child Study*, 9(6) (October 1916), 79–83.

Eddy, Matthew, 'The child writer: graphic literacy and the Scottish educational system, 1700–1820', *History of Education*, 45 (2016), 695–718.

'The interactive notebook: how students learned to keep notes during the Scottish Enlightenment', *Book History*, 19 (2016), 87–131.

'The shape of knowledge: children and the visual culture of literacy and numeracy', *Science in Context*, 26 (2013), 215–45.

Eddy, Matthew Daniel, *Media and the Mind: Art, Science, and Notebooks as Paper Machines, 1700–1830* (University of Chicago Press, Chicago, 2023).

Edgcumbe, Rose, *Anna Freud: A View of Development, Disturbance and Therapeutic Techniques* (Routledge, London, 2000).

Edwards, Elizabeth, *The Camera as Historian: Amateur Photographers and Historical Imagination* (Duke University Press, Durham, 2012).

Raw Histories: Photographs, Anthropology and Museums (Bloomsbury Academic, London, 2001).

Edwards, Elizabeth and Janice Hart, *Photographs, Objects, Histories: On the Materiality of Photography* (Routledge, London, 2004).

Ekman, Paul, *Emotions Revealed: Recognizing Faces and Feelings to Improve Communication and Emotional Life* (Times Books, New York, 2003).

Pictures of Facial Affect (Consulting Psychologists Press, Palo Alto, CA, 1976).

Ekman, Paul and Wallace Friesen, 'Constants across cultures in the face and emotion', *Journal of Personality and Social Psychology*, 17 (1971), 124–29.

Ellenberger, Henri, *The Discovery of the Unconscious* (Basic Books, New York, 1970).

Engel, G., '"Psychogenic" pain and the pain-prone patient', *American Journal of Medicine*, 26 (1959), 899–918.

Engelmann, Lukas, 'Photographing AIDS: on capturing a disease in pictures of people with AIDS', *Bulletin of the History of Medicine*, 90 (2016), 250–78.

Epstein, Julia L., 'Writing the unspeakable: Fanny Burney's mastectomy and the fictive body', *Representations*, 16 (1986), 131–66.

Erb, Wilhelm Heinrich, *Handbook of Electro-Therapeutics* (William Wood & Company, New York, 1883).

Esquirol, Jean Etienne Dominique, *Mental Maladies: A Treatise on Insanity* (Lea and Blanchard, Philadelphia, PA, 1845).

Evans, Elida, *The Problem of the Nervous Child* (Kegan Paul, Trench Trubner, London, 1919).

Evans, Erie, 'Problems of evacuation', Letter to the editor, *British Medical Journal* 2 (28 October 1939), 884.

Evanson, Richard Tonson, *A Practical Treatise on the Management and Diseases of Children* (Fannin & Co., Dublin; Renshaw and Longman, London, 1842).

Fallace, Thomas D., *Race and the Origins of Progressive Education, 1880–1929* (Teachers College Press, New York, 2016).

Faulkner, Robert, 'Graduated backgrounds', *British Journal of Photography* (25 October 1872), 513.

'Producing stippled grounds', *British Journal of Photography* (7 March 1873), 111.

Favazza, Armando R., *Bodies under Siege: Self-Mutilation and Body Modification in Culture and Psychiatry* (Johns Hopkins University Press, Baltimore, 1996).

Febvre, Lucien, 'Sensibility and history: how to write the emotional life of the past', in Peter Burke (ed.), *A New Kind of History from the Writings of Lucien Febvre* (Routledge & Kegan Paul, London, 1973), 12–26.

Ferenczi, S., K. Abraham, E. Simmel and E. Jones, *Psycho-Analysis and the War Neuroses* (International Psychoanalytical Press, London, 1921).

Fernández-Fontecha, Leticia, 'The language of children's pain (1870–1950)', in Dolores Martin Moruno and Beatriz Pichel (eds.), *Emotional Bodies: Studies on the Historical Performativity of Emotions* (University of Illinois Press, Urbana-Champaign, 2019), 77–96.

'Little patients: photography and the configuration of the sick child in Victorian Britain', in Jutta Ahlbeck, Paäivi Lappalainen, Kati Launis and Kirsi Tuohela (eds.), *Childhood, Literature and Science: Fragile Subjects* (Routledge, London, 2017), 110–27.

'Signos, legibilidad y diagnóstico: El problema del dolor en la infancia, 1870–1920', *Cuadernos de Historia Contemporánea*, 36 (2014), 89–112.

Festini, Filippo and Edward Alan Glasper, 'The contribution of Dr Charles West to the development of contemporary health care for sick children', *Comprehensive Child and Adolescent Nursing*, 39 (2016), 84–93.

Fildes, Valerie (ed.), *Women as Mothers in Pre-Industrial England: Essays in Memory of Dorothy McLaren* (Routledge, London, 1990).

Finger, Stanley, *Origins of Neuroscience: A History of Explorations into Brain Function* (Oxford University Press, Oxford, 2001).

Finlay, Roger, 'Gateways to death? London child mortality experience, 1570–1653', *Annales de Démographie Historique* (1978), 105–34.

Fisher, Katherine E., *Writing (in) the Spaces of the Blitz: Spatial Myths and Memory in Wartime British Literature* (University of Michigan Press, Ann Arbor, 2014).

Fitzgerald, M., C. Millard and N. MacIntosh, 'Cutaneous hypersensitivity following peripheral tissue damage in newborn infants and its reversal with topical anaesthesia', *Pain* 39 (1989), 31–36.

Fleming, Donald, 'Charles Darwin: the anaesthetic man', *Victorian Studies*, 4 (1961), 219–36.

Fletcher, Anthony, *Growing Up in England: The Experience of Childhood 1600–1914* (Yale University Press, London, 2008).

Fluger, John Carl, *Man, Morals and Society: A PsychoAnalytical Study* (International Universities Press, New York, 1945).

Forbes, John, (ed.), *The Cyclopaedia of Practical Medicine: Comprising Treatises on the Nature and Treatment of Disease, Materia Medica and Therapeutics, Medical Jurisprudence*, vol. 1 (Sherwood, Gilbert, and Piper, and Baldwin and Craddock, London, 1833–35), 578.

Ford, Julienne et al., *Special Education and Social Control: Invisible Disasters* (Routledge and Kegan Paul, London, 1982).

Fordham, M., 'Diurnal enuresis', *British Medical Journal*, 1 (13 January 1940), 73.

Forsyth, David, *Children in Health and Disease: A Study of Child-Life* (John Murray, London, 1909).

Foss, Brian, *War Paint: Art, War, State and Identity in Britain, 1939–1945* (Yale Books, New Haven, CT, 2007).

Foss, Brian Frederick, 'British artists and the Second World War. With particular reference to the War Artists', Advisory Committee of the Ministry of Information' (PhD thesis, University College London, 1991).

Foucault, Michel, *The Birth of the Clinic* (Taylor & Francis, Abingdon, 2002).

Discipline and Punish: The Birth of the Prison (Allen Lane, London, 1977).

Power, Lectures at the Collège de France 1973–1974 (Palgrave Macmillan, Basingstoke, 2008).

Foyster, Elizabeth, 'Boys will be boys? Manhood and aggression, 1660–1800', in Tim Hitchcock and Michele Cohen (eds.), *English Masculinities, 1660–1800* (Longman, London, 1999), 151–66.

Manhood in Early Modern England: Honour, Sex, and Marriage (Longman, London, 1999).

Freeman, Hugh and German, Berrios (eds.), *150 Years of British Psychiatry, Volume II: The Aftermath* (Athlone, London, 1996).

Freud, Anna, *The Writings of Anna Freud* (International Universities Press, New York, 1951).

Freud, Anna and Dorothy T. Burlingham, *Infants without Families* (International Universities Press, New York, 1944).

War and Children (Medical War Books, New York, 1943).

Young Children in War-Time: A Year's Work in a Residential War Nursery (George Allen & Unwin, London, 1942).

Freud, Anna and Sophie Dann, 'An experiment in group upbringing', in *The Writings of Anna Freud*, vol. 4, (International Universities Press, New York, 1951), 163–229.

Freud, Sigmund, *Freud, The Standard Edition of the Complete Psychological Works* (Hogarth Press, London, 1955).

'Introduction', in S. Ferenczi, K. Abraham, E. Simmel and E. Jones, *Psycho-Analysis and the War Neuroses* (International Psychoanalytical Press, London, 1921), 1–5.

'On the psychical mechanism of hysterical phenomena' (1893), in Freud, *The Standard Edition of the Complete Psychological Works*, vol. II (Hogarth Press, London, 1955), 8–13.

Frevert, Ute, 'Piggy's shame', in U. Frevert, P. Eitler, S. Olsen, et al. (eds.), *Learning How to Feel: Children's Literature and the History of Emotional Socialization, 1870–1970* (Oxford University Press, Oxford, 2014), 134–54.

Frevert, Ute et al., *Learning How to Feel: Children's Literature and the History of Emotional Socialization, 1870–1970* (Oxford University Press, Oxford, 2014).

Fulop-Mueller, René (trans. C. Paul), *Triumph over Pain* (Literary Guild of America, New York, 1938).
Furst, Lilian R., *Before Freud: Hysteria and Hypnosis in Later Nineteenth-Century Psychiatric Cases* (Bucknell University Press, Lewisburg, 2008).
Galton, Francis, *Inquiries into the Human Faculty and Its Development* (Macmillan, London, 1883).
Garrison, F. and A. Abt, *Abt-Garrison History of Paediatrics, with New Chapters on the History of Paediatrics in Recent Times* (W. B. Saunders, Philadelphia, PA, 1965).
Garrison, H. Fielding, *A System of Pediatrics*, vol. 1 (W. B. Saunders, Philadelphia, PA, 1931).
Garrod, Archibald Edward, Frederick E. Batten and Hugh Thursfield (eds.), *Diseases of Children* (Edward Arnold, London, 1913).
Gatchel, Robert J. et al., 'The biopsychosocial approach to chronic pain, scientific advances and future directions', *Psychological Bulletin*, 133 (2007), 581–624.
Gates, Barbara T., *Victorian Suicide: Mad Crimes and Sad Histories* (Princeton University Press, Princeton, NJ, 1988).
Gatty, Alfred (ed.), 'Report of the "*Aunt Judy's Magazine Cots*" at the Great Ormond Street Children's Hospital', in *Aunt Judy's Christmas Volume for Young People*, vol. 8 (Bell and Daldy, London, 1870), 447–749.
Gaukroger, Stephen, *Descartes: An Intellectual Biography* (Clarendon Press, Oxford, 1995).
Gay, Peter, *Freud: A Life for Our Time* (Papermac, London, 1995).
Geissmann, Claudine and Giessemann, Pierre, *A History of Child Psychoanalysis* (Routledge, London, 1998).
Genzmer, Alfred, *Untersuchugen Ueber die Sinneswahrhehumugen des Neugeborenen Menschen*, Inaugural Dissertation (Plötzche Buchhandlung, Halle, 1873).
Gere, Cathy, *Pain, Pleasure and the Greater Good* (University of Chicago Press, Chicago, 2017).
Geroulanos, Stefanos and Todd Meyers, *The Human Body in the Age of Catastrophe: Brittleness, Integration, Science, and the Great War* (University of Chicago Press, Chicago, 2018).
Gesell, Arnold, *An Atlas of Human Behavior: A Systematic Delineation of the Forms and Early Growth of Human Behavior Patterns. In two volumes. Illustrated with 3,200 Action Photographs* (Yale University Press, New Haven, CT, 1934).
Infant Behavior: Its Genesis and Growth (McGraw-Hill Book Company, New York, 1934).
The Mental Growth of the Pre-school Child (The MacMillan Company, New York, 1925).
Gibson, Ian, *The English Vice* (Duckworth, London, 1978).
Gijswijt-Hofstra, M. and H. Marland (eds.), *Cultures of Child Health in Britain and the Netherlands in the Twentieth Century* (Rodopi, New York, 2003).
Gijswijt-Hofstra, Marijke and Roy Porter (eds.), *Cultures of Neurasthenia from Beard to the First World War* (Rodopi, Amsterdam, 2001).
(eds.), *Cultures of Psychiatry and Mental Health Care in Postwar Britain and the Netherlands* (Rodopi, Amsterdam, 1998).

Gill, S. E., 'Nocturnal enuresis: experiences with evacuated children', *British Medical Journal*, 2 (10 August 1940), 199.

Gillis, J., 'Not just small adults: the metaphors of paediatrics', *Archives of Disease in Childhood*, 92 (2007), 946–47.

'Taking a medical history in childhood illness: representations of parents in pediatric texts since 1850', *Bulletin of the History of Medicine*, 79 (2005), 393–429.

Gilman, Sander L., Helen King, Roy Porter, G. S. Rousseau and Elaine Showalter (eds.), *Hysteria Beyond Freud* (University of California Press, Berkeley, 1993).

Gingell, K., 'The forgotten children: children admitted to a county asylum between 1854 and 1900', *Psychiatric Bulletin*, 25 (2001), 432–34.

Glaser, Brigitte, 'Gendered childhoods: on the discursive formation of young females in the eighteenth century', in Anja Müller (ed.), *Fashioning Childhood in the Eighteenth Century, Age and Identity* (Ashgate, Aldershot, 2006), 189–98.

Gleason, Mona Lee, *Small Matters: Canadian Children in Sickness and Health, 1900–1940* (McGill-Queen's University Press, Montreal, 2013).

Glover, Edward, *War, Sadism and Pacifism* (George Allen & Unwin, London, 1947).

Goldberg, Daniel, 'Pain without lesion: debate among American neurologists, 1850–1900', *19: Interdisciplinary Studies in the Long Nineteenth Century*, 15 (2012), 1–24.

Goldstein, S. and M. Goldstein, *Managing Attention Deficit Disorders in Children: A Guide for Practitioners* (John Wiley & Sons, New York, 1990)

Managing Attention and Learning Disorders in Late Adolescence and Adulthood (Wiley, New York, 1997).

Gontard, Alexander von, 'The development of child psychiatry in 19th century Britain', *Journal of Child Psychology and Psychiatry*, 29 (1988), 569–88.

Goodhart, James Frederic, *The Diseases of Children* (J & A Churchill, London, 1899).

Gordon, I., 'Allergy, enuresis, and stammering', *British Medical Journal* (14 March 1942), 357.

Gordon, R. G., On behalf of the Child Guidance Council (ed.), *A Survey of Child Psychiatry: Contributed by Contemporary British Authorities* (Oxford University Press and Humphrey Milford, London, 1939).

Gould, Stephen Jay, *Ontogeny and Phylogeny* (Harvard University Press, Cambridge, MA, 1977).

Graebner, William, 'The unstable world of Benjamin Spock: social engineering in a democratic culture, 1917–1950', *The Journal of American History*, 67 (1980), 612–29.

Grahek, Nikola, *Feeling Pain and Being in Pain* (MIT Press, Cambridge, MA, 2007).

Grayzel, Susan R., *At Home and under Fire: Air Raids and Culture in Britain from the Great War to the Blitz* (Cambridge University Press, Cambridge, 2014).

Greven, Philip, *Spare the Child: The Religious Roots of Punishment and the Psychological Impact of Physical Abuse* (Random House, New York, 1991).

Griesinger, Wilhelm, 'Ueber psychische Reflexactionen: Mit einem Blick auf das Wesen der psychischen Krankheiten', reprinted in *Gesammelte Abhandlungen, Ersters Band: Psychiatrische Abhandlungen* (E. J. Bonset, Amsterdam and Berlin, 1968 [1843]), 76–113.

Griffin, William, *An Essay on the Nature of Pain* (J. Moir, Edinburgh, 1826).

Griffith, Edward F., *Doctors by Themselves: An Anthology* (Cassell, London, 1951).

Gross, Daniel M., 'Defending the humanities with Charles Darwin's *The Expression of the Emotions in Man and Animals* (1872)', *Critical Inquiry*, 37 (2010), 34–59.

Grosskurth, Phyllis, *Melanie Klein and Her Work* (Alfred A. Knopf, New York, 1986).

Gruner, Cameron, *A Treatise on the Canon of Medicine of Avicenna Incorporating a Translation of the First Book* (Luzac, London, 1930).

Grunau, R. E., 'Early pain in preterm infants: a model of long-term effects', *Clinics in Perinatology*, 29 (2002) 373–94.

Guthrie, Leonard, *Functional Nervous Disorders in Childhood* (Henry Frowde and Oxford University Press, London, 1907).

Gutman, Marta and Ning de Coninck-Smith, *Designing Modern Childhoods: History, Space, and the Material Culture of Children* (Rutgers University Press, New Brunswick, NJ, 2008).

Hacking, Ian, *Historical Ontology* (Harvard University Press, Cambridge, MA, 2002).

Mad Travelers: Reflections on the Reality of Transient Mental Illnesses (Harvard University Press, Cambridge, MA, 2002).

Rewriting the Soul: Multiple Personality and the Sciences of Memory (Princeton University Press, Princeton, NJ, 1998).

Haggard, Howard W., *Devils, Drugs and Doctors: The Story of the Science of Healing from Medicine Man to Doctor* (Heinemann, London, 1929).

Haggett, Ali, *Desperate Housewives: Neurosis and the Domestic Environment, 1945–1970* (Pickering & Chatto, London, 2012).

Hall, G. Stanley, *Adolescence: Its Psychology and Its Relations to Physiology, Anthropology, Sociology, Sex, Crime, Religion and Education* (D. Appleton and Company, New York, 1904).

Aspects of Child Life and Education (D. Appleton and Company, New York, 1921).

The Contents of Children's Minds on Entering Education (E. L. Kellogg & Co., New York, 1893).

Haraway, Donna, 'Modest witness', *British Journal for the History of Science*, 10(2) (1977), 271–72.

Hardcastle, D. N., 'Personal environment and enuresis', *British Medical Journal*, 2 (10 August 1940), 206.

Hardy, Anne, *The Epidemic Streets: Infectious Disease and the Rise of Preventive Medicine, 1856–1900* (Clarendon Press, Oxford, 1993).

Hardyment, Christina, *Dream Babies: Childcare Advice from John Locke to Gina Ford* (Frances Lincoln, London, 2007).

Perfect Parents: Baby-Care Advice, Past and Present (Oxford University Press, Oxford, 1985).

Harris, Bernard, *The Health of the Schoolchild: A History of the School Medical Service in England and Wales* (Open University Press, Buckingham, 1995).

Harris, Walter (trans. William Cockburn), *An Exact Enquiry into, and Cure of the Acute Diseases of Infants* (E. L. Kellogg, London, 1693).

Harris, Walter, *A Full View of All the Diseases Incident to Children* (A. Millar, London, 1742).

Harrison, Tom, *Bion, Rickman, Foulkes and the Northfield Experiments: Advancing on a Different Front* (Jessica Kingsley Publishers, London, 2000).

Hartenberg, Paul, *Treatment of Neurasthenia* (Joint Committee of Henry Frowde and Hodder & Stoughton, Edinburgh, 1914).

Hayes, Sarah, 'Rabbits and rebels: the medicalisation of maladjusted children in mid-twentieth century Britain', in Mark Jackson (ed.), *Health and the Modern Home* (Routledge, New York, 2007), 128–52.

Hefler, Mary Edna and Ruth S. Kempe, *The Battered Child* (University of Chicago Press, Chicago, 1968).

Hellal, Paula and Marjorie Lorch, 'Charles West: a 19th century perspective on acquired childhood aphasia', *Journal of Neurolinguistics*, 18 (2005), 345–60.

Hellman, Ilse, 'Work in the Hampstead War Nurseries', *International Journal of Psychoanalysis*, 64 (1983), 435–36.

Henderson, J. L., 'The relief of pain in childhood', in Sir Heneage Ogilvie and William A. R. Thomson (eds.), *Pain and Its Problems* (Eyre and Spottiswoode, London, 1950), 171–72.

Hendrick, Harry, 'Child labour, medical capital, and the school medical service, c. 1890–1918', in Roger Cooter (ed.), *In the Name of the Child, Health and Welfare, 1880–1940* (Routledge, London, 1992), 45–71.

Child Welfare: England 1872–1989 (Routledge, London, 1994).

Child Welfare: Historical Dimensions, Contemporary Debate (Policy, Bristol, 2003).

Children, Childhood and English Society (Cambridge University Press, Cambridge, 1997).

'Children's emotional well-being and mental health in early post-Second World War Britain: the case of unrestricted hospital visiting', in M. Gijswijt-Hofstra and H. Marland (eds.), *Cultures of Child Health in Britain and the Netherlands in the Twentieth Century* (Rodopi, London, 2003), 213–42.

Hess, A., 'On the necessity of practical instruction in the treatment of diseases of children', *The Lancet*, 10 (1849), 341–42.

Hess, S. J. 'Civilian evacuation to Devon in the Second World War' (Unpublished PhD thesis, University of Exeter, 2006).

Heywood, Colin, *A History of Childhood: Children and Childhood in the West from Medieval to Modern Times* (Polity Press, Cambridge, 2001).

Hide, Louise, 'Making sense of pain: delusions, syphilis and somatic pain in London County Council asylums, c.1900', *19: Interdisciplinary Studies in the Long Nineteenth Century*, 15 (2012), 1–20.

Hide, Louise, Joanna Bourke and Carmen Mangion, 'Introduction: perspectives on pain', *19: Interdisciplinary Studies in the Long Nineteenth Century*, 15 (2012), 1–8.

Hinton, James, *Social Leadership, and the Second World War: Continuities of Class* (Oxford University Press, Oxford, 2002).

Hippocrates (trans. J. Chadwick and W.N. Mann), *The Medical Works of Hippocrates: A New Translation from the Original Greek Made Especially for English Readers* (Blackwell Scientific Publications, Oxford, 1950).

Hitchcock, Tim and Michele, Cohen (eds.), *English Masculinities, 1660–1800* (Longman, London, 1999).

Hodgkiss, Andrew, *From Lesion to Metaphor: Chronic Pain in British, French and German Medical Writings, 1800–1914* (Rodopi, Amsterdam, 2000).

Hodgson, Jack, 'Historians, emotions, and children's trauma in the archives', *Qualitative Inquiry*, https://journals.sagepub.com/doi/full/10.1177/10778004231200265

Holman, Robert, *The Evacuation: A Very British Revolution* (Lion, Oxford, 1995).

Holmes, Tarquin, 'Science, sensitivity and the sociozoological scale: constituting and complicating the human–animal boundary at the 1875 Royal Commission on Vivisection and beyond', *Studies in History and Philosophy of Science*, Part A, 90 (2021), 194–207.

Holmes, Tarquin and Carrie Friese, 'Making the anaesthetised animal into a boundary object: an analysis of the 1875 Royal Commission on Vivisection', *History and Philosophy of the Life Sciences*, 42(50) (2020), 1–28.

Holt, Luther Emmett, *The Diseases of Infancy and Childhood: For the Use of Students and Practitioners of Medicine* (New York, Appleton, 1987).

Horn, Margo, *Before It's Too Late: The Child Guidance Movement in the United States, 1922–1945* (Temple University Press, Philadelphia, PA, 1989).

Horst, Frank C. P. van der, *John Bowlby – From Psychoanalysis to Ethology: Unraveling the Roots of Attachment Theory* (Wiley-Blackwell, Chichester, 2011).

Houlbrooke, Ralph, *The English Family* (Longman, London, 1984).

Hulbert, Ann, *Raising America: Experts, Parents, and a Century of Advice about Children* (Knopf, New York, 2003).

Hume, David, *A Treatise of Human Nature* (Clarendon Press, Oxford, 1978).

Humphries, Stephen and Pamela Gordon, *Out of Sight: The Experience of Disability, 1900–1950* (Northcote House, Plymouth, 1992).

Hunt, David, *Parents and Children in History: The Psychology of Family Life in Early Modern France* (Basic Books, London, 1972).

Hunt, Lynn, 'The experience of revolution', *French Historical Studies*, 32 (2009), 671–78.

Hutchison, Robert, *Lectures on Diseases of Children* (Edward Arnold, London, 1904).

Ingle, 'Cambridge Medical Society: Hysteria', *The Lancet*, 2 (21 July 1883), 106.

Illich, Ivan, *Medical Nemesis: The Expropriation of Health* (Calder & Boyars, London, 1975).

Ireland, William, *The Mental Affections of Children: Idiocy, Imbecility and Insanity* (J & A Churchill, London, 1898).

Isaacs, Susan, 'Cambridge evacuation survey', *The Fortnightly* (June 1940), 619–30.

The Cambridge Evacuation Survey: A Wartime Study in Social Welfare and Education (Methuen & Co., London, 1941).

Childhood and After: Some Essays and Clinical Studies (Agathon Press, New York, 1970).

'Children of Great Britain in wartime', in S. M. Gruenberg (ed.), *The Family in a World at War* (Harper, New York, 1942).

'The nursery as a community', in John Rickman (ed.), *On the Bringing Up of Children* (Paul, Trench, Trubner, London, 1936).

Jackson, Mark, *Health and the Modern Home* (Routledge, London, 2007).

(ed.), *The Oxford Handbook of the History of Medicine* (Oxford University Press, Oxford, 2011).

Jacyna, L. S., 'The physiology of mind, the unity of nature, and the moral order in Victorian thought', *The British Journal for the History of Science*, 14 (1981), 109–32.

'Somatic theories of mind and the interests of medicine in Britain, 1850–1879', *Medical History*, 26 (1982), 233–58.

James, Allison and Prout, Alan, *Constructing and Reconstructing Childhood: Contemporary Issues in the Sociological Study of Childhood* (Routledge, London, 1997).

James, William, *Psychology* (Macmillan, London, 1892).

Jansson, Åsa, 'The creation of "disordered emotion": melancholia as biomedical disease, c.1840–1900' (Unpublished PhD thesis, Queen Mary University of London, 2014).

From Melancholia to Depression: Disordered Mood in Nineteenth-Century Psychiatry (Palgrave Macmillan, Cham, 2021).

'Mood disorders and the brain: depression, melancholia, and the historiography of psychiatry', *Medical History*, 55 (2011), 393–99.

'From statistics to diagnostics: medical certificates, melancholia, and suicidal propensities in Victorian Psychiatry', *Journal of Social History*, 46 (2013), 716–31.

Jersild, A. T. and M. F. Meigs, 'Children and war', *Psychological Bulletin*, 40 (1943), 541–73.

Jewson, Nicholas D., 'The disappearance of the sick-man from medical cosmology, 1770–1870', *Sociology*, 10 (1976), 225–44.

John, Enid M., 'A study of the effects of evacuation and air raids on children of pre-school age', *British Journal of Educational Psychology*, 11 (1941), 173–82.

Johnston, C. C., J. M. Collinge, S. J. Henderson and K. J. Anand, 'A cross-sectional survey of pain and pharmacological analgesia in Canadian neonatal intensive care units', *Clinical Journal of Pain*, 13 (1997), 308–12.

Jones, Ernest, 'How can civilization be saved?', *International Journal of Psychoanalysis*, 24 (1942), 1–7.

'Pain', *International Journal of Psychoanalysis*, 38 (1957), 255.

'The psychology of quislingism', *International Journal of Psychoanalysis*, 22 (1941), 1–12.

Jones, Greta, *Social Hygiene in Twentieth-Century Britain* (Croom Helm, London, 1986).

J. S., *Paidon Nosemata; or Childrens Diseases Both Outward and Inward* (Printed by W. G., London, 1664).

Kahr, Brett, *D. W. Winnicott: A Biographical Portrait* (Karnac, London, 1996).

Kaufman Shelemay, Kay (edited by Sarah Coakley), *Pain and Its Transformations: The Interface of Biology and Culture* (Harvard University Press, Cambridge, MA, 2007).

Keele, K. D., *Anatomies of Pain* (Blackwell, Oxford, 1957).

'Some historical concepts of pain', in C. A. Keele and D. Smith (eds.), *Proceedings of the International Symposium held under the auspices of the University Federation for Animal Welfare* (Middlesex Hospital, London, 1962), 2–27.

Keir, I. C., 'Evacuation', Letter to the editor, *British Medical Journal*, 2 (7 October 1939), 745–46.

Key, Ellen, *The Century of the Child* (G. P. Putnam's Sons, New York, 1909).

Khan, Murad Ahmad, Fauzia Raza and Iqbal Akhtar Khan, 'Pain: history, culture, and philosophy', *Acta Medico-Historica Adriatica*, 13 (2015), 113.

Kidd, W., 'The prehensile power of the hands of the human infant', *The Lancet*, 150 (1897), 1010.

King, Andrew, Alexis Easley and John Morton, *The Routledge Handbook to Nineteenth-Century British Periodicals and Newspapers* (Routledge Taylor & Francis Group, London, 2016).

King, Peter, 'The rise of juvenile delinquency in England, 1780–1840: changing patterns of perception and prosecution', *Past and Present*, 160 (1998), 116–66.

King, Pearl, 'Activities of British psychoanalysts during the Second World War and the influence of their interdisciplinary collaboration on the development of psychoanalysis in Great Britain', *International Journal of Psychoanalysis*, 16 (1989), 15–32.

Klein, Melanie, 'Early stages of the Oedipus conflict and of super-ego formation', in Melanie Klein (ed.), *The Psychoanalysis of Children* (The Hogarth Press, London, 1975), 123–48.

'Symposium on child-analysis', *International Journal of Psychoanalysis*, 8 (1927), 339–70.

'Weaning', in John Rickman (ed.), *On the Bringing Up of Children* (Paul, Trench, Trubner, London, 1936), 32–33.

Kleinman, Arthur, *The Illness Narratives: Suffering, Healing and the Human Condition* (Basic Books, New York, 1988).

Kosky, Jules, *Mutual Friends: Charles Dickens and Great Ormond Street Hospital* (Weidenfeld & Nicolson, London, 1989).

Koselleck, Reinhart, 'Is there an acceleration of history?' in Hartmut Rosa and William Scheuerman (eds.), *High-Speed Society: Social Acceleration, Power and Modernity* (Pennsylvania State University, University Park, 2009), 113–34.

'Transformation of experience and methodological change: a historical-anthropological essay', in Reinhart Koselleck (trans. Todd Samuel Presner and others), *The Practice of Conceptual History* (Stanford University Press, Stanford, 2002), 45–83.

Kotowicz, Zbigniew, 'Children, insanity and child psychiatry c.1800–1935', *Kairos: Revista de Filosofia Ciencia*, 3 (2011), 7–37.

Kottek, Samuel, 'Citizens! Do you want children's doctors?: an early vindication of "paediatric" specialists', *Medical History*, 35 (1991), 103–16.

Koven, S. 'Remembering and dismemberment: crippled children, wounded soldiers and the Great War in Great Britain', *American Historical Review*, 99 (October 1994), 1167–202.

Kristeva, Julia (trans. Ross Guberman), *Melanie Klein* (Columbia University Press, New York, 2002).

Kroner, Traugott, 'Uber die sinnesempfindungen der neugeborenen', *Separat-Abzug aus der Breslauer arztl. Zt.*, 4 (1882), 14

Kuhn, Thomas, *The Structure of Scientific Revolutions* (University of Chicago Press, Chicago, 1962).

Kundanis, Rose M., '"Baby riots" and "Eight-hour orphans": a comparison of the images of child care in British and US popular magazines during World War II', *Women's Studies International Forum*, 19 (1996), 239–42.

Kushner, Howard I., 'Suicide, gender and the fear of modernity in nineteenth-century medical and social thought', *Journal of Social History*, 26 (1993), 461–90.

Kussmaul, Adolf, *Untersuchungenüber das Seelenleben des Neugeborenen Menschen* (Winter, Leipzig, 1859).

Lancaster, E. G., 'The psychology and pedagogy of adolescence', *The Pedagogical Seminary: An International Record of Educational Literature, Institutions and Progress*, 5 (1897–98), 61–128.

Lane, Joan, *A Social History of Medicine: Health, Healing and Disease in England, 1750–1950* (Routledge, London, 2001).

Lane, Penelope et al. (eds.), *Women, Work and Wages in England, 1600–1850* (Boydell Press, Woodbridge and Rochester, NY, 2004), 15–46.

Langwill, H. G., 'Case of hysteria in a child, with remarkable psychical symptoms', *Edinburgh Hospital Reports* 2 (1894), 426.

Lawrence, Christopher, *Medicine in the Making of Modern Britain 1700–1920* (Routledge, London, 1994).

'Still incommunicable: clinical holists and medical knowledge in interwar Britain', in C. Lawrence and G. Weisz (eds.), *Greater than Their Parts: Holism in Biomedicine, 1920–1950* (Oxford University Press, Oxford, 1998), 94–111.

Lawrence, C. and G. Weisz (eds.), *Greater than their Parts: Holism in Biomedicine, 1920–1950* (Oxford University Press, Oxford, 1998).

Laycock, Thomas, 'On the reflex function of the brain', *British and Foreign Medical Review*, 19 (1845), 298–311.

Leahey, Thomas, *A History of Psychology* (Routledge, London, 2015).

Le Breton, David, *Anthropologie de la Douleur* (Métailié, Paris, 1995).

Leigh, M. D. and M. K. Belton, *Pediatric Anesthesiology* (Macmillan, New York, 1948).

Lesch, J., *Science and Medicine in France: The Emergence of Experimental Physiology, 1790–1855* (Harvard University Press, Cambridge, MA, 1984).

Levene, Alysa, 'Childhood and adolescence', in Mark Jackson (ed.), *The Oxford Handbook of the History of Medicine* (Oxford University Press, Oxford, 2012), 321–37.

et al. (eds.), *Illegitimacy in Britain, 1700–1920* (Palgrave Macmillan, Basingstoke, 2005).

'The mortality penalty of illegitimate children, foundlings and poor children in eighteenth-century England', in Alysa Levene, Samantha Williams and Thomas Nutt (eds.), *Illegitimacy in Britain, 1700–1920* (Palgrave Macmillan, Basingstoke, 2005), 34–49.

Levene, Alysa and William Reinarz, 'Child Patients and voluntary hospitals in eighteenth-century England', *Family and Community History*, 15 (2012), 15–33.

Levy, David M., 'The infant's earliest memory of inoculation: a contribution to public health procedures', *Journal of Genetic Psychology*, 96 (1960), 3–46.

Lewis, Jane, *The Politics of Motherhood: Child and Maternal Welfare in England 1900–1939* (Croom Helm, London, 1980).

'Providers, "consumers", the state and the delivery of health-care services in twentieth-century Britain', in Andrew Wear (ed.), *Medicine in Society: Historical Essays* (Cambridge University Press, Cambridge, 1992), 317–46.

Lewis, Michael and Alan Slater, 'A brief history of infancy research', in Alan Slater and Michael Lewis (eds.), *Introduction to Infant Development* (Oxford University Press, Oxford, 2002), 5–7.

Lewis, William Bevan, *Text-Book of Mental Diseases* (Charles Griffin and Company, London, 1899).

Leys, Ruth, *From Sympathy to Reflex: Marshall Hall and His Opponents* (Garland Pub., New York, 1990).

'The turn to affect: a critique', *Critical Inquiry*, 37 (May 2011), 434–72.

Likierman, Meira, *Melanie Klein: Her Work in Context* (Continuum, London, 2001).

Liskowski, F. P., 'Prehistoric and early history of trepanation', in D. Brothwell and A. T. Sandison (eds.), *Diseases of Antiquity: A Survey of the Diseases, Injuries and Surgery of Early Populations* (Charles T. Thomas, Springfield, IL, 1967), 651–67.

Lomax, Elizabeth, *Small and Special: The Development of Hospitals for Children in Victorian Britain, Medical History*, 16 (Wellcome Institute for the History of Medicine, London, 1996).

Long, Vicky, *The Rise and Fall of the Healthy Factory: The Politics of Industrial Health in Britain, 1914–60* (Palgrave-Macmillan, Basingstoke, 2011).

Lorch, Marjorie and Paula Hellal , 'Darwin's "natural science of babies"', *Journal of the History of the Neurosciences*, 19 (2010), 140–57.

Lowenfeld, Margaret F., 'A new approach to the problem of psychoneurosis in childhood' (Paper read to the Medical Section of the British Psychological Society on March 25, 1931), *British Journal of Medical Psychology*, 11 (November 1931), 177–214.

Maater, Florence, *Child Behavior: A Critical and Experimental Study of Young Children by the Method of Conditioned Reflexes* (The Gorham Press, Boston, 1918).

MacDonald, Geoff and Lauri A. Jensen-Campbell (eds.), *Social Pain, Neuropsychological and Health Implications of Loss and Exclusion* (American Psychological Association, Washington, DC, 2011).

MacDonald, M. W., 'Impact of war on children and youth intensification of emotional problems', *American Journal of Public Health*, 33 (1943), 336–38.

Mackintosh, J. Stewart, 'The nervous child', *British Medical Journal*, 2 (15 December 1923), 1183–84.

Macnicol, John, 'The effect of the evacuation of school children on official attitudes to state intervention', in Harold L. Smith (ed.), *War and Social Change: British Society in the Second World War* (Manchester University Press, Manchester, 1986), 3–31.

Mahnke, C. B., 'The growth and development of a specialty: the history of pediatrics', *Clinical Pediatrics*, 39 (2000), 705–14.

Mai, C. M. and M. Yaster, 'Pediatric anesthesia: a historical perspective', *American Society of Anesthesiologists*, 75 (2011), 10–13.

Malloy, J., 'Enuresis', *British Medical Journal* (17 February 1940), 277.

Mangion, Carmen, '"Why, would you have me live upon a gridiron?": pain, identity, and emotional communities in nineteenth-century English convent culture', *19: Interdisciplinary Studies in the Long Nineteenth Century*, 15 (2012), 1–16.

Marland, Hilary, *Health and Girlhood in Britain, 1874–1920* (Palgrave Macmillan, Berkshire, 2013).

Martensen, Robert L., *The Brain Takes Shape: An Early History* (Oxford University Press, Oxford, 2004).

Martín Moruno, Dolores, 'Pain as practice in Paolo Mantegazza's science of emotions', *Osiris*, 31 (2016), 137–62.

Martin, Mary Clare, 'Disabled children and domestic living spaces in Britain, 1800–1900', in M. S. Romero, E. A. Garcia and G. A. Jimenez (eds.), *Children, Spaces and Identity: Childhood in the Past Monograph Series* (Oxbow Books, Oxford, 2015), 136–54.

Matthews, Jill, 'They had such a lot of fun: the women's league of health and beauty between the wars', *History Workshop Journal*, 30 (1990), 22–54.

Maudsley, Henry, 'The genesis of mind', *Journal of Mental Science*, 7 (1862), 461–94.

The Pathology of Mind: A Study of Its Distempers, Deformities and Disorders, 2nd ed. (Macmillan and Co., London, 1895).

The Physiology and Pathology of the Mind (Macmillan, London, 1867).

Mazumdar, Pauline M. H., *Eugenics, Human Genetics and Human Failings: The Eugenics Society, Its Sources and Its Critics in Britain* (Routledge, London, 1992).

McBride, Mary M., 'Can you tell me where it hurts?', *Pediatric Nursing*, 3–4 (July/August 1977), 7–8.

McGlynn, Sean, *By Sword and Fire: Cruelty and Atrocity in Medieval Warfare* (Weidenfeld and Nicolson, London, 2008).

McGrath, Patrick, 'Science is not enough: the modern history of pediatric pain', *Pain*, 152 (2011), 2457–59.

McGrath, Patrick J. (ed.), *Oxford Textbook of Paediatric Pain* (Oxford University Press, Oxford, 2013).

McGraw, Myrtle B., 'Neural maturation as exemplified in the changing reaction of the infant to pin prick', in Myrtle B. McGraw (ed.), *The Neuromuscular Maturation of the Human Infant* (Hafner, New York, 1969), 42–47.

The Neuromuscular Maturation of the Human Infant (Hafner, New York, 1969).

A Study of Johnny and Jimmy (Appleton Century Crofts, New York, 1935).

Mediratta, Sangeeta, 'Beauty and the breast: the poetics of physical absence and narrative presence in Frances Burney's mastectomy letter (1811)', *Women: A Cultural Review*, 19 (2008), 188–207.

Meigs, John Forsyth, *A Practical Treatise on the Diseases of Children* (Lindsay and Blackiston, Philadelphia, PA, 1853).

Meldrum, Marcia, 'A capsule history of pain management', *Journal of the American Medical Association*, 290 (2003), 2470–75.

Mellett, D., *The Prerogative of Asylumdom: Social, Cultural and Administrative Aspects of the Institutional Treatment of the Insane in Nineteenth Century Britain* (Garland, New York, 1982).

Melling, J., R. Adair and B. Forsythe, '"A proper lunatic for two years": pauper lunatic children in Victorian and Edwardian England: child admissions to the Devon County Asylum, 1845–1914', *Journal of Social History*, 31 (1997), 371–405.

Melzack, Ronald, 'Evolution of the neuromatrix theory of pain', *Pain Practice*, 5 (2005), 85–94.

'Pain, past, present and future', *Canadian Journal of Experimental Psychology*, 4 (1992), 615–29.

The Puzzle of Pain (Penguin Education, Harmondsworth, 1973), 147–62.

Melzack, Ronald and Richard Wall, *The Challenge of Pain* (Penguin, London, 1982).

'Pain mechanisms: a new theory', *Science*, 150 (1965), 971–79.

Mendelson, Sara and Patricia Crawford, *Women in Early Modern England, 1550–1720* (Oxford University Press, Oxford, 2003).

Merback, Mitchell B., *The Thief, the Cross, and the Wheel: Pain and the Spectacle of Punishment in Medieval and Renaissance Europe* (University of Chicago Press, Chicago, 1999).

Merskey, Harold, 'On the development of pain', *Headache*, 10 (1970), 116–23.

'Pain in terms: a list with definitions and notes on usage', *Pain*, 6 (1979), 249.
'Response to editorial "New perspectives on the definition of pain"', *Pain*, 66 (1996), 209.
Mettler, C. C. and F. A. Mettler, *History of Medicine* (The Blakiston Co., Philadelphia, PA, 1947).
Micale, Mark, *Hysterical Men: The Hidden History of Male Nervous Illness* (Harvard University Press, Cambridge, MA, 2008).
Middleton, Dorothy, *Sir Francis Galton, 1822–1911* (Eugenics Society, London, 1982).
Midgley, Nick, 'Anna Freud: the Hampstead War Nurseries and the role of the direct observation of children for psychoanalysis', *International Journal of Psychoanalysis*, 88 (2007), 939–59.
Reading Anna Freud (Routledge, London, 2013).
'Test of time: Anna Freud's *Normality and Pathology in Childhood* (1965)', *Clinical Child Psychology and Psychiatry*, 16 (2011), 475–82.
Midmer, Deana K., 'Pain perception in the neonate: a matter of opinion', *Canadian Family Physician*, 35 (1989), 1049–54.
Miller, Emmanuel (ed.), *The Growing Child and Its Problems* (Routledge, Trench, London, Trubner & Co, London, 1937).
Miller, James, *Surgical Experience of Chloroform* (Sutherland & Knox, Edinburgh, 1848).
Miller Beard, George, 'Neurasthenia, or nervous exhaustion', *Boston Medical and Surgical Journal*, 3 (1869), 45–53.
Mintz, Steven, 'Reflections on age as a category of historical analysis', *The Journal of the History of Childhood and Youth*, 1 (2008), 91–94
Mitchell, Juliet, *Psychoanalysis and Feminism* (Basic Books, New York, 1974).
Money-Kyrle, Roger, 'Towards a common aim: psychoanalytic contribution to ethics', *British Journal of Medical Psychology*, 20 (1944), 105–17.
Psychoanalysis and Politics: A Contribution to the Psychology of Politics and Morals (Duckworth, London, 1951).
Mons, W. E. R., 'Air raids and the child', *British Medical Journal*, 2 (1 November 1941), 625.
Moodie, William, *The Doctor and the Difficult Child* (Commonwealth Fund, New York, 1947).
Moricca G. (ed.), *Advances in the Management of Pain: Advances in Pain Research and Therapy* (Raven, New York, 1984).
Morris, David, *The Culture of Pain* (University of California Press, Berkeley, 1991).
Illness and Culture in the Postmodern Age (University of California Press, Berkeley, 1998).
'An invisible history of pain: early 19th-century Britain and America', *Clinical Journal of Pain*, 14 (1998), 191–96.
Morus, Iwan Rhys, 'Marketing the machine: the construction of electrotherapeutics as viable medicine in early Victorian England', *Medical History*, 36 (1992), 34–37.
Moscoso, Javier, 'El dolor crónico en la historia', *Revista de Estudios Sociales*, 47 (2013), 171–77.
Pain: A Cultural History (Palgrave Macmillan, Basingstoke, 2012).
Pain: Passion, Compassion, Sensibility (Wellcome Trust, London, 2004).

'Politics of pain: "A good subject for eminent amateurs"', *Rubrica Contemporanea*, 4 (2015), 67–76.

Mott, Frederick W., summary of Paul Flechsig conference, 'Cerebral development and function', *British Medical Journal*, 1 (9 April 1921), 529.

Muller, Johannes (trans. William Baly), *Handbuch der Physiologie des Menschen*, vol. 2 (Taylor & Walton, London, 1839–42).

Müller, Anja (ed.), *Fashioning Childhood in the Eighteenth Century: Age and Identity* (Ashgate, Aldershot, 2006).

Murrell, William and Frederick Albert Castle, *A Manual of Pharmacology and Therapeutics* (W. Wood & Company, New York, 1896).

National Federation of Women's Institutes, *Town Children through Country Eyes* (Dorking, 1940).

Neve, M. and T. Turner, 'History of child and adolescent psychiatry', in M. Rutter and E. Taylor (eds.), *Child and Adolescent Psychiatry* (Blackwell, Oxford, 2002), 382–95.

Newton, Hannah, *The Sick Child in Early Modern England, 1580–1720* (Oxford University Press, Oxford, 2012).

Nichols, B. L., A. Ballabriga, and N. Kretchmer (eds.), *History of Pediatrics 1850–1950* (Nestlé Nutrition, New York, 1991).

Nietzsche, Friedrich, *On the Advantage and Disadvantage of History for Life* (Hackett Publishing Company, Oxford, 1980).

Nuremberg, David, *Communities of Violence: Persecution of Minorities in the Middle Ages* (Princeton University Press, Princeton, NJ, 1996).

Nye, Robert A., 'The rise and fall of the eugenics empire: recent perspectives on the impact of biomedical thought in modern society', *Historical Journal*, 36 (1993), 687–700.

Odlum, D. M., 'Enuresis', *British Medical Journal*, 1 (27 January 1940), 151.

'Nocturnal enuresis', *British Medical Journal*, 1 (6 January 1940), 8.

Oertzen, Christine von, 'Science in the cradle: Milicent Shinn and her home-based network of baby observers, 1890–1910', *Centaurus*, 55 (2013), 175–95.

Ogilvie, Sir Heneage and William A. R., Thomson (eds.), *Pain and Its Problems* (Eyre and Spottiswoode, London, 1950).

Olsen, Stephanie, *Childhood, Youth and Emotions in Modern History: National, Colonial and Global Perspectives* (Palgrave Macmillan, Basingstoke, 2015).

'The history of childhood and the emotional turn', *History Compass*, 15 (2017), e12410.

Juvenile Nation: Youth, Emotions and the Making of the Modern British Citizen, 1880–1914 (Bloomsbury Academic, New York, 2014).

'The limits of experience? A case study on children's dreams', *Digital Handbook of the History of Experience* (2022), https://researchportal.tuni.fi/en/publications/the-limits-of-experience-a-case-study-on-childrens-dreams.

Oppenheim, Janet, *'Shattered Nerves': Doctors, Patients, and Depression in Victorian England* (Oxford University Press, Oxford, 1991).

Osler, William, *The Principles and Practice of Medicine* (D. Appleton and Company, New York, 1920).

Pabis, E., M. Kowalczyk and T. B. Kulik, 'Pain in children in historical perspective', *Anestezjol Intens Ter*, 42 (2010), 37–41.

Padley, Richard and Margaret Cole (eds.), *Evacuation Survey: A Report to the Fabian Society* (Routledge, London, 1940).
Page, Gayle Giboney, 'Are there long-term consequences of pain in newborn or very young infants?', *Journal of Perinatal Education*, 13 (2004), 10–17.
Palmegiano, Eugenia M., *Perceptions of the Press in Nineteenth-Century British Periodicals: A Bibliography* (Anthem Press, London, 2013).
Paris, Leslie, 'Through the looking glass: age, stages, and historical analysis', *The Journal of the History of Childhood and Youth*, 1 (2008), 106–13.
Parliamentary Debates (Hansard), vol. 336, col 1380 (1928).
Parry-Jones, William Ll., 'The history of child and adolescent psychiatry: its present-day relevance', *Journal of Child Psychology and Psychiatry*, 1 (1989), 3–11.
Parsons, Martin, *I'll Take That One: Dispelling the Myths of Civilian Evacuation, 1939–1945* (Beckett Karlson, Peterborough, 1998).
Payne, Linda Ellen Stephenson, *With Words and Knives: Learning Medical Dispassion in Early Modern England* (Ashgate, Aldershot, 2007).
Peirson, A. L., 'Early operation for harelip', *The American Journal of Medicine*, 24 (1852), 576.
Pernick, Martin, *A Calculus of Suffering: Pain, Professionalism, and Anesthesia in Nineteenth-Century America* (Columbia University Press, New York, 1985).
Perry, Mr, *Perry's Treatise on the Prevention and Cure of the Tooth-Ache with Directions for Preserving the Teeth and Gums from Disease and Discolouration to the Latest Period in Life. Also, Instructions to Mothers on the Management and Cutting of Teeth in Children* (Messrs Butler, London, 1827).
Pearson, Wilfred J. and W. G. Wyllie, *Recent Advances in Diseases of Children* (P. Blakiston's Son & Co. Inc., Philadelphia, PA, 1935).
Pichel, Beatriz, 'From facial expressions to bodily gestures: passions, photography and movement in French 19th century sciences', *History of the Human Sciences*, 29 (2016), 27–48.
Picturing the Western Front: Photography, Practices and Experiences in First World War France (Manchester University Press, Manchester, 2021).
Pick, Daniel, *Faces of Degeneration: A European Disorder, c.1848–c.1918* (Cambridge University Press, Cambridge, 1989).
Pollock, Linda, '"Teach her to live under obedience", the making of women in the upper ranks of early modern England', *Continuity and Change*, 4 (1989), 231–58.
Pooley, Siân, '"All we parents want is that our children's health and lives should be regarded": child health and parental concern in England, *c.*1860–1910', *Social History of Medicine*, 23 (2010), 528–48.
Poovey, Mary, *Uneven Developments: The Ideological Work of Gender in Mid-Victorian England* (Chicago University Press, Chicago, 1988).
Preyer, William, *The Mind of the Child: The Development of the Intellect* (Arno Press, New York, 1889).
Prichard, J. C., *A Treatise on Insanity and Other Disorders Affecting the Mind* (Sherwood, Gilbert and Piper, London, 1835).
Pritchard, Michael, *A Directory of London Photographers, 1841–1908* (PhotoResearch, Watford, 1994).
Pritcherd, R. and S. Rosenzweig, 'The effects of war stress upon childhood and youth', *Journal of Abnormal Psychology*, 37 (1942), 329–44.

Procacci, Paolo and Marco Maresca, 'The pain concept in western civilization: a historical review', in G. Moricca (ed.), *Advances in the Management of Pain. Advances in Pain Research and Therapy* (Raven, New York, 1984), 1–11.

Prodger, Phillip, *Darwin's Camera: Art and Photography in the Theory of Evolution* (Oxford University Press, Oxford, 2009).

'Rejlander, Darwin, and the evolution of 'Ginx's Baby', *History of Photography*, 23 (1999), 260–68.

Radbill, Samuel X., 'Pediatrics', in Allen G. Debus (ed.), *Medicine in Seventeenth Century England* (University of California Press, London, 1974), 237–82.

Raja, Srinivasa N. et al., 'The revised International Association for the Study of Pain definition of pain: concepts, challenges, and compromises', *Pain*, 161 (2020), 1977.

Rankin, Guthrie, 'Neurasthenia: the wear and tear of life', *British Medical Journal*, 1 (2 May 1903), 1017–20.

Ray, M. B., 'Case of acute mania occurring in a boy', *Journal of Mental Science*, 44 (1898), 320–22.

'A case of acute melancholia occurring in a child', *The Quarterly Medical Journal: A Quarterly Review of the Medical Sciences for Yorkshire and Adjoining Counties*, 5 (October 1896–July 1897), 242.

Razzell, Peter Ernest and Christine Spence, 'The history of infant, child and adult mortality in London, 1550–1850', *London Journal*, 32 (2007), 271–92.

Rebok Rosenthal, Amy, 'Insanity, family and community in late-victorian Britain', in Anne Borsay and Pamela Dale (eds.), *Disabled Children: Contested Caring, 1850–1979* (Pickering & Chatto, London, 2012), 29–42.

Rees, Jackson, 'Anaesthesia in the newborn', *British Medical Journal*, 2 (23 December 1950), 1419–22.

'An early history of paediatric anaesthesia', *Pediatric Anesthesia*, 1 (1991), 3–11.

Rey, Roselyne (trans. Louise Elliott Wallace), *The History of Pain* (Harvard University Press, Cambridge, MA, 1995).

Richards, Stewart, 'Anaesthetics, ethics and aesthetics: vivisection in the late nineteenth-century British laboratory', in Andrew Cunningham and Perry Williams (eds.), *The Laboratory Revolution in Medicine* (Cambridge University Press, Cambridge, 1992), 142–69.

Rickman, John, 'Evacuation and the child's mind', letter to the editor, *The Lancet*, 234 (2 December 1939), 1192.

Riley, Denise, *War in the Nursery: Theories of the Child and Mother* (Virago, London, 1983).

Ritter von Reuss, August, *The Diseases of the Newborn* (John Bale, Sons & Danielsson Ltd., London, 1920).

Roberts, Hilary, *Cecil Beaton: Theatre of War* (Jonathan Cape, London, 2012).

Robinson, Louis, 'Darwinism in the nursery', *Nineteenth Century*, 30 (1891), 831–42.

'Reflex action (physiological)', in D. H. Tuke (ed.), *A Dictionary of Psychological Medicine*, 2 vols. (Churchill, London, 1892), 1074–76.

Robson, Charles, 'Anesthesia in children', *Anesthesia and Analgesia*, 4 (1925), 235–40.

Rodkey, Elissa N. and Rebecca Pillai Riddell, 'The infancy of infant pain research, the experimental origins of infant pain denial', *The Journal of Pain*, 14 (2013), 338–50.

Rollin, Bernard E., *The Unheeded Cry: Animal Consciousness, Animal Pain and Scientific Change* (Oxford University Press, Oxford, 1989).
Roper, Michael, 'From the shell-shocked soldier to the nervous child: psychoanalysis in the aftermath of the First World War', *Psychoanalysis and History*, 18 (2016), 39–69.
Rose, Jacqueline, *The Case of Peter Pan, or the Impossibility of Children's Fiction* (Macmillan, London, 1984).
Rose, Nikolas, *Governing the Soul: The Shaping of the Private Self* (Routledge, London, 1998).
The Psychological Complex: Psychology, Politics and Society in England, 1869–1939 (Routledge and Kegan Paul, London, 1985).
Rose, Sonya O., *Which People's War? National Identity and Citizenship in Wartime Britain 1939–1945* (Oxford University Press, Oxford, 2003).
Rosenberg, Charles E., *Explaining Epidemics and Other Studies in the History of Medicine* (Cambridge University Press, Cambridge, 1992).
Rosenwein, Barbara H., *Emotional Communities in the Early Middle Ages* (Cornell University Press, Ithaca, NY, 2006).
'Worrying about emotions in history', *The American Historical Review*, 107 (2002), 821–45.
Ross, Dorothy, *G. Stanley Hall: The Psychologist as Prophet* (University of Chicago Press, Chicago, 1972).
Ross, T. A., *An Enquiry into Prognosis in the Neuroses* (Cambridge University Press, Cambridge, 1936).
Rotch, T., 'Iconoclasm and original thought in the study of pediatrics', *Archives of Pediatrics*, 7 (1891), 806–11.
Romanes, George, *Mental Evolution in Man: Origin of Human Faculty* (Kegan Paul, London, 1888).
Ruhrah, John, *Pediatrics of the Past* (P. B. Hoeber, New York, 1925).
Russell, Brock C., *The Life and Work of Astley Cooper* (E. & S. Livingstone, Edinburgh, 1952).
Safford, P. L. and E. J. Safford, *A History of Childhood and Disability* (Teachers College Press, New York, 1996).
Salaman, Naomi and Ronnie Simpson (eds.), *Postcards on Photography: The Handmade Copy in production* (Cambridge Darkroom Galley, Cambridge, 1998).
Salisbury, Laura and Andrew Shail (eds.), *Neurology & Modernity: A Cultural History of Nervous Systems, 1800–1950* (Palgrave Macmillan, Basingstoke, 2010).
Sampson, Olive, *Child Guidance: Its History, Provenance and Future* (British Psychological Society, London, 1980).
Samways, Richard (ed.), *We Think You Ought to Go* (London Metropolitan Archives, City of London, 1995).
Savage, George, 'Case of marked hysteria in a boy of eleven years', *The Journal of Mental Science*, 31 (1885), 201–2.
'Locomotor Ataxy, Tabes Dorsalis, Ataxie Locomotrice Progressive', in D. Hack Tuke (ed.), *A Dictionary of Psychological Medicine*, 2 vols. (Churchill, London, 1892), II, 750.
Scarry, Elaine, 'Among schoolchildren: the use of body damage to express physical pain in pain and its transformations', in Sarah Coakley and Kay Kaufman

Shelemay (eds.), *Pain and Its Transformations: The Interface of Biology and Culture* (Harvard University Press, Cambridge, MA, 2007), 279–317.
The Body in Pain: The Making and Unmaking of the World (Oxford University Press, Oxford, 1985).
Schatz, Stephanie L., 'Lewis Carroll's dream-child and Victorian child psychopathology', *Journal of the History of Ideas*, 76 (2015), 93–114.
Schrag, P. and D. Divoky, *The Myth of the Hyperactive Child and Other Means of Child Control* (Pantheon, New York, 1975).
Schweitzer, Albert, *On the Edge of the Primeval Forest* (Macmillan, New York, 1931).
Scofield, R. S. and E. A. Wrigley, 'Infant and child mortality in England in the Late Tudor and Early Stuart Period', in C. Webster (ed.), *Health Medicine and Mortality* (Cambridge University Press, Cambridge, 1979), 61–95.
Scull, Andrew, *Museums of Madness: The Social Organization of Insanity in Nineteenth Century England* (Penguin Books, London 1979).
The Most Solitary of Afflictions: Madness and Society in Britain, 1700–1900 (Yale University Press, New Haven, CT, 1993).
Scullin, Sarah E., 'Hippocratic pain', Publicly Accessible Penn Dissertations, Paper 578 (ScholarlyCommons, University of Pennsylvania, Philadelphia, PA, 2012).
Searle, G. R., *Eugenics and Politics in Britain, 1900–1914* (Noordhoff International, Leyden, 1976).
The Quest for National Efficiency: A Study in British Politics and Political Thought, 1899–1914 (University of California Press, Berkeley, 1971).
Sennert, Daniel et al., *Practical Physick the Fourth Book in 3 Parts: Section 2: of Diseases and Symptoms in Children* (Peter Cole, London, 1664).
Sgarbi, Marco, *La logica dell'irrazionale. Studio sul significato e sui problemi della Kritik der Urteilskraft* (Mimesis, Milan, 2010).
Shapira, Michal, 'The psychological study of anxiety in the era of the Second World War', *Twentieth Century British History*, 1 (2012), 31–57.
The War Inside: Psychoanalysis, Total War, and the Making of the Democratic Self in Post-War Britain (Cambridge University Press, Cambridge, 2013).
Sheehan, Tanya, *Doctored: The Medicine of Photography in Nineteenth-Century America* (Pennsylvania State University Press, University Park, 2011).
Sheer, Monique, 'Are emotions a kind of practice (and is that what makes them to have a history)? A Bourdieuian approach to understanding emotion', *History and Theory*, 51 (May 2012), 193–220.
Sheldon, W. and P. Evans, 'Town children in the country', *The Lancet* (13 January 1940), 94.
Sherman, M. and I. Sherman, 'Infant behavior', *Comparative Psychology Monographs*, 12 (1936), 1–107.
'Sensori-motor responses in infants', *Journal of Comparative Psychology*, 5 (1925), 53–68.
Shinn, Milicent Washburn, *The Biography of a Baby* (Houghton Mifflin, Boston, 1900).
Notes on the Development of a Child (University of California Press, Berkeley, 1893–99).
Shmuely, Shira, *The Bureaucracy of Empathy: Law, Vivisection, and Animal Pain in Late Nineteenth-Century Britain* (Cornell University Press, Ithaca, NY, 2023).

Shore, H., '"Inventing" the juvenile delinquent in nineteenth-century Europe', in B. S. Godfrey, C. Emsley and G. Dunstall (eds.), *Comparative Histories of Crime* (Willan Publishing, Devon, 2003), 110–24.

Shorter, Edward, *A History of Psychiatry: From the Era of the Asylum to the Age of Prozac* (John Wiley & Sons, New York, 1997).

How Everyone Became Depressed: The Rise and Fall of the Nervous Breakdown (Oxford University Press, Oxford, 2013).

The Making of the Modern Family (Collins, London, 1976).

'Paralysis: the rise and fall of a "hysterical" symptom', *Journal of Social History*, 19 (1986), 549–82.

Showalter, Elaine, *The Female Malady: Women, Madness and English Culture, 1830–1980* (Virago, London, 1987).

Shuttleworth, Sally, 'Childhood, severed heads, and the uncanny: Freudian precursors (Critical essay)', *Victorian Studies*, 58 (2015), 84–110.

The Mind of the Child: Child Development in Literature, Science, and Medicine, 1840–1900 (Oxford University Press, Oxford, 2010).

'Night terrors: medical and literary representations of childhood fear', in Anne-Julia Zwierlein (ed.), *Unmapped Countries: Biological Visions in Nineteenth Century Literature and Culture* (Anthem Nineteenth-Century Series) (Anthem Press, London, 2005), 193–206.

'The psychology of childhood in Victorian literature and medicine', in Helen Small and Trudi Tate (eds.), *Literature, Science, Psychoanalysis, 1830–1970: Essays in Honour of Gillian Beer* (Oxford University Press, Oxford, 2003), 86–101.

Siegel, Alexander W. and Sheldon H. White, 'The Child Study Movement: early growth and development of the symbolized child', *Advances in Child Development and Behavior*, 17 (1982), 233–85.

Skey, Frederick, *Operative Surgery* (John Churchill, London, 1850).

Slater, Alan and Michael Lewis (eds.), *Introduction to Infant Development* (Oxford University Press, Oxford, 2002), 5–7.

Sloan, D. C., 'A better home away from home: the emergence of children's hospitals in an age of women's reform', in M. Gutman and N. De Coninck-Smith (eds.), *Designing Modern Childhoods: History, Space, and the Material Culture of Children* (Rutgers University Press, New Brunswick, NJ, 2008), 42–60.

Smail, Daniel Lord, *On Deep History and the Brain* (University of California Press, Berkeley, 2008).

Smiles, Samuel, *Physical Education or the Nurture and Management of Children* (Oliver and Boyd, Edinburgh, 1838).

Smith, Harold L. (ed.), *War and Social Change: British Society in the Second World War* (Manchester University Press, Manchester, 1986).

Smith, Jonathan, *Charles Darwin and Victorian Culture* (Cambridge University Press, Cambridge, 2006).

Smith, P., 'Case of hysteria in a boy', *Journal of Mental Science*, 31 (October 1885), 370.

Smith, Richard, 'The trouble with medical journals', *Journal of the Royal Society of Medicine*, 99 (2006), 115–19.

Smith, Roger, *Inhibition: History and Meaning in the Sciences of Mind and Brain* (Free Association Books, London, 1992).

Smith, T. N., 'Observations on hysteria', *Boston Medical and Surgical Journal*, 3 (1831), 541.

Snow, John, *On Chloroform and Other Anaesthetics: Their Action and Administration* (John Churchill, London, 1858).

Solomon, J. C., 'Reaction of children to blackouts', *American Journal of Orthopsychiatry*, 12 (1942), 62.

Soloway, Richard, *Demography and Degeneration: Eugenics and the Declining Birthrate in Twentieth-Century Britain* (University of North Carolina Press, Chapel Hill, 1990).

Sontag, Susan, *Illness as Metaphor* (Allen Lane, London, 1979).

Regarding the Pain of Others (Hamish Hamilton, London, 2003).

Spanos, Nicholas P. and Jack Gottlieb, 'Demonic possession, mesmerism, and hysteria: a social psychological perspective on their historical interrelations', *Journal of Abnormal Psychology*, 88 (1979), 527–46.

Spurgin, William H., 'Case of hysteria in a child aged ten years', *British Medical Journal*, 2 (2 October 1875), 555.

Starr, Louis, 'The clinical investigation of disease and the general management of children', in Louis Starr and T. S. Westcoote (eds.), *An American Text-Book of the Diseases of Children* (Saunders, Philadelphia, PA, 1985), 1–36.

Starr, Louis and T. S. Westcoote, *An American Text-Book of the Diseases of Children* (Saunders, Philadelphia, PA, 1985).

Starobinski, Jean, *Action and Reaction: The Life and Adventures of a Couple* (Zone Books, New York, 2003).

Starobinski, Jean (trans. Judith P. Serafini-Saul), 'The word reaction: from physics to psychiatry', *Psychological Medicine*, 7 (1977), 373–86.

Steedman, Carolyn, 'Bodies, figures and physiology: Margaret McMillan and the late nineteenth century remaking of working class childhood', in Roger Cooter (ed.), *In the Name of the Child: Health and Welfare, 1880–1940* (Routledge, London, 1992), 19–44.

Childhood, Culture, and Class in Britain: Margaret McMillan, 1860–1931 (Virago Press, London, 1990).

Strange Dislocations: Childhood and the Idea of Human Interiority, 1780–1930 (Virago Press, London, 1995).

Stearns, Peter, 'Challenges in the history of childhood', *The Journal of the History of Childhood and Youth*, 1 (2008), 35–42.

Childhood in World History (Routledge, London, 2009).

Stevens, Bonnie J., Gareth Hathway and William T. Zempsky (eds.), *Oxford Textbook of Pediatric Pain*, 2nd ed., Oxford Textbook (Oxford Academic, Oxford, 2021; online ed., 1 June 2021), 5.

Stevenson, John, *British Society 1914–1945* (Penguin, London, 1984).

Stewart, John, *Child Guidance in Britain, 1918–1955: The Dangerous Age of Childhood* (Pickering & Chatto, London, 2013).

'"I thought you would want to come and see his home": child guidance and psychiatric social work in inter-war Britain', in Mark Jackson (ed.), *Health and the Modern Home* (Routledge, London, 2007), 111–27.

'The scientific claims of British Child Guidance, 1918–1945', *British Journal for the History of Science*, 42 (2009), 407–32.

Stewart, John and John Welshman 'Culture, behaviour and poverty: the evacuation of children in Scotland, 1939–1945', *Journal of Scottish Historical Studies*, 26 (2006), 100–20.

Still, George, *The History of Paediatrics: The Progress of the Study of Diseases of Children up to the End of the 18th Century* (Hodder & Stoughton, Oxford, 1931).

'On some abnormal psychical conditions in children: the Goulstonian Lectures', *The Lancet*, 159 (1902), 1077–82.

Still, George Frederic, 'A clinical lecture on infantile scurvy: delivered at the Hospital for Sick Children, Great Ormond Street', *British Medical Journal*, 2 (28 July 1906), 186–90.

Common Disorders and Diseases of Childhood (Henry Frowde, London, 1910).

Stones, R. Y., 'Medical problems of a reception area', *British Medical Journal*, 1 (8 March 1941), 370.

Strange, Julie-Marie, *Death, Grief and Poverty in Britain, 1870–1914* (Cambridge University Press, Cambridge, 2005).

Strauss, Murray A., *Beating the Devil out of Them: Corporal Punishment in American Families* (Free Press, New York, 1994).

Sully, James, *Studies of Childhood* (D. Appleton and Company, New York, 1896).

Tanner, Andrea, 'Choice and the children's hospital: Great Ormond Street hospital patients and their families, 1855–1900', in A. Borsay and P. Shapely (eds.), *Medicine, Charity and Mutual Aid: The Consumption of Health and Welfare in Britain, c.1550–1950* (Ashgate, Aldershot, 2007), 135–62.

'Too many mothers? Female roles in metropolitan Victorian children's hospital', in J. Henderson and A. Pastore (eds.), *The Impact of Hospitals* (Peter Lang, Oxford, 2007), 135–66.

Tanner, T. H., *A Practical Treatise on the Diseases of Infancy and Childhood* (Henry Renshaw, London, 1858), 276–79.

Taylor, James, *Paralysis and Other Diseases of the Nervous System in Childhood and Early Life* (J & A Churchill, London, 1905).

Taylor, Steven '"All his ways are those of an idiot": the admission, treatment and social reaction to two idiot children of Northampton Pauper Lunatic Asylum, 1877–1883', *Family & Community History*, 15 (2012), 34–43.

Child Insanity in England, 1845–1907 (Palgrave Macmillan, London, 2016).

'Insanity, philanthropy and emigration: dealing with insane children in late-nineteenth-century North-West England', *History of Psychiatry*, 25 (2014), 224–25.

Thane, Pat, *Old Age in English History: Past Experiences, Present Issues* (Oxford University Press, 2000).

Thom, Deborah, 'Wishes, anxiety, play, and gestures: child guidance in inter-war England', in Roger Cooter (ed.), *In the Name of the Child, Health and Welfare, 1880–1940* (Routledge, London, 1992), 200–19.

Thomas, Alan, *The Expanding Eye: Photography and the Nineteenth-Century Mind* (Croom Helm, London, 1978).

Thomson, Mathew, 'Before anti-psychiatry: "Mental Health" in wartime Britain', in Marijke Gijswijt-Hofstra and Roy Porter (eds.), *Cultures of Psychiatry and Mental Health Care in Postwar Britain and the Netherlands* (Rodopi, Amsterdam, 1998), 43–59.

Lost Freedom: The Landscape of the Child and the British Post-War Settlement (Oxford University Press, Oxford, 2013).
'Neurasthenia in Britain: an overview', in Marijke Gijswijt-Hofstra and Roy Porter (eds.), *Cultures of Neurasthenia from Beard to the First World War* (Rodopi, Amsterdam, 2001), 77–95.
The Problem of Mental Deficiency: Eugenics, Democracy, and Social Policy in Britain c.1870–1959 (Oxford University Press, Oxford, 1998).
Psychological Subjects: Identity, Culture and Health in Twentieth-Century Britain (Oxford University Press, Oxford, 2006).
'"The solution to his own enigma": connecting the life of Montague David', *Medical History*, 55 (2011), 61–84.
Thorek, Max, *Modern Surgical Technique*, vol. III (Lippincott, Montreal, 1938).
Titmuss, Richard M., *Problems of Social Policy (History of the Second World War United Kingdom Civil Series)* (His Majesty's Stationary Office, London, 1950).
Tousignant, Noémi, 'Pain and the pursuit of objectivity: pain-measuring technologies in the United States *c.*1890–1975' (Unpublished PhD thesis, McGill University, 2006).
Tucker, Beverley R., *Nervous Children: Prevention and Management* (R. G. Badger, Boston, MA, 1916).
Tucker, Jennifer, 'Entwined practices, engagements with photography in historical inquiry', special theme issue of *History and Theory*, 48 (2009), 1–12.
Nature Exposed: Photography as Eyewitness in Victorian Science (Johns Hopkins University Press, Baltimore, 2005).
Tuke, D. Hack (ed.), *A Dictionary of Psychological Medicine*, 2 vols. (Churchill, London, 1892).
Turda, Marius, 'Recent scholarship on race and eugenics', *Historical Journal*, 51 (2008), 1115–24.
Turner, Trevor, 'The early 1900s and before', in Hugh Freeman (ed.), *A Century of Psychiatry: Vol I* (Mosby-Wolfe, London, 1999), 3–29.
'James Crichton-Browne and the anti-psychoanalysts', in Hugh Freeman and German Berrios (eds.), *150 Years of British Psychiatry, Volume II: The Aftermath* (Athlone, London, 1996), 144–55.
Underwood, Michael, *A Treatise on the Diseases of Children, with Directions for the Management of Infants from the Birth; Especially Such as Are Brought up by Hand* (J. Mathews, London, 1784).
Unruh, Anita, 'Voices from the past: ancient views of pain in childhood', *The Clinical Journal of Pain*, 8 (1992), 247–54.
Urwin, Cathy and John Hood-Williams (eds.), *Child Psychotherapy, War, and the Normal Child: Selected Papers of Margaret Lowenfeld* (Free Association Books, London, 1988).
Urwin, Cathy and Elaine Sharland, 'From bodies to minds in childcare literature: advice to parents in inter-war Britain', in Cooter, Roger (ed.), *In the Name of the Child: Health and Welfare, 1880–1940* (Routledge, London, 1992), 174–99.
Varga, Donna, 'Look – normal: the colonized child of developmental science', *History of Psychology*, 14 (2011), 137–57.
Vernon, M. D., 'A study of some effects of evacuation on adolescent girls', *British Journal of Educational Psychology*, 10 (1940), 114.

Vernon, Philip E., 'Psychological effects of air-raids', *Journal of Abnormal and Social Psychology*, 36 (1941), 469.
Vesalius, *De Humani Corporis Fabrica* (Johannes Oporinus, Basel, 1543).
Vicedo, Marga, *The Nature and Nurture of Love: From Imprinting to Attachment in Cold War America* (University of Chicago Press, Chicago, 2013).
Vincent, Ralph, *The Nutrition of the Infant*, 4th ed. (Bailliere, Tindall and Cox, London, 1913).
Viner, Russell, 'Melanie Klein and Anna Freud: the discourse of the early dispute', *Journal of the History of the Behavioural Sciences*, 32 (January 1996), 4–15.
Vittoz, Roger, *Treatment of Neurasthenia by Teaching of Brain Control* (Longmans, Green, London, 1911).
Voss, Julia, *Darwin's Pictures: Views of Evolutionary Theory, 1837–1874* (Yale University Press, New Haven, CT, 2010).
Waddington, Keir, *An Introduction to the Social History of Medicine: Europe since 1500* (Palgrave-Macmillan, Basingstoke, 2011).
Wailoo, Keith, *Pain: A Political History* (Johns Hopkins University Press, Baltimore, 2014).
Wake, J., 'Babies', *British Journal of Photography* (26 April 1872), 195–96.
Wall, Patrick, *Pain: The Science of Suffering* (Columbia University Press, New York, 2002).
Walton, J. K., 'Casting out and bringing back in Victorian England: pauper lunatics, 1840–70', in W. F. Bynum, R. Porter and M. Shepherd (eds.), *The Anatomy of Madness: Essays in the History of Psychiatry*, vol. 2 (Tavistock, London, 1985), 132–46.
Wear, Andrew, 'Perceptions of pain in seventeenth century England', *Society for the Social History of Medicine Bulletin*, 36 (1985), 7–9.
Webster, C. (ed.), *Health Medicine and Mortality* (Cambridge University Press, Cambridge, 1979).
Welshman, John, *Churchill's Children: The Evacuee Experience in Wartime Britain* (Oxford University Press, Oxford, 2010).
'Evacuation and social policy during the Second World War: myth and reality', *Twentieth Century British History*, 9 (1998), 28–53.
'Evacuation, hygiene, and social policy: our towns report of 1943', *The Historical Journal*, 42 (1999), 781–807.
From Transmitted Deprivation to Social Exclusion: Policy, Poverty and Parenting (The Policy Press, Bristol, 2012).
Wertheimer, Michael, 'The evolution of the concept of development in the history of psychology', in G. Eckardt, W. G. Bringmann and L. Sprung (eds.), *Contributions to a History of Developmental Psychology: International William T. Preyer Symposium* (Mouton Publishers, New York, 1982), 13–26.
West, Charles, 'On the mental peculiarities and mental disorders of childhood', *Medical Times and Gazette*, 1 (1860), 133–37.
Lectures on the Diseases of Infancy and Childhood (Longman, Brown, Green & Longmans, London, 1852).
White, Paul S., 'The experimental animal in Victorian Britain', in Lorraine Daston and Gregg Mitman (eds.), *Thinking with Animals: New Perspectives on Anthropomorphism* (Columbia University Press, New York, 2005), 59–81.

'Sympathy under the knife: experimentation and emotion in late victorian medicine', in Fay Bound Alberti (ed.), *Medicine, Emotion and Disease, 1700–1950* (Palgrave, Basingstoke, 2006), 100–24.
Wilder, Kelley, *Photography and Science (Exposures)* (Reaktion Books, London, 2009).
'Visualizing radiation: the photographs of Henry Becquerel', in Lorraine Daston and Elizabeth Lunbeck (eds.), *Histories of Scientific Observation* (Chicago University Press, Chicago, 2011), 349–68.
Williams, Andrew, 'Eighteenth-century child health care in a Northampton infirmary, a provincial English hospital', *Family and Community History*, 10 (2007), 153–66.
'Gowers Young Physicians Prize 2000 Winner, Thomas Willis, childhood stroke, neonatal convulsions and infanticide', *Seizure*, 10 (2001), 471–83.
'"To observe . . . and thence to make himself rules", John Locke's principles and practice of child health care', *Journal of Medical Ethics; Medical Humanities*, 33 (2007), 22–34.
'Thomas Willis' paediatric general practice', *British Journal of General Practice*, 57 (2007), 70–73.
Winnicott, Donald W., *The Child and the Outside World* (Tavistock, London, 1957).
'Children's hostels in war and peace', *British Journal of Medical Psychology*, 21 (1948), 175–80.
Clinical Notes on Disorders of Childhood (William Heinemann (Medical), London, 1931).
Deprivation and Delinquency (Tavistock, London, 1984).
'Evacuation of small children', in D. W. Winnicott, R. Shepherd and M. David (eds.), *Deprivation and Delinquency* (Routledge, London, 1941), 11–12.
'Hate in the counter-transference', *The Journal of Psychotherapy Practice and Research*, 3 (1994), 348–56.
'The psychology of Juvenile Rheumatism', in R. G. Gordon, On behalf of the Child Guidance Council (ed.), *A Survey of Child Psychiatry: Contributed by Contemporary British Authorities* (Oxford University Press and Humphrey Milford, London, 1939), 28–44.
'Some thoughts on the meaning of the word democracy', *Human Relations*, 3 (1950), 175–86.
Winnicott, Donald W. and Clare Britton, 'The problem of homeless children', in *Children's Communities: Experiments in Democratic Living* (NEF Monograph, London, 1944), 155–61.
Wolf, Katharine M., 'Evacuation of children in wartime – a survey of the literature, with bibliography', *Psychoanalytic Study of the Child*, 1 (1945), 389–404.
Women's Group on Public Welfare, *Our Towns* (Oxford University Press, Oxford, 1943).
Wood, Diana (ed.), *The Church and Childhood (Studies in Church History, Vol. 31)* (Blackwell, Oxford, 1994).
Wood, Whitney, '"When I think of what is before me, I feel afraid." Narratives of fear, pain and childbirth in late Victorian Canada', in Rob Boddice (ed.), *Pain and Emotions in Modern History* (Palgrave Macmillan, Basingstoke, 2014).
Woolf, Virginia, *On Being Ill* (Paris Press, Ashfield, MA, 2002).

Wright, D., *Mental Disability in Victorian England: The Earlswood Asylum, 1847–1901* (Clarendon Press, Oxford, 2001).

Würtz, Felix, 'An experimental treatise of surgerie in four parts. . . the children's book', in L. Fox (translator) and J. Ruhrah (ed.), *Pediatrics of the Past* (P. B. Hoeber, New York, 1925), 198–220.

Wynne Smith, Lisa, 'An account of an unaccountable distemper: the experience of pain in early eighteenth century England and France', *Eighteenth-Century Studies*, 41 (2008), 459–80.

Yates, S. L., 'Problems of evacuation', Letter to the editor, *British Medical Journal*, 2 (28 October 1939), 883–84.

Yeo, R., 'Scientific method and the image of science, 1831–1891', in R. MacLeod and P. Collins (eds.), *The Parliament of Science: The British Association for the Advancement of Science, 1831–1981* (Science Reviews, Norwood, 1981), 65–88.

Young, Robert M., *Mind, Brain, and Adaptation in the Nineteenth Century: Cerebral Localization and Its Biological Context from Gall to Ferrier* (Oxford University Press, New York, 1990).

Young Simpson, James, *Answer to the Religious Objections Advanced against the Employment of Anaesthetic Agents in Midwifery and Surgery* (Sutherland and Know, Edinburgh, 1849).

Young-Bruehl, Elisabeth, *Anna Freud: A Biography* (London, Macmillan, 1988).

Zelizer, Viviana, *Pricing the Priceless Child: The Changing Social Value of Children* (Princeton University Press, New York, 1985).

Zornado, Joseph L., *Inventing the Child: Culture, Ideology, and the Story of Childhood* (Routledge, Oxford, 2006).

Index

Abraham, Karl, 140
Achylia Gastrica Nervosa, 130
ADHD (attention deficit hyperactivity disorder), 122
adolescence
  and criminal behaviour, 105
  as marker of adulthood, 8
  as specific developmental phase, 105
adult world, child's role in construction of
  and evolution, 23–27, 32, 58
  overview of, 6–9
  and research motivation, 66, 199
adults. *See also* mothers; parents
  age of adulthood, 8
  child as adult-in-training and citizenship, 177, 196
  child as adult-in-training and evolution, 23–27, 32
  economic and political interest in children, 8
  reactions to air raids, 188
aesthetics of pain, 154
age
  of adulthood, 8
  and air-raid shock, 187
  as variable in child pain, 11, 201
'Air raid shock' (Brend), 156, 186
'Air raids and the child' (Mons), 184
air-raid shock, 183–90
Alcock, Theodora, 156, 181, 183, 191
alcoholism, 116
Allen, Clifford, 146
anaesthesia, 59, 74–77
Anderson, John, 170
animals, children as similar to
  and behavioural psychology, 69
  and denial of pain, 58
  and evolutionary approaches, 25, 32, 62
  and paediatric practice, 72
animals, cruelty to, 105
anthropology
  and child as adult-in-training, 24
  evolutionary approach to childhood and child pain, 22, 24
  recapitulation theory, 58
Ariès, Philippe, 13
articulation of pain. *See also* crying
  accounts by children, 40
  as challenge, 17, 198
  as challenge in diagnosis and treatment, 6, 19, 34, 71
  as challenge in research, 4
  disciplinary differences in understanding of, 22
  and metaphors, 17
  in photography, 21
  and politics of pain, 202
  screaming, 22
Ashby, Henry, 40
Aspects of Child Life and Education (Hall), 64
atropine, 75
attention deficit hyperactivity disorder (ADHD), 122
Aunt Judy's Magazine, 51–52

Ballet, Gilbert, 116, 119
Beard, George Miller, 113
Beaton, Cecil, 160–67
bed-wetting. *See* enuresis
behaviourism
  denial of pain and, 67–70, 198
  rise of, 68
Bending, Lucy, 18, 78, 202
'biographical sketch of an infant, A' (Darwin), 2, 23–27
biographies of babies, 24, 62
Biography of a Baby, The (Shinn), 62
Blandford, G. Fielding, 88
Blanton, Margaret Gray, 68
Boddice, Rob, 19
Bodman, Frank, 187
body
  First World War and shifts in understanding of, 113

and hysteria, 100
and melancholia, 96
mental pain as having physical causes, 81, 88, 97, 125
mind–body overlap in early approaches to child pain, 11, 80
mind–body separation, 11, 19, 79, 108
and nervous disorders, 125
and night terrors, 87–93
Body in Pain, The (Scarry), 17
Bohannon, E. W., 106
Boismont, Alexandre Brière de, 98, 107
Bourke, Joanna
on challenges of studying pain, 14
on cultural aspects of pain, 16, 18
on denial of infant pain, 15, 22, 57
on metaphors for pain, 17
Bowlby, John, 144, 179
Brend, William A., 186
Breuer, Josef, 109
Britton, Clare, 180
Brown, Felix, 186
Brown, Paterson, 147
Bucknill, Dr, 99
Budin, Pierre, 71
Burbury, Mary, 176, 187, 191
Burlingham, Dorothy, 153, 186
Burt, Cyril, 189

Calder, Ritchie, 175
Cambridge Evacuation Survey, 157, 193
Cameron, Hector, 136–39
Canestrini, Silvio, 27, 30
Carling, Esther, 173
Carmichael, James, 39
cartes de visite, 23, 46–51
Cattell, Raymond B., 181
Cautley, Edmund, 72, 127, 131
Centuries of Childhood (Ariès), 13
century of the child, 25, 57
cerebral neurasthenia, 117
Chain of Feeling, 11
Chamberlain, Alexander Francis, 59, 66
Chamberlain, David, 15
Chapin, Henry Dwight, 71, 134
child. *See also* adult world, child's role in construction of
as adult-in-training and citizenship, 177, 196
as adult-in-training and evolution, 23–27, 32
as category, 10
child development
behaviourism studies, 70
language development, 61
maturation concept, 66
and observation during Second World War, 194
paediatrics' interest in, 73
post-Second World War understanding, 195, 200
rise of discipline, 57, 66
Child Guidance Clinics, 113–14, 140, 181
Child Guidance Council, 143
child pain. *See also* articulation of pain; evacuees; infant pain denial; mental pain; nervous child concept; politics of pain
background and concepts, 3–12
emotional expressions of, 19
lack of historical personal narratives, 6
scholarship lacking, 21
scholarship overview, 3–6, 12–16
child study movement
approach to pain, 59–67
and child as adult-in-training, 24
development of, 58
and evolution, 60–67
and 'normal' child, 60
recapitulation theory, 63–67
Child: A Study in the Evolution of Man. The (Chamberlain), 59
childhood
and cultural power, 201
scholarship on, 9, 12–16
variations in cultural concepts of, 7
variations in disciplinary concepts of, 6
Children's Clinic for the Treatment Study of Nervous and Difficult Children, 114
'Children's communities: experiments in democratic living' (Winnicott and Britton), 180
children's hospitals. *See* hospitals
Christmas Under Fire (1941), 166
chronic pain
articulating, 18
and nervous disorders, 130
and neurasthenia, 117
Churchill, Winston, 160, 162
citizens, children as future, 8, 177, 196
Clark, Kenneth, 160, 168
Clarke, J. Michell, 100–3, 118
class
and evacuees, 155–59, 168, 172–75
and juvenile delinquency, 181
and mental pain, 93, 107
and pain sensitivity, 11
and photography for hospital fundraising, 41, 46, 53–54
and photography for Second World War propaganda, 164, 168

Clinical Lectures on Neurasthenia (Savill), 116
Clinical Notes on the Disorders of Childhood (Winnicott), 143
Clouston, Thomas, 90, 93, 96–97
Cobb, Ivo Geikie, 120
Coghill, George, 70
Colman, Dr, 91
Commercial & General Photographic Co., 42
Common Disorders and Diseases of Childhood (Still), 123
communication of pain. *See* articulation of pain
Conolly, John, 84, 99
context and performative nature of pain, 4
Coombes, Robert, 106
Cooter, Roger, 13
corporal punishment, 147
Crichton-Browne, James
  and melancholia, 94, 96
  and night terrors, 81, 84, 87, 90, 92
  and suicide in children, 98
Crichton-Miller, Hugh, 114, 146
crying
  attempts to distinguish types of, 38
  and child study movement, 61
  and denial of infant pain, 31
  as diagnostic tool, 36–40
  as innate in Darwin, 25
  photographs of, 21, 25
Culpin, Millais, 141
culture
  concept of childhood and, 8
  cultural power and childhood, 201
  pain as cultural experience, 16–20
Culture of Pain, The (Morris), 19
Cultures of Child Health in Britain and the Netherlands in the Twentieth Century (Gijswijt-Hofstra and Marland), 13

Darwin, Charles
  emotions and evolution, 21, 32
  infant research, 2, 23
  pain as reflex action, 23–27, 96, 198
Darwin, William, 23
Day of Rest, 51
daydreams, 81, 84, 92
degeneration, theory of, 83, 115
democracy
  and children in the Second World War, 156, 159, 167, 180, 182, 194
  and mother–child bond, 167, 194
denial of infant pain. *See* infant pain denial
'Developmental Insanities and Psychoses' (Clouston), 90
diagnosis
  challenges of, 19, 36, 97
  crying as diagnostic tool, 36–40
  different diagnoses for same symptoms, 1, 6, 139
  emotions as tool in, 135
  mothers as cause of ailments, 39
  mothers as sources of information, 39
  and night terrors, 90
  pain as diagnostic tool, 22, 36–40, 71
  pain as diagnostic tool and nervous disorders, 126, 128–31, 141–46
  politics of diagnosis, 6
Dickens, Charles, 34, 41
Dickinson, W. H., 89
Die Seele des Kindes (Preyer), 30
diet and nervous disorders, 119, 127
digestion
  and neurasthenia, 120
  and night-terrors, 87, 90
disciplines. *See also* infant pain denial
  and childhood concept, 6
  lack of unity on child pain, 2, 6, 11, 19, 197, 199
  methodological differences, 3
  political use of child pain, 78, 197
Diseases of Children (Garrod), 128
Diseases of Infants and Children, The (Cautley), 131
Doctor and the Difficult Child, The (Moodie), 144
Donkin, H. B., 90
Down, John Langdon, 107
Drummond, William Blackley, 73
Duckworth, Dyce, 129
Dunne, Eileen, 160–67
Dunsdon, M. I., 187

Eastland, Annie Kezia, 46, 51
economic interest in children, 8
Eder, David, 140
'Effects of evacuation and of air raids on city children' (Bunbury), 176
Elliot, Walter, 170
embryology
  denial of infant pain and, 22, 68
  German experiments in, 28–31
emotions
  connection to pain, 19
  evolutionary approaches to, 21–27
  shift to focus on, 125, 132
enuresis
  and evacuees, 156, 175–76
  as focus of child psychiatry, 144

environmental factors and nervous disorders, 115, 120–21, 124–27, 146
epilepsy, 126
Esquirol, Jean Étienne Dominique, 83, 105
ether, 75
eugenics
  children as future citizens, 9
  defined, 60
  and evacuees, 173
  and mental pain, 97
evacuees
  and class, 155–59, 168, 172–75
  criticism of policy, 168
  and democracy, 156, 159, 180, 182
  health issues of, 172–75
  medical understanding/approaches to, 154–55
  as natural experiment, 192–94
  and observation, 186, 190, 192
  pain of, 152–59
  planning and logistics of evacuation, 170–73
  scholarship on, 153, 175–82
  and schools, 181
  and shock of separation, 2, 153, 190
Evans, Elida, 147
Evanson, Richard Tonson, 37
evolution
  and child study movement, 58, 60–67
  child's role in construction of adult world, 23–27, 58
  and emotional development, 21–27
  and inheritability of mental illness, 85
  Maudsley and child development theory, 92
  neurological development in infants, 30–33
  and night terrors, 92
  recapitulation theory, 58, 63–67, 73
Expression of the Emotions in Man and Animals, The (Darwin), 21, 24–27
expressions, facial
  crying as diagnostic tool, 38
  localisation of pain with, 71

family. *See also* evacuees; parents
  psychoanalysis and understanding of family, 194
  subjectification of, 157
fathers, loss of, 192, *See also* parents
Faulkner, Robert, 42, 46–51, 53–54
Ferenczi, Sandor, 133
Flechsig, Paul Emil, 28
Forsyth, David, 71
Foucault, Michel, 157
France, first children's hospitals in, 34
free will, 24
Freud, Anna
  on air-raid anxiety, 189
  evacuation policy criticism, 191
  evacuees and pain of separation, 2, 152, 190
  evacuees, observation of, 186, 190, 192
  influence of, 133
  as resource, 157
  on rise of child analysis, 140
Freud, Sigmund
  and child analysis, 134
  and hysteria, 109
  influence on nervous child concept, 113
  and instinct theory, 148
  and neurosis, 132
Functional Nervous Disorders in Childhood (Guthrie), 124

Galton, Francis, 60
Garrod, Archibald, 72, 126, 128–30
Garrow, R. P., 192
gastralgia, 130
gender
  and hysteria, 82
  and neurasthenia, 116
  pain sensitivity and, 11
  roles and Second World War, 158
  as variable in child pain, 11, 201
genetics
  and homicidal monomania, 106
  and mental pain, 85, 97, 106, 115
  and nervous disorders, 115, 119, 127, 134
Genzmer, Alfred, 27, 29
Georget, Étienne-Jean, 101
Germany, infant pain experiments in, 27–33
Gesell, Arnold, 66, 69
gestures, as diagnostic tool, 38
Gijswijt-Hofstra, Marijke, 13
Gillespie, R. D., 145
'Ginx's Baby', 21, 25
Goodhart, James Frederic, 130
Gordon, Ronald, 143
Great Ormond Street Hospital
  cartes de visite, 23, 46–51
  development of, 34–36, 41
  diagnosis and history-taking in, 39
  and hysteria, 100
  photography and fundraising, 41–54
  photography and Second World War, 164
  and Still, 121
grief, 16, 98, 190
Griesinger, Wilhelm, 94
Guthrie, Leonard, 93, 124–26

Haeckel, Ernst, 64
Hall, Granville Stanley, 105
hallucinations. *See also* night terrors
  as having physical causes, 88
  and melancholia, 96

Hampstead War Nurseries, 1, 152, 186, 190, 193
Hans (patient of Freud), 134
Harris, Percy, 174
Hartenberg, Paul, 117, 119
'Hate in the countertransference' (Winnicott), 148
Hellman, Ilse, 186
Henderson, J. L., 76
Hendrick, Harry, 159
Heredity and Child Culture (Chapin), 134
Hess, A., 35
History of Paediatrics, The (Still), 14
Hoare, Samuel, 170
Holt, Luther, 38, 130
homicidal monomania, 82, 105–7
hospitals. *See also* Great Ormond Street Hospital
  acceptance of, 36
  attitudes towards mothers, 39
  bed sponsorships, 51–52
  communication with parents, 44
  photography and fundraising, 23, 40–54, 89
  photography and Second World War, 164
  postcards, 42, 44
  resistance to, 34, 36
  rise of, 33–36
Hug-Hellmuth, Hermine, 140
Hutchison, Robert, 72, 129
hygiene
  and evacuees, 172–75
  and schools, 116, 135
  shift from to focus on emotions, 125
  social hygiene movement, 9
  treatments for nervous disorders, 127
hyperactivity
  attention deficit hyperactivity disorder (ADHD), 122
  and neurasthenia, 117
hyperesthesia, 129
hysteria
  conflation with neurasthenia, 128
  as diagnosis, 79–83, 99–104
  false vs. true, 104
  and Freud, 109
  pain as symptom of, 144
  and women, 82, 100
'Hysteria in children' (Bowlby), 144
hysterical paralysis, 129

IASP (International Association for the Study of Pain), 77, 198
ideational insanity, 94
idiocy, as classification, 82
Illustrated London News, 162
Infant Behavior, Its Genesis and Growth (Gesell), 67
infant pain denial
  and anaesthesia, 59, 74–77
  consolidation of theories, 57–59
  development of theories, 14, 22, 27–33
  experiments on, 27–33, 70
  and pain as reflex, 23–27, 58, 67, 73, 198
  and politics of pain, 78, 202
infantile paralysis, 129
infants
  biographies of babies, 24, 62
  crying as diagnostic tool, 38
  emotional expression as reflex in, 23–27, 58, 67, 73
  as evolutionary mirror, 23–27
  melancholia in, 95
insanity. *See also* mental pain
  affective, 94
  as classification, 82
  defining in children, 83–87
  ideational, 94
  in utero, 85
  moral, 81, 95, 104–7
  resistance to labeling children as insane, 83
  stigma of, 135
Insanity and Its treatment (Blandford), 88
instinct theory, 148
International Association for the Study of Pain (IASP), 77, 198
Introduction to Child Study (Drummond), 73
Introduction to the Technique of Child Analysis (Freud), 133
Investigations on the Psychic Function of the Newborn (Genzmer), 29
Ireland, William, 85, 96
Isaacs, Susan, 149, 184, 192–93

John, E. M., 188
Jones, Ernest, 76
Jones, Sydney, 46, 49, 52
juvenile delinquency
  and class, 181
  and evacuation, 155–56, 176–82
  increase in criminal behaviour and adolescence, 105
  school concerns about, 135
  and war strain, 183–86

ketonzemia (cyclical vomiting), 138
Kimber, W. J. T., 192
King's College Hospital, 121
Klein, Melanie, 133, 148
Kroner, Traugott, 27, 30
Kuhn, Thomas, 118
Kussmaul, Adolf, 28

Langley & Sons, Ltd, 44
language development, 61
Laycock, Thomas, 94
Lectures on the Diseases of Infancy and Childhood (West), 81, 86
Leigh, Digby, 76
Levy, David M., 76
LIFE, 159–62
Lowenfeld, Margaret, 110, 114, 142

MacDonald, Martha W., 182
Mackintosh, J. Stewart, 138
maladjustment
  and evacuees, 155
  and Still, 122
  and Sully, 60
malingering, 104
Marland, Hilary, 13
masochism, 147
masturbation, 119
maturation concept, 66
Maudsley, Henry
  and affective vs. ideational insanity, 94
  and children who inflict pain, 92–93, 106–7
  and emotions as reflexes, 96
  and eugenics, 97
  and melancholia, 94
  and moral insanity, 95
  and night-terrors, 82, 85, 88, 90
McGrath, Patrick, 15
McGraw, Myrtle, 69
Meigs, John Forsyth, 39
melancholia, 81, 93–99
memory
  inherited memories and night terrors, 93
  and pain, 65, 76
Mental Maladies: A Treatise on Insanity (Esquirol), 105
mental pain. *See also* evacuees
  and bombed child, 156, 183–90
  and children who inflict pain, 82, 105–7
  and class, 93, 107
  classification of mental disorders, 82
  and daydreams, 81, 84, 92
  defining insanity in children, 83–87
  Guthrie's consolidation of, 126
  melancholia, 81, 93–99
  moral insanity, 81, 95, 104–7
  night-terrors, 81, 87–93, 100
  overview of approaches to, 79–83
  pain as symptom of, 144
  physical manifestation/cause of, 81, 88, 97, 101, 111–13, 118, 134–39
  psychosis, 145
  resistance to labeling children as insane, 83
  shift from insanity concept to nervous concept, 115
  shift to unconscious mind concept, 113, 131–35
  suicide and suicidal ideation, 96, 98
  treatment challenges in interwar period, 145
  treatment in asylums vs. treatment at home, 89
Merskey, Harold, 77, 198
methodology and resources
  evacuees, 157
  mental illness in children, 80, 82, 114
  overview of, 197
  physicians' variations in and child's inability to communicate, 6
Miller, Emanuel, 178
Ministry of Information, 160–68
modernity and nervous disorders, 115, 120, 147
Mons, W. E., 156, 183–86
Moodie, William, 144
moral insanity, 81, 95, 104–7
morality
  and evacuees, 175
  moral insanity, 81, 95, 104–7
  and nervous disorders, 122
Morris, David, 19
Moscoso, Javier, 18, 112, 128
mothers
  anger at/hatred of, 148, 190
  blame on for ailments, 39, 127
  blame on for evacuees' problems, 173–75
  and children's hospitals, 39
  mother–child bond and democracy, 167, 194
  mother–child bond in psychoanalysis and Second World War, 158, 182
  nurses as surrogate mothers, 42
  reactions to air raids, 188
  as resource in diagnosis, 39, 58
  separation anxiety in evacuees, 190
Müller, Johannes, 28
In the Name of the Child (Cooter), 13

nerve fatigue, 113
Nervous Child at School, The (Cameron), 136, 138
nervous child concept. *See also* hysteria; neurasthenia
  environmental factors, 115, 120–21, 124–27, 146
  hereditary factors, 115, 127
  nervousness as term, 114, 135
  and New Psychology, 113, 132–35
  overview of, 110–14
  pain as diagnostic tool in, 126, 128–31
  and repression, 146
  shifts in understanding of, 115–31

'nervous child, The' (Culpin), 141
nervous system
  German experiments in, 28–31
  neurological development in infants, 30–33
  pathologisation of in interwar period, 115–21
  as seat of disease, 114
neurasthenia
  decline of diagnosis, 131
    and gender, 128
  hereditary factors, 116, 119
  vs. neurosis, 126, 141
  precocious, 116
  as term, 113, 128
  treatment of, 119
neurologists, conflicts with psychologists over nervous pain, 113, 134
neurosis
  acceptance of concept for children, 121–31
  development of concept, 132
  vs. neurasthenia, 126, 141
  and parents, 146
'Neurosis in schoolchildren' (Burns), 143
'new approach to the problem of psychoneurosis in childhood, A' (Lowenfeld), 142
New Psychology
  and nervous child concept, 113, 132–35
  vs. psychoanalysis, 140
  rise of, 132–35
New Psychology and the Teacher, The (Crichton-Miller), 146
newborns
  and anaesthesia, 74
  crying as diagnostic tool, 38
  denial of pain, 23–27, 58, 70, 74
Newton, Hannah, 11, 13, 17, 201
night terrors, 81, 87–93, 100
'nursery as a community, The' (Isaacs), 149
Nursery Years, The (Isaacs), 185
nurses
  class of as corrupting factor, 93
  as surrogate mothers, 42

'On Being Ill' (Woolf), 18
'On the peculiarities and mental disorders of childhood' (West), 86
opiates, 75
Osler, William, 130

Pabis, Emilia, 15
paediatrics
  acceptance of psychogenic pain, 114
  and anaesthesia, 74–77
  and bombed children, 155
  conflicts with neurologists and psychologists over nervous pain, 113, 121–31
  and denial of pain, 22, 57–59, 74–77
  development of discipline, 71–74, 123
  diagnostic use of mental pain, 128–31
  diagnostic use of pain, 22
  as disconnected from other disciplines, 10
  and evacuees, 154, 175
  explorer metaphor, 35, 58
  histories of, 14
  increase in pyschotherapeutic role, 132
  overview of approaches to child pain, 6
  and photography of children, 41
  rise of, 33
  rise of children's hospitals, 33–36
  shifts in understanding of nervous pain, 121–31
  West on role of paediatrician, 35, 58
pain. *See also* articulation of pain; evacuees; infant pain denial; mental pain; nervous child concept; politics of pain
  acceptable vs. unacceptable, 16, 169
  as cultural experience, 16–20
  challenges of studying, 14, 198
  definitions of, 77, 198
  as diagnostic tool, 22, 36–40, 71
  as diagnostic tool and nervous disorders, 126, 128–31, 136, 141–46
  and emotional affect, 19
  and memory, 65, 76
  metaphors for, 17
  subjectivity of, 14, 17
  tests for, 37
  as unstable object, 2, 7
Pain: A Cultural History (Moscoso), 18
pantophobia, 81, 92
paralysis, 129
Paralysis and Other Diseases of the Nervous System in Childhood and Early Life (Taylor), 129
parents. *See also* mothers
  anger at/hatred of, 148, 190
  blame on for nervous disorders, 121, 124, 127, 141
  challenges of modernity, 147
  communication with hospitals, 44
pattern theory, 28
Pediatric Anesthesiology (Digby and Smith), 76
Pediatrics of the Past (Ruhrah), 14
performative nature of pain and and contexts, 4
'Personality deviations in children' (Allen), 146
photography and child pain
  cartes de visite, 23, 46–51
  clinical, 41

and Darwin, 21, 25
and hospital fundraising, 23, 40–54
representation without showing pain, 46–56, 163
and World Second World War, 154, 159–67
toys and happy child imagery in, 42, 46, 51–52, 54
'physiological approach to psychiatric problems, The' (Gordon), 144
physiology
and denial of pain, 22, 27–31
as disconnected from other disciplines, 10
overview of approaches to child pain, 6
pattern theory, 28
shift to psychological explanations for mental pain, 111
specificity, theory of, 28
Pillai Riddell, Rebecca, 14
play
and evacuees, 190
and recapitulation theory, 64
pleasure
and masochistic pain, 147
recapitulation theory, 65
politics of pain
and democracy, 156, 159
and denial of pain, 78, 202
and differing diagnoses for same symptoms, 6
and disciplinary prestige and conflict, 19, 78, 198
images of children's suffering in Second World War, and bombed children, 159–67
images of children's suffering in Second World War, and evacuated children, 5, 154–59
political significance of children, 8
and power dynamics, 78, 197
uses of, 202
postcards, 42, 44
post-traumatic stress disorder (PTSD), 156
poverty
and evacuees, 155–59, 172–75
and homicidal monomania, 107
hospital fundraising and middle-class values, 41
and mental pain, 107, 140
and rheumatism, 142
precocious neurasthenia, 116
Preyer, William Thierry, 30, 198
Prichard, James Cowles, 81, 95
Pritchart, Rosemary, 183
Problem of the Nervous Child, The (Evans), 147
Problems of Social Policy (Titmuss), 192
propaganda and images of children's suffering in Second World War, 154, 159–67
psychasthenia, 131
psychiatry
child psychiatry, development of as discipline, 84, 86, 144
child psychiatry, term, 144
conflicts with neurology and psychology over nervous pain, 121–31
consolidation of discipline, 84, 121
disconnect from other disciplines, 10
evolutionary psychiatry, 26, 85
overview of approaches to child pain, 6, 79–83
shift to neurosis concept, 121–31
and West, 86
'Psychical Diseases of Early Life' (Chricton-Browne), 84
psychoanalysis
and air-raid shock, 189
development of discipline, 111–14, 133, 140
as disconnected from other disciplines, 10
and evacuees, 153–59, 166–70, 175–82
increased interest in with Second World War, 167
influence on social policy, 176, 182, 194
influence on understanding of family, 194
and nervous child concept, 111–14, 146–47
vs. New Psychology, 140
observation and, 186
overview of approaches to child pain, 6
psychogenic pain. *See* mental pain
psychology
and bombed child, 186–92
conflicts with neurology and paediatrics over nervous child, 113, 121–31
consolidation of discipline, 84, 121
denial of pain, 22, 57–59, 66–70
development of discipline, 66, 97, 111–14
disconnect from other disciplines, 10
and evacuees, 155, 175–82
evolutionary psychology, 26, 85
overview of approaches to child pain, 6
shift to neurosis concept, 121–31
'psychology of juvenile rheumatism, The' (Winnicott), 144
'Psychoses in children' (Gillespie), 145
psychosis, 145
PTSD (post-traumatic stress disorder), 156
puberty
gender as variable and, 12
and increase in criminal behaviour, 105
as marker of adulthood, 8

race
  and pain sensitivity, 11, 66
  and pathologisation of developmental differences, 59
Ray, M. B., 83, 98
recapitulation theory
  child study movement, 63–67
  in paediatrics, 73
  rise of, 26, 58
Rees, Gordon Jackson, 75
reflex and melancholia, 94
reflex, pain as
  and anaesthesia, 75
  and emotional expression as reflex in infants, 23–27, 58, 67, 96, 198
  in paediatrics, 73
Rejlander, Oscar, 21, 25–27
'Relief of Pain in Childhood, The' (Henderson), 76
Representation of Bodily Pain in Late Nineteenth-Century English Culture, The (Bending), 18
repression of trauma, 146
rheumatism, 1, 128, 142–44
Rickman, John, 149, 178
Ritter von Reuss, August, 74
Robinson, Louis, 62
Robson, Charles, 76
Rodkey, Elissa N., 14
Romanes, George, 32, 61
Rorschach test, 184
Rosenzweig, Saul, 183
Rotch, Thomas, 36
Ruhrah, John, 14

sanitation and hospital fundraising, 41
savage, child as
  and child study movement, 61
  and evolutionary approaches, 26, 31, 61
  and politics of pain, 78
Savill, Thomas D., 110, 116–18
Scarry, Elaine
  and mental vs. physical pain, 79
  and political use of pain, 78, 202
  and subjectivity of pain, 17
'school and the child guidance clinic, The' (Cattell), 181
schools
  and delinquency, 135, 181
  and evacuees, 181
  and hygiene, 116, 135
  and neurasthenia/nervous child, 116–19, 127
self-consciousness
  and pain in recapitulation theory, 65
  as preceding language development, 61
sentimentalism, 41
separation anxiety, 190, *See also* evacuees
Shapira, Michal, 159, 167, 177, 182
shell shock, 133
Sherman, Irene, 69
Sherman, Mandel, 69
Shinn, Millicent Washburn, 62
Sick Child in Early Modern England, 1580–1720, The (Newton), 13, 17
Smith, Robert, 76
Social Conditions and Acute Rheumatism (Lowenfeld), 142
social hygiene movement, 9, *See also* hygiene
social policy. *See also* welfare state
  concerns about emotional harm to children, 192
  influence of psychoanalysis on, 176, 182
  lessons from evacuation program, 193
Solomon, Joseph C., 188
specificity, theory of, 28
Spurgin, William H., 1, 79, 101
Starr, Louis, 37
Stereoscopic Company, 42
Still, George Frederic, 14, 74, 121–24, 127
Story of Pain, The (Bourke), 15, 57
Studies of Childhood (Sully), 61
subjectification, 157
suicide and suicidal ideation, 96, 98
Sully, James, 60, 105
Survey of Child Psychiatry, A (Gordon), 143
syphilis, 139

tactile thresholds and pain, 28
Tavistock Clinic, 114, *See also* Alcock, Theodora; Mons, W. E.
Taylor, James, 91, 129
teething, 91
tests for pain, development of, 37
Thomas, André, 76
Thorek, Max, 75
tics, 153
Tilney, Frederick, 70
Titmuss, Richard, 192
trauma
  and air raids, 184
  and child mental pain, 98, 102, 146
  and hysteria, 102
Treatise on Insanity and Other Disorders Affecting the Mind (Prichard), 81, 95
treatment of mental pain
  in asylums vs. treatment at home, 89
  challenges of, 145

hygiene treatments, 127
inconsistency of, 201
for neurasthenia, 119
Treatment of Neurasthenia (Hartenberg), 117, 119
Treatment of Neurasthenia by Teaching of Brain (Vittoz), 119
trust, 202
Tucker, Beverley, 139
Tuke, Daniel, 90

unconscious mind
bombed child and, 184
shift in focus to, 113, 131–35
'unconscious mind in the child, The' (Eder), 140
United States
and British Second World War propaganda, 161
first children's hospitals, 34
Unruh, Anita, 15
Untersuchungen über Das Seelenleben des Neugeborenen Menschen (Kussmaul), 28

Vernon, Philip Ewart, 185
Vincent, Ralph, 38
violence and abuse against children, 12
Vittoz, Roger, 119
vomiting, cyclical (ketonzemia), 138

Wallace, Nellie, 46–49
War Artists' Advisory Committee (WAAC), 160, 168
War Nurseries. *See* Hampstead War Nurseries
war strain, 156, 183–90
Watson, John Broadus, 68–69
Weber, Ernst, 28
welfare state
influence of psychoanalysis on, 182
interest in children's emotional welfare post-First World War, 140, 167
and role of state, 177
West, Charles
and diagnosis and history-taking, 39, 135
and Great Ormond Street Hospital development, 34–36, 41
and mental disorders, 85
and night terrors, 81, 87–93, 100
and rheumatism, 1
and role of paediatrician, 35, 58
Winnicott, Donald, 143–44, 146, 148, 179, 192
women
and hysteria, 82, 100
and nervous disorders, 128
and nervousness, 113
Women's Voluntary Service, 158
Woods twins, 70
Woolf, Virginia, 17
First World War, shift in understanding of the body and selfhood, 113
Second World War. *See also* evacuees
bombed child, 155–59, 183–90
child pain and national resistance, 5, 154, 162–67
images of children's suffering and propaganda, 154, 159–67
research experiments, 192–94
shift in perception of pain, 2
and subjectification of family, 157
Wundt, Wilhelm, 60

For EU product safety concerns, contact us at Calle de José Abascal, 56–1°, 28003 Madrid, Spain or eugpsr@cambridge.org.

www.ingramcontent.com/pod-product-compliance
Lightning Source LLC
LaVergne TN
LVHW011811200926
848484LV00005B/1151
9781009558730